Table of Contents

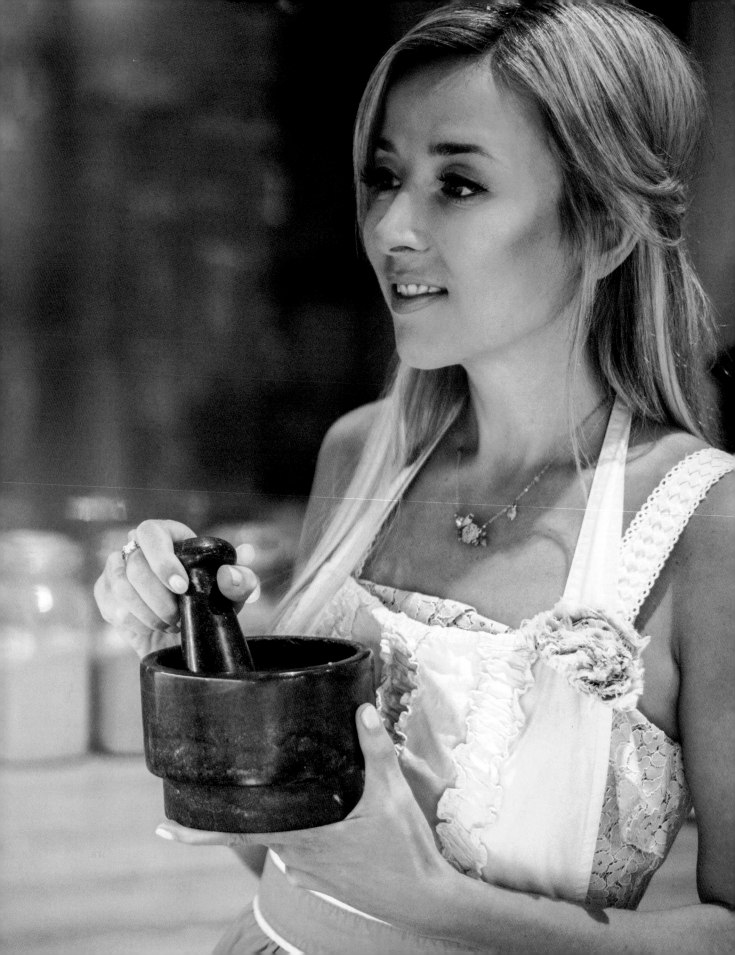

KETO
Essentials

Vanessa Spina

Victory Belt Publishing Inc.

Las Vegas

First Published in 2017 by Victory Belt Publishing Inc.

ISBN-13: 978-1-628602-64-7

The author is not a licensed practitioner, physician, or medical professional and offers no medical diagnoses, treatments, suggestions, or counseling. The information presented herein has not been evaluated by the U.S. Food and Drug Administration, and it is not intended to diagnose, treat, cure, or prevent any disease. Full medical clearance from a licensed physician should be obtained before beginning or modifying any diet, exercise, or lifestyle program, and physicians should be informed of all nutritional changes.

The author/owner claims no responsibility to any person or entity for any liability, loss, or damage caused or alleged to be caused directly or indirectly as a result of the use, application, or interpretation of the information presented herein.

Author photo taken by Lucie Vysloužilová
Recipe photos by Diana Mocanu
Interior design by Justin-Aaron Velasco
Photos shot at My Raw Café, Prague

Printed in Canada

TC 0518

Keto: What's All the Buzz About?

As a young woman, I had two lofty personal diet and health goals:

- To lose weight
- To eat food

My passion for eating delicious food bested my passion for losing weight, and it wasn't hard to see which goal was dominant. But through years of frustration with my poor health, the one mainstay—aside from unwanted body fat—was hope. Despite feeling exasperated, I never gave up hope that one day I would discover the secret to having the pain-free, healthy body of my dreams, without daily deprivation from a constant cycle of dieting and punishing exercise. I knew I would find a way to have the wellness and body confidence I'd always dreamed of while also enjoying life and feeling at peace around food. Even when things seemed bleak, I had a single-minded obsession.

This obsession eventually drove me all the way to my personal nirvana of enjoying inflammation-free health. I am satisfied and happy without feeling deprived or being chained to a treadmill. And the cherry on top of my high-fat health sundae is that I am able to have all that while enjoying real, delicious foods. I call it having my keto cake and eating it, too.

Through my business, Ketogenic Girl, I've had the privilege of guiding thousands of people to having their own keto cakes and eating them, too. And now, with this book, I'm here to do the same for you! Let's dig in.

Keto versus Other Low-Carb Diets

The ketogenic diet gets its name from ketone bodies, which are water-soluble molecules that circulate in the body when fat is broken down. In the absence of carbohydrates or during fasting, the body breaks down stored or consumed fat for energy. In other words, when you limit your carb intake, your body is forced to burn the fat you're already storing as well as the fat in your food. Keto is defined as a very-low-carbohydrate diet. There are varying approaches, but I recommend that your total carbohydrate intake not exceed 5 percent of your total food intake, with the other 95 percent coming from fat and protein.

On the spectrum of low-carbohydrate diets, keto is the most carb-restrictive. Atkins and LCHF (Low Carb High Fat) are in the mid-range, and the Whole30 and Paleo diets are the least carb-restrictive. Whole30 and Paleo diets restrict certain processed foods and refined sugars but allow higher amounts of carbohydrates as well as unrefined sugars such as beets, sweet potatoes, and fresh and dried fruits. These unrefined sugars are completely restricted from the approach to the diet that I ascribe to, which is known as the therapeutic approach to keto. For the most part, they contain too much fructose and starch per serving to stay within the keto diet's maximum of 5 percent carbohydrate.

Another central feature that differentiates the ketogenic diet from other low-carb diets is that it moderates protein and features healthy fats as a core staple. It also differs from other low-carb diets because of the presence of ketones.

There are three main reasons why ketogenic diets are so effective:

- Nutritional ketosis (a state of being fueled by ketones) mimics the state of fasting and generates many of the same beneficial effects, such as autophagy (whereby the body "burns off" old cells, tissues, and even cysts while also burning body fat), increased production of human growth hormone, and restored insulin sensitivity. (See page 52 for more on fasting.)

- A keto diet optimizes health by properly nourishing the body with fat and protein, which are essential macronutrients, and limits the intake of carbohydrates, which are not essential. (See page 63 for more on macros.)

- A keto diet generates results via the endocrine theory of weight loss rather than the energy balance theory of weight loss. (See page 43 for more on these two theories of weight loss.)

Your Ketogenic Cake

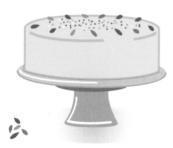

Welcome to the wonderful world of being fat-fueled! I use the word *wonderful* because my path to the ketogenic lifestyle has been full of wonder and amazement. You might have several reasons for wanting to learn more about the ketogenic diet. You might be looking for a solution to illness, relief from pain caused by chronic inflammation, help with an autoimmune condition, or weight loss. Or perhaps you are attracted by the buzz you have heard about the ketogenic way of eating and its many benefits, which include mental clarity, high energy, and optimized health. Astoundingly, a ketogenic diet can assist with all of these goals. When it comes to optimizing health, nutrition is the most underrated aspect of all. In my opinion, what we eat (or do not eat) is the single most important factor in our overall physical health. Our cells are formed from and nourished (or not nourished) by the foods we eat.

Although the current and predominant approach to a "healthy" diet in the Western world can be classified as low-fat and high-carb, this manner of eating, in my opinion, is far from healthy or ideal. We have been led to believe that eating large amounts of carbohydrates—grains, beans, starches, and certain vegetables and fruits—is healthy. Carbs have been touted as the most nutritious foods, and fats are regarded as being the least nutritious and most detrimental to health. We've also been erroneously taught that the total calorie count is more important than which types of foods are supplying those calories. This thinking leads us to believe that we can eat as many french fries, snack cakes, and pizzas as we want as long as we keep total calories in check. This kind of thinking has also led people to ingest food products made in factories that emphasize flavor as opposed to real foods that emphasize health.

However, current science explains the perils of sugar consumption and shows that saturated fats do not cause heart disease. Current science also supports the effectiveness of low-carbohydrate diets. (See page 61 for a few examples.) Consuming large amounts of carbs generates persistent high blood sugar levels, which lead to chronic inflammation and contribute to insulin resistance. Insulin-resistant cells require the pancreas to secrete more and more insulin, potentially leading to type 2 diabetes and a crescendo of negative health effects and other conditions, including nonalcoholic fatty liver disease (NAFLD), which is a precursor to type 2 diabetes, or, worse, stroke or heart disease caused by elevated triglycerides in the blood.

Consuming large amounts of carbohydrates (especially sugars) can lead to chronic high blood sugar, which in turn can lead to persistent inflammation, insulin resistance, metabolic disorders, excessive fat tissue generation and fat storage, and, most dangerous of all, contribute to elevated triglycerides because the body converts excess blood sugar into denser forms called blood lipids (fats), commonly referred to as triglycerides. Having high triglycerides is a precursor to heart disease and stroke.

Eating a low-fat diet also deprives our bodies of the essential fatty acids that they cannot make on their own; our bodies must get these essential fatty acids from outside food sources to function optimally and survive. Combine these excessively high blood sugar levels with a lack of essential nutrients and you have the basis for our current epidemic of malnourishment, leading to obesity, type 2 diabetes, autoimmune conditions, heart disease, and many more. The causes of disease are multifactorial and are affected by diet, as well as genetic and environmental factors. However, as I've stated, I believe that what we eat is the single most significant and overlooked factor in how our bodies look, feel, and function.

I will explore the reasons I took on the ketogenic diet a little later in this Introduction. For now, let's focus on what brought *you* to the ketogenic diet. My clients often tell me that they first heard about keto from colleagues, friends, or family members who have experienced remarkable results. It is one thing to read about the benefits of a diet, but seeing someone you know experience those benefits is much more compelling!

Digging into the Cake

It's important to define what you consider to be good health. When your health and weight are the way you want them to be, you barely think about them. Your body is invisible to you because you feel comfortable in your clothing and confident in your body. You are at peace with your daily food intake. You eat to live rather than live to eat. You enjoy your food without overanalyzing it. You feel alive and vibrant; you are energized, ready to take on physical demands, and inspired to engage in good-feeling movement, such as a bike ride in the park or a sunset walk on the beach. These forms of exercise are not an obligation or a means to an end; the idea is simply to experience the pure joy of inhabiting your body.

On the other hand, if your health and/or weight are not what you want them to be, you probably take notice of that fact more often than not. Like it or not, we take our bodies with us wherever we go, and we interact with our bodies all day long. When our bodies are not in good health or are carrying excess fat, every interaction can generate feelings of discomfort.

I know from experience how unpleasant it can be to feel uncomfortable every day. I know how it feels when simple routines like showering and finding clothes to wear become much more difficult than they ought to be. When you aren't comfortable in your own body, dieting can become a constant part of life, and mealtimes can be filled with anxiety. This anxiety can be especially bad at social gatherings involving meals when you end up bargaining and negotiating with yourself while keeping score of calories. Going off your diet plan or indulging leads to feelings of guilt and regret. Depending on how you feel, you either avoid exercise or exercise excessively as a form of punishment for overindulging. Even when you've done the best you can or accepted your discomfort, you can't escape the reality that your health is not where you want it to be any more than you can escape your own skin. Worse still, all this is not for lack of effort or doing the best you can. In my opinion, it is the result of a faulty approach to health and weight loss that is based entirely on energy balance (calories in versus calories out), which leads to a lack of results and to food fixation.

Keto differs because it is not a diet; it is a long-term lifestyle based on eating real, whole foods, and it generates real results. If your experience with health and diet to date has been less than ideal, don't fret! The ketogenic lifestyle has arrived.

Feeling on top of the world [and] ready to tackle my day. Day 68 of my keto journey, down 41 pounds. Woot woot. My goal was to hit 40 by Sept. 30. Next short-term goal? 5 more by Oct. 15! Shouldn't be difficult as there are so many nummy new recipes [in Vanessa's meal plans] to keep me focused.

—Karen S.

Taking the First Bite

What is your picture of glowing and vibrant health? Is it feeling like your best possible self, loving the experience of being in your body, having a sense of boundless physical and mental energy, being at your ideal weight, and feeling confident and comfortable without compromise? I can tell you that no matter the current condition of your health and body, you can begin to change it now. No matter how far you are from where you want to be, there is hope. The ketogenic lifestyle is a powerful healing protocol that can dramatically transform your physical state. By picking up this book, you've already set the gears in motion, and you can begin making your way toward your ideal health and body. Just keep putting one foot in front of the other and read this book along with me to learn why the ketogenic diet is so effective.

Before starting on your journey, it's critical to know why you are taking the time to invest in and learn about keto. The people who experience the greatest success are the ones who have their reasons—their "whys"—defined. I am here to help you get to where you want to be. However, to get there, we first need to know what your goals are and what kind of vision you have for your physical health and well-being. Knowing your "whys" will propel you forward with massive inertia; having a grip on your "whys" will also sustain you when you hit roadblocks.

The good news is that the ketogenic diet has been a runaway success for thousands of people around the world because long-term compliance is easy. When a diet is difficult to sustain over time, it is less successful. Deprivation diets—the most common model today—often fail because they are hard to maintain over the long haul. Deprivation diets are looked upon as temporary restrictions. The word *diet* itself implies that this way of eating is a time-limited undertaking after which "normal" life will resume.

As I mentioned, keto is generally referred to as a *diet*, but I truly think of it as a long-term *lifestyle*. Once you learn how to do it properly, you will see how easy it is to follow, regardless of your circumstances.

So, before you go any further, take a moment to define what you see as your dream health and body. Close your eyes, form a picture in your mind, and think about why making the effort is worth it to you. Write down your reasons and keep them where you can see them every day; they will add fuel to your fire when you need it most. Your goals will play a big part in propelling you forward on your journey to ideal health.

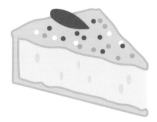

Biohacking Our Way to Good Health

Biohacking is a relatively new practice that has exciting possibilities for your health and, therefore, your quality of life. Who doesn't love getting more of what you want with less effort? Who doesn't love faster, more efficient ways of reaching your goals? By picking up this book, you have taken a step toward leveraging your health with biohacking—also known as life hacking—which is the latest social movement of citizen or "do-it-yourself" health. Biohacking is about using the latest tools and technology to learn about your body and how it is affected by your daily food, exercise, and sleep choices.

When it comes to health, there has never been a more exciting time to be alive. We are at the forefront of incredible discoveries that will drastically alter our quality of life. Researchers, scientists, and health advocates around the world have begun to democratize health by questioning the mainstream consensus of what makes a diet and body healthy. This health revolution is also being propelled by solo biohackers who are willing to venture into new territory. I hope that includes you! When you are armed with hope, determination, and a sense of responsibility for yourself, the health of your dreams is not just some mirage; it is a real and attainable possibility.

The ketogenic diet is one of the most exciting new fields of research in the realm of health. The latest scientific studies showing the health benefits of keto are staggering, as is the growing wealth of empirical data from people doing keto for themselves, often not heeding their doctors' advice to avoid dietary fat, to great success. (You can read about the positive experiences of some of my clients in the margins of this book.) And these discoveries and the benefits derived from them are no longer confined to labs; they can now be accessed by anyone with a glucometer, a device that fits in the palm of your hand. At one time, glucometers were used only by diabetics to monitor blood sugar; today, however, anyone can buy these monitors without a prescription. Glucometers allow us to monitor our blood sugar levels and track the effects of various foods on our bodies. Apps for our phones and other devices enable us to easily track our diets and macronutrient breakdowns.

A ketogenic diet makes use of these fantastic tools so that we can see with our own eyes how processed foods and real foods affect us differently. This kind of testing is eye-opening for many people, and it is part of what makes following a ketogenic diet a biohacking activity. Testing your blood sugar and ketone levels is not a requirement for following the keto diet, but the information that testing provides is very useful. See page 66 for more on testing with a glucometer.

My Story

"Tired? How can you possibly be so tired? At your age, I was full of energy!" I still remember hearing this from my well-meaning parents when I visited them as a young adult. And I vividly recall how terrible I felt in my body. In my twenties, I claimed to feel like an old soul. Unfortunately, the fact of the matter was that I felt like an old soul trapped in an even older body. Every day, something in my body didn't feel good. I dealt with fatigue, brain fog, headaches, and inflammation. In 2011, I reached the peak of my physical discomfort. My hands were often stiff and cramped, and they throbbed with arthritic pain. I suffered from intolerable digestive pain from ulcerative colitis, for which a common treatment is invasive intestinal surgery. At the time, I was a vegetarian (and former strict vegan).

I had begun avoiding sugar in the early 2000s after the low-carb/Atkins phenomenon had taken off. I tried to eat as healthfully as possible, but I had a hard time shaking off the prevailing advice that whole-wheat bread and pasta needed to form the foundation of my "healthy" diet. I believed my diet was healthy, and I never thought to examine it until my then-partner (now husband) told me a story about his cousin who had learned that she had a gluten sensitivity and suggested that I look into whether I had the same sensitivity. I had a gluten test done by an accredited laboratory in Texas, and it came back positive. This led me to try eliminating gluten from my diet. Within weeks, the inflammation in my hands had dissipated, and after a few months, my sharp intestinal pains had started to subside. I confirmed that the pain in my hands and abdomen was tied to my consumption of gluten by noting that it returned only when I had accidentally consumed gluten within the past two days. This miraculous discovery sparked my low-carb journey, which eventually led me to the ketogenic diet.

Removing gluten from my diet dramatically improved my overall health. However, I still experienced low energy, headaches, and brain fog and carried an extra 30 pounds. I'd been saddled with that extra weight for most of my life—from a chubby child and teenager to an adult who never felt comfortable in her skin. What I didn't realize was that I had developed insulin resistance over the years from eating a high-carb, high-protein, low-fat diet.

I was born in the 1980s, and I was a product of the belief that a diet of fat-free foods, such as whole grains, brown rice, potatoes, and fruit, was the way to go. My grandfather died of type 2 diabetes, and I inherited a predisposition to being more sensitive to sugar and carbohydrates than the average person. Both of these issues have been a constant in my life for as long as I can remember.

I had been a vegetarian for fifteen years (between the ages of seventeen and thirty-two) and was a vegan for a brief stint, too. I had been seeing a naturopath about my lethargy, brain fog, and general anxiety, and he prescribed some remedies for leaky gut and *Candida* overgrowth. The naturopath also suggested that I consider adding some animal proteins, such as fish and poultry, back into my diet. I decided to give it a try, although it was challenging for me to eat animal foods after going without them for so long. However, I was desperate.

I knew something wasn't quite right about my persistent exhaustion and feeling generally unwell, so I started researching adrenal fatigue. I learned that my adrenal glands were likely depleted due to stress and high anxiety. What I probably didn't realize at the time was that I was likely experiencing symptoms related to underactive thyroid. I visited doctor after doctor but did not find relief from the lethargy, regular headaches, and excess weight. I read scores of health and diet books and restricted my eating to large vegetarian salads. I was told that the way to lose weight was to eat low-fat and high-carb and to exercise, so I avoided dietary fat and did cardio daily on my quest to get healthy. I even saved up to buy a treadmill and placed it in my living room, facing the television so that I could watch shows while running for 30 to 120 minutes every day. But despite diet after diet, cleanse after cleanse, and hour after hour on the treadmill, my weight didn't budge, and my low energy levels, brain fog, and headaches persisted. I tried everything to lose weight and feel better in my body, including even extended juice fasting. The caloric restriction resulted in temporary weight loss, but the weight piled back on when my metabolism slowed down. I started to accept that being anxious, overweight, groggy, and tired was going to be my life.

I studied nutrition in college. While the courses were insightful, they reinforced the high-carb, low-fat dietary regimen that was blasphemous to question at that time. Until, that is, Dr. Robert Atkins and other brave doctors and authors such as Gary Taubes (*Why We Get Fat*), sparked a low-carbohydrate revolution.

Until then, my vegetarian diet was centered around salads, legumes, and fat-free yogurt and salad dressings. As my efforts continued to fail, I kept hearing about the amazing results people were seeing on the low-carbohydrate or Atkins diet, which was rising in popularity. I was determined to shed my post-college weight, which was creeping up, and to improve my overall health, so I decided to give Atkins a try. I loved the high-fat foods I was allowed on the Atkins diet, but I did not lose the weight I wanted to lose, have the energy I hoped to have, or experience any of the other results I hoped to experience.

My health struggles continued until that fateful day I discovered the ketogenic diet. At first, the concept seemed so foreign to me. The idea of a diet full of fat flew in the face of everything I thought I knew about healthy eating. And yet I had to ask: if everything I had done until now hadn't worked, what would happen if I did the opposite? The more I read, the more outlandish the ketogenic diet seemed, but the more confident in

July 2016: Eating "clean," 5 meals a day [of] measured protein and carbs with heavy mood swings and no movement on the scale!! July 2017: Eating keto since middle of January with more energy, no mood swings and 45 lbs weight loss!!! #ketoworks #thankfulforvanessasplan

—Bethany W.

it I became. I began to think that it might be crazy enough to work. Little did I know that my life and health were about to change dramatically. The person I would become was nearly unrecognizable to me at the time!

Becoming the Ketogenic Girl

When I first started the keto diet, I made a *lot* of mistakes—that is, until I studied and tested it enough for it to all make sense. It felt like I had been searching for most of my adult life for the plan or program that would finally release me from food and weight fixation, heal my body, and enable me to lose that extra 30 pounds. I was excited about keto and wanted to learn everything I could about it.

You can find a wealth of information about keto on the Internet. However, too much information can lead to confusion and paralysis. The only way to know whether something is working for you is to assess your results. If your goal is to lose fat, you want to see the numbers on the scale moving down; you also want to feel more comfortable in your clothing and become more body confident.

When I decided to take the plunge and try keto, I was overwhelmed by all the information I came across. I started out using urine test strips, as many people do. Initially, it was exciting to see the bright purple readings indicating the presence of ketones in my urine. I wanted more proof, so I purchased a breath meter, which also confirmed the presence of ketones in my breath. I thought this must mean that I was in nutritional ketosis and that the fat would start melting off. I made the mistake of relying on inaccurate data from the urine test strips and the breath meter, which were giving me only part of the picture.

Because I was measuring my ketone levels and getting positive confirmation, I didn't weigh myself for the first few months. This was the first mistake that I made. I thought that high ketones meant that I was in fat-burning mode because that's what I had read and seen online. I "knew" that I was on my way to the weight of my dreams because I was following the advice of keto experts I had found on the internet and was getting high ketones. I believed it was only a matter of time before I would see the results I wanted. I was having a blast making delicious high-fat keto recipes and indulging in keto cheesecake, keto ice cream, and bulletproof coffee.

However, a few things were nagging at me. First, I never felt full. Despite all the fat I was eating, I was still fixating on food, and I found myself going back to the refrigerator multiple times a day. Second, I was not feeling especially energetic, and my mental clarity had not improved. Lastly, my clothes were getting tighter and tighter. I felt uncomfortable, but I believed so much in what I was doing that I thought I had to be succeeding. My carb intake was next to nonexistent, and my ketones were consistently in the 2.0 to 5.0 range.

My husband and I went to Las Vegas for a getaway in the desert, and my swimsuit was not fitting well. The bottoms were tight, and I thought they must have shrunk. One evening, we went out to dinner and wandered by a place where we'd had our picture taken two years prior. We had our picture taken in the same place doing a similar pose. When we returned to the hotel, I opened my phone to see the photo, and I could not believe my eyes. I put the two photos side by side and saw a shocking difference in my body size. It dawned on me that I might have gained weight, but it seemed impossible considering how well I was following keto—even going to the grocery store to buy ingredients for homemade omelets with cream cheese during our trip! I measured my ketone levels morning and night. How could this be?

When we returned home, I got on the scale, and my eyes bulged. I weighed 168 pounds. I had gained about 20 pounds since I'd last weighed myself a few months prior, after I'd done some extreme calorie restricting. I could not believe this had happened!

I realized that despite my best efforts and the fact that I was seeing the numbers I wanted to see, I was still gaining weight. I didn't know that it is possible to gain weight in nutritional ketosis (a state in which the body burns fat instead of carbs). However, I was eating too much food, even though it was the right kind of food.

Clearly, something was way off, and I was doing some major things wrong. Despite this, I still believed in keto. The premise of converting the body from a sugar burner to a fat burner appealed to my sense of logic and ignited my interest. I wanted to be a fat burner more than anything, and I wasn't ready to throw in the towel. I believed that being a fat burner was going to be *the* solution for me, and I loved eating high-fat after living most of my life feeling deprived of flavor and being stuck eating low-fat foods.

My mistakes were starting to reveal themselves, but I wasn't quite there yet. I invested in a glucometer and tested my blood ketones. From the start, my ketones were high. My readings were between 4.0 and 5.2 mmol/L, and I knew that 1.0 to 3.0 is the optimal range for nutritional ketosis. I was so excited to see the high ketones reflected on the screen. I tested my husband for comparison, and his ketones were 0.2 mmol/L. Wow! I was in the ketone zone, and it was incredibly exciting. However, I made the third mistake of not measuring my blood glucose along with my blood ketones.

Even though I had read several books and blogs and listened to podcasts on the topic, I missed a lot of key information. Success on keto comes down to several important rules, in addition to the 80/15/5 macronutrient formula that we will explore later in this book.

One of my main mistakes was eating too much protein, which can take you out of ketosis if you eat more than protein your body can use for energy or store. The body treats excess protein as excess sugar in the bloodstream. I did not realize that I was overconsuming protein because I was not testing my blood glucose.

Another mistake I made was using a lot of artificial *as well as* natural noncaloric sweeteners, such as stevia and erythritol, to replace sugar. I had a major candy addiction for years, so I needed to replace candy and sugar with anything that could replicate it. Also, I read that these artificial sweeteners were completely acceptable on a low-carb diet. I fell for a lot of products that pretended to be "sugar-free" only to discover that they contained maltodextrin, polydextrose, or agave, all of which are sugar by another name. These ingredients were hard to pinpoint because when I saw something advertised as being "sugar-free" or containing stevia, I believed that it was indeed sugar-free. Unfortunately, in many cases, products labeled as being "sugar-free" or containing other sugar substitutes are really only free of cane sugar. The product might contain sugar in the form of fructose, sucrose, or sugars going by dozens of other names. I will discuss sweeteners in their own section later in the book.

The last major mistake I made was not eating enough fat. When I started keto, the most difficult part was embracing the idea of eating fat at all, let alone consuming a lot of it. Fat still terrified me because I had long believed that it was artery-clogging and I literally believed that if I ate any food containing fat, it would deposit itself directly on my thighs or elsewhere. Years of fat fearmongering made switching to eating so much fat a scary proposition at first, and it took me a while to work up to retooling my diet from scratch and basing it on eating fat.

My weight had still not really started to trend downward until I broadened my research and redoubled my efforts by reading every book I could find. I watched videos and expert panels online, attended low-carb conferences, and listened to every podcast and audio book on the subject. I started to realize that blood sugar levels—not just ketone levels—are a huge part (if not the more important part) of the equation. I also started to understand that high-fat dairy could prevent weight loss.

I began measuring my blood glucose levels in addition to my blood ketone levels, and combined that with daily, detailed macronutrient tracking. I made some key changes to my diet, and I finally started seeing the results I wanted! The weight started trending down. I started feeling truly satisfied from meals for the first time in my life and began to experience what I have come to know and refer to as "food peace," which is exactly what it sounds like. It's freedom from constant fixation on food and where my next snack or meal was going to come from. My body was finally being fully nourished by real food and receiving essential fatty acids from the healthy fats and high-quality proteins that it had been deprived of for so many years. I was astonished by how sharp and clear my focus and thoughts were becoming. I went from constant exercise and punishing

Thought I'd share a milestone that I've been striving for—hit a weight loss of 35 lbs this morning and have been on the life-changing 'Vanessa train' since end of Feb. I'm pretty close to my goal weight — just want [to lose] a few more pounds before I start easing into maintenance.

—Colleen H.

workouts with no results on the scale to working out only when I felt like it and shedding weight without any regular, scheduled time at the gym. Instead of steady-state cardio, I started going for delightful walks and embracing good-feeling movement, like yoga.

My clothes were getting so loose that I had to keep buying smaller and smaller sizes, which is probably the best problem ever. I ended up losing more than 40 pounds and getting down to my goal weight of 125 for my wedding in July 2016. I got to wear my dream wedding dress, which was very form-fitting, when I always thought I would have to wear a giant cupcake-style ball gown to hide my out-of-shape form. Feeling so body confident and comfortable in my skin for the most special week of my life was a dream come true.

Through trial and error, I learned from my mistakes. At the same time, I developed a formula that was effective for getting into nutritional ketosis. I was able to apply this formula time and time again to get others into ketosis. Being very carb-sensitive and having struggled with my weight for most of my life, I personally tested my blood glucose and ketone levels with every single recipe in my programs. I knew that if the recipes helped *me* achieve high ketone levels, low blood sugar, and weight loss, they would work for most people.

The increased energy and mental clarity I also gained in addition to the weight loss helped me accomplish my goal of leaving the online finance news reporting role which I enjoyed, to having the energy and confidence to launch my dream, passion-based business with Ketogenic Girl! While this almost seems too good to be true, it isn't—and you can do it, too. I always believed I would be depriving myself for my entire life. I had accepted living without much fat or flavor in my food, to keep my calorie intake as low as possible. The irony is that all that sacrifice resulted in me feeling deprived, always hungry, tired, and constantly preoccupied with food. That is, until I found the ketogenic lifestyle!

Taking the Ketogenic Girl Online

I started sharing videos online explaining my early mistakes and what I had learned on my way to enjoying success. Spreading the word about the harmful effects of sugar in the diet and the incredible benefits of keto was quickly becoming my life's purpose, despite the fact that I was running a finance business and serving as an anchor for a finance news web series. I would wake every day at around 4 a.m. to create as many blog posts as I could before I needed to turn my attention to my finance work. Each day, people sent me messages about how they had been doing keto for a while but were struggling to see results. People were requesting one-on-one help in greater and greater numbers. I felt so driven by my passion and loved it so much that I was working on my blog early in the morning and late into the night, losing track of time.

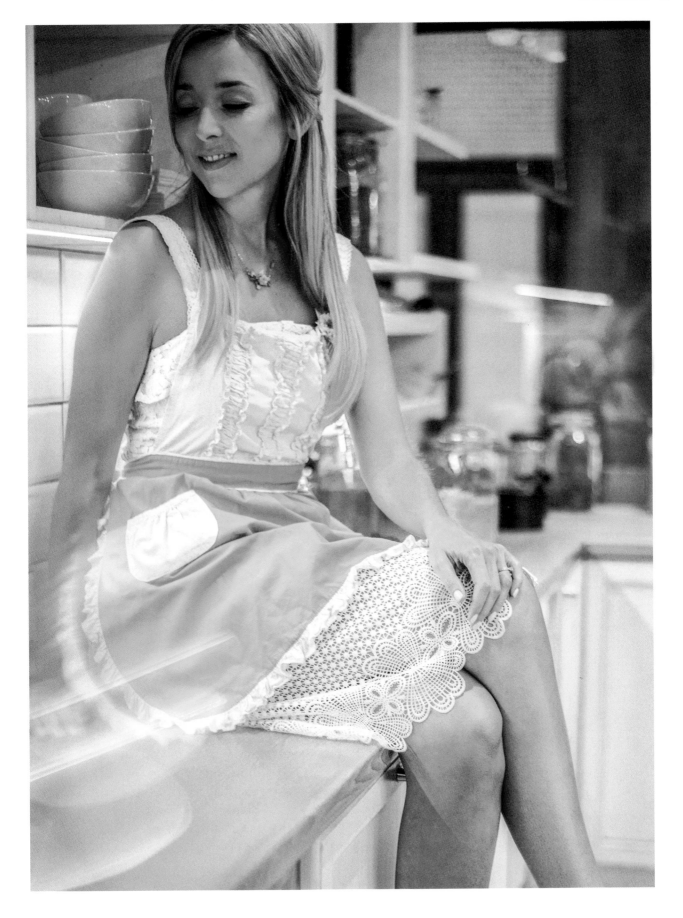

I realized that to serve the greatest number of people, I needed to leave the finance world and transition to working on Ketogenic Girl full-time. I wanted to be able to provide wonderful 24/7 support to the people following my program. I also wanted to create an encouraging and loving community of people who wanted to make keto a lifestyle instead of just a means of losing a few pounds. Based on what I had learned was the most effective path to getting into nutritional ketosis and losing weight, I created the Ketogenic Girl Challenge. The challenge features my 28-Day Meal Plans along with online coaching to support people as they follow the program. My coaching includes answering questions and making personalized dietary modifications as needed. I also teach how to test for ketosis, how to maintain a keto diet while traveling and eating out, and how to eat a proper keto diet for life.

Because a high-fat, low-carb keto diet is contrary to what we have been conditioned to believe is optimal for health, it's critical to have the support of family members and/or a community around you—especially when you make a misstep or lose hope along the way. I have had the privilege of playing a part in the health journeys of thousands of people, and I have witnessed nothing short of miraculous health transformations.

To date, the Ketogenic Girl Challenge has grown to include over 2,300 participants whom I actively coach on a daily basis, with new daily sign-ups of anywhere from five to thirty people.

My Mission Statement

Ketogenic Girl is deeply committed to excellence and serving you with love, kindness, skill, refinement, and compassion so that you may reach your goals and inspire others to do the same for themselves! We believe in vibrant health, confidence, and energy for all through the healing power of nourishing, whole foods. We believe in democratizing health care by upholding a sense of self-responsibility for our health, and healing and restoring the body (and spirit) with love and nutrition. We are honored to serve you and play a part in your health journey, as well as that of hundreds of thousands of people worldwide. Our passion is championing you in living your life to the fullest!

My approach has been extremely effective because it adheres to the science behind nutritional ketosis. I refer to my approach as strict keto, but without going over the edge. For a program to work, it has to be relatively easy to follow on a day-to-day basis, even during travel and at social events.

When you are on a deprivation diet, attending a special event or going to a restaurant can feel like an experiment in willpower. When you are depriving your body of essential nutrients, as well as over-exercising with the goal to "burn fat," you will easily succumb to temptation and sabotage your efforts. Don't waste effort resisting treats, counting and restricting calories, and forcing yourself into an intensive exercise regimen that you don't enjoy. Doing these things will rob you of the willpower to make the choices that will support your goals when it comes to eating, which is the most important factor when it comes to weight loss and health. You will literally run out of willpower juice! We have to conserve our willpower and use it only when we need it most, and in this case it is selecting what goes on your plate and what stays off of it.

Carbs have a hedonic effect as well because sugar has addictive properties that make it difficult to limit ourselves to a small amount. Sugar's effects on the body bring on massive cravings for more. On keto, your body and cells are continuously satisfied from the abundance of nourishing, delectable whole foods and healthy fats. You are never in a state of deprivation. Because you also have unlimited fuel derived from ketones from your own sources of body fat, you don't have to fear losing progress when traveling or during special occasions. You don't have to worry about carbs triggering an addictive response that will drive you to eat more and more of them with no end in sight. This unlimited supply of fuel puts the odds of success on your side and generates long-term sustainable results!

At the end of the day, weight loss comes from the kinds of foods we eat, when we choose to eat, and how frequently we eat, not from restricting calories and overtraining. The most important thing you can do is to make good choices about *what* to eat and *when* to eat it.

My Before-and-After Photos

I've spoken at length about the benefits I've gained from following a ketogenic diet. The keto lifestyle has improved my quality of life, giving me more energy and vitality, and I live pain-free without autoimmune discomfort. Although weight loss might have motivated me to try keto, the "side effects" have been wonderful, too. My focus has mostly been centered on my physical health. I love how good it feels being in my body and enjoying life to the fullest. However, I know all too well the emotional toll that being overweight can take. You suffer feelings of shame, embarrassment, and worst of all, self-loathing. Learning to love myself

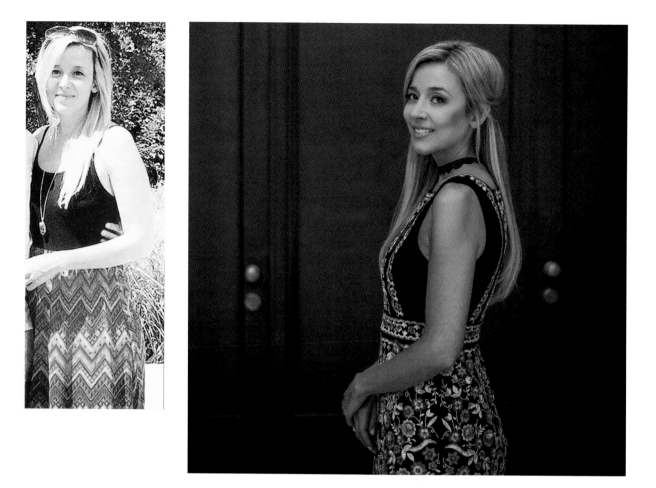

is probably the single most important thing that has come out of this journey. Once I was willing to give keto a try, I realized just how much our bodies do for us, and I began to appreciate all the hard work my body does to keep me as healthy as possible. I also learned to love and appreciate myself for who I am.

My Passion for Democratizing Health

To me, keto is a health revolution because many aspects of the ketogenic lifestyle emphasize the responsibility to take charge of our own health. The democratization of health is about increasing access for everyone so that we all can nourish ourselves to the best of our abilities while taking the time to learn about our bodies and how they respond to the foods we eat. We have more and more tools at our disposal, and at lower and lower costs. We are empowered to become our own health advocates, especially when it comes to our daily eating and physical activity choices.

We are fortunate to have unprecedented access to data; we're also fortunate because the health technology revolution is just beginning. Never before have we had access to small handheld devices that could calculate the amount of sugar in our bloodstream following meals. This data is valuable because it helps us learn how our bodies metabolize food. It also helps us understand how insulin-sensitive our bodies are. Insulin sensitivity (or resistance) is a measure of the body's sensitivity to "hearing" insulin and its ability to actively respond. If a person overconsumes glucose over a prolonged period, the effectiveness of insulin starts to become compromised, and more and more insulin is required to clear the bloodstream, resulting in hyperinsulinemia. Hyperinsulinemia is characterized by excessive levels of insulin in the bloodstream, as insulin's effectiveness at clearing glucose from the blood is lowered. Eventually, the pancreas can no longer keep up with the demand as it rises. When a person is no longer sensitive to insulin, otherwise known as being resistant to insulin, or "insulin resistant." In advanced cases, a person cannot produce enough insulin (or any at all), requiring supplementation with insulin, resulting in a diagnosis of type 2 diabetes. Years of overconsumption of sugar impedes the body's ability to detect and appropriately respond to sugar in the blood. When you choose to eat a ketogenic diet of whole foods instead of refined or processed foods and you avoid excess carbohydrates and sugar, you lower your blood glucose and restore your pancreas' ability to respond, as it is no longer being overstrained by ever-increasing demands to generate insulin to clear the bloodstream. It will then be able to respond with appropriate amounts of insulin and thereby restore sensitivity. This restored insulin sensitivity has a massive impact on your present and future health.

If you are ill, I can relate. If you have ever experienced the fear and uncertainty that come with illness, I know exactly how you feel. Diet-derived illness can trigger much uncertainty and fear because it is often difficult for traditional medicine to pinpoint the cause. I have a high regard for modern medicine and am thankful that we have access to well-trained surgeons and sophisticated medical technology. However, I believe that our healthcare system could be greatly enhanced if we returned to viewing whole-food nutrition as being paramount in both preventing and treating disease; nutrition should come before prescription drugs and surgeries. This approach is key for addressing the cause of disease instead of treating the symptoms. When I was suffering from painful inflammation, an expert recommended that I resort to drugs and surgery. However, drugs and surgery never would have addressed the actual cause—an autoimmune reaction from ingesting gluten. Not only would the effects from drugs and surgery have been temporary—because the actual cause would not have been fixed—but I might have ended up taking more drugs, having additional surgeries, and living with part of my colon removed. Instead, I stopped eating gluten and all the pain went away. Not only was it effective, but it was free, too! And after a bit of research into gluten-free foods, I found it relatively easy to do.

Health is the first wealth, and without it, there is no point or purpose to do or have anything else. Without health, we cannot live, much less enjoy life. I have always been interested in learning about health and nutrition. Much of what I have learned comes from my burning desire to have the health, weight, and body confidence of my dreams. This desire has driven me my entire life to seek and understand the food, exercise, and body connection. Like many of you, I listened to the predominating health advice proclaimed by the government, health organizations, and the media, and I followed it to a T. I was told that eating fat was bad, and I avoided even a single gram of it. I was told to eat my five to six servings of fruit and vegetables a day, and I did just that. I juiced greens and made "healthy" fruit smoothies. I avoided junk food except for an occasional fat-free frozen yogurt or artificially sweetened ice cream. I did everything I was told, and I never saw the results that I wanted. But I never gave up. I knew that my pursuit of health would eventually yield results if I found that one real solution or answer. I believed it was out there, and I was going to attempt anything and everything to find it, including quite a bit of self-experimentation.

Before I found keto, I tried nearly every health and body treatment under the sun. I've tried IV chelation therapy to remove heavy metals, cold baths with hydrotherapy, colonics, extreme calorie restriction, hot yoga, spinning, daily running, personal trainers, workouts using power plates, the Zone Diet, juice fasting, the Atkins Diet, vegetarianism, and veganism. I've tried being a raw foodist, being a fruitarian, being a pescatarian, and eating only fish and poultry. I've gone high-carb, low-fat, and high-protein. You name it, I have read and/or tried it. If it offered some glimmer of hope for improved health and weight loss, I was on board. Everything was worth trying, and everything gave me hope. However, nothing I'd found previously transformed my health and life until I found my way to keto!

Today, there is a revived interest in low-carb dieting. People following the keto lifestyle are reporting incredible results, and functional medicine, which incorporates all aspects of health by making diet a central pillar of its approach to healing, is on the rise. I believe we are facing a nationwide and worldwide health crisis. Diabetes, obesity, heart disease, nonalcoholic fatty liver disease (NAFLD), Alzheimer's disease, cancer, and many more conditions are on the rise. These conditions have been firmly linked to persistent inflammation, insulin resistance, and poor metabolic health, which is linked to eating excess carbohydrates (and in some cases excess protein). Fear of eating fat still grips our society despite the advances in science that prove otherwise.

We must take responsibility for our health and the choices we make, starting with our food. The sugar awareness movement has been increasingly successful and is gaining traction thanks to increased mainstream media coverage and the growing popularity for a return to our ancestral way of eating. We are returning to the way our great-grandparents ate, when nobody feared eating lard and eating whole foods from the land rather than candy and soda was commonplace.

The ketogenic diet is rooted in therapeutic applications. It was used as a powerful healing protocol for epilepsy (and was very effective until that treatment was replaced by pharmaceutical drugs). The keto diet has been proven to effectively manage seizures, in some cases more effectively than drugs. The keto diet and fasting also have shown success in halting—and in some cases reversing—type 2 diabetes. Because carb intake is dramatically reduced, both keto and fasting rapidly diminish the requirement for exogenous insulin (injected or infused insulin). This approach is much more effective than allowing patients to continue consuming carbohydrates and managing type 2 diabetes with higher and higher doses of insulin. Alzheimer's disease, which is the most common form of dementia and is a neurodegenerative disease, is now being referred to in certain scientific circles as type 3 diabetes. The most significant risk factor for Alzheimer's disease is lifestyle choices, and there have been links made to an inability of the brain to metabolize glucose, which leads to impaired brain function and neurotransmitter action, which decreases memory, processing speed, and overall function. Therapeutic use of medium-chain triglycerides (MCT) oil has seen tremendous success in halting and treating the disease because ketones can pass through the blood-brain barrier (a semipermeable membrane separating the brain and extracellular fluid in the central nervous system from circulating blood), thereby providing an alternative energy source for the brain. We have known for some time that sugar feeds cancerous tumors. We also know that excess blood glucose contributes to high triglycerides. Stroke, heart disease, and deep vein thrombosis are caused by blockages in the bloodstream and have been linked to excessively high blood triglycerides. Because many modern diseases are connected to excessive sugar consumption and to high-carb, low-fat diets, it is time to democratize health for all. We can do so by healing our bodies with nourishing whole foods and limiting our intake of sugars, grains, and processed foods.

I hit a 49-pound weight loss today!!!! Feeling good!! Started at 239, down to 190. Started at a tight size 20, and now 12s are loose. I have 9 friends who have started your program. Thank you, Vanessa Spina, for all that you do! I was going to wait to post until I hit 50, but it's just a number and I am feeling great so wanted to share.

—Lori D.

PART ONE

The Science of Keto

Chapter 1

The Ketogenic Diet

The Basics in a Nutshell

There are three macronutrients: fat, protein, and carbohydrate. The food we eat is made up of varying combinations of these macronutrients, or "macros." A state of nutritional ketosis is achieved by adhering to a diet with a macronutrient distribution of 80 percent fat, 15 percent protein, and 5 percent carbohydrate. To illustrate this distribution, let's start with the basics.

Don't Eat

Limit or eliminate the following foods:

- sugar, including processed, refined, unrefined, and natural or raw forms
- candy
- beets, carrots, corn, and peas
- bread, pasta, and other wheat flour–based products
- fruits and fruit juices (an occasional serving of berries and small amounts of lemon and lime juice are okay)
- milk
- legumes
- processed foods
- starchy vegetables, such as plantains, potatoes, and sweet potatoes
- sugary vegetables, such as beets, carrots, corn, and peas

Eat Instead

Include plenty of these foods in your ketogenic diet:

- healthy fats for cooking, such as avocado oil, coconut cream, coconut oil, lard, duck fat, and butter
- nourishing fats for eating, such as avocados, olives, and olive oil
- high-quality proteins that have a higher fat content, such as bacon, chicken thighs, and eggs
- low-carb vegetables, including asparagus, broccoli, cabbage, and leafy greens

- fermented foods, which feed and support the healthy gut bacteria: sauerkraut, kimchi, homemade fermented yogurt, full-fat Greek yogurt, and so on

Easing the Transition with Smart Swaps

If you need to transition gradually, as I did, work on sweetness first. Replace sugar, honey, and fructose with noncaloric natural sweeteners in their pure forms (for instance, stevia, erythritol, and monk fruit). These natural sweeteners do not raise blood sugar as significantly and tend to stimulate insulin less in most people. However, sweeteners still do have an effect on blood sugar and insulin and can cause cravings for carbohydrates. When I transitioned off sugar, I needed to do it gradually rather than take a cold-turkey approach, and natural sweeteners helped me at first. I also still drank a lot of naturally sweetened (with stevia and erythritol) beverages to help me make the transition from artificially sweetened diet soda. The final step in my keto journey was to quit using sweeteners altogether, as I found that they were causing cravings for sweet drinks and foods. Halting my daily consumption of them has enabled me to eliminate cravings and fully restore my insulin sensitivity.

It is important to eliminate all foods and condiments that contain added sugars and replace them with unsweetened options. Here are some examples:

- Replace reduced-fat and fat-free mayonnaise and salad dressings with full-fat mayonnaise and dressings with no added sugars.

- Replace candy with 99% dark chocolate.

- Replace breads and other wheat flour-based baked goods with almond flour or coconut flour–based breads and muffins.

- Replace egg white omelets with omelets made from whole eggs, and enjoy breakfasts such as Eggs Benedict (page 128).

- Enjoy pasta guilt-free with zero-carb shirataki noodles.

- Instead of nonfat milk and fat-free dairy products, enjoy coconut cream, heavy whipping cream, and full-fat plain yogurt (count the carbs in Greek-style yogurt), cheeses, and sour cream.

- Replace vegetable oils with real butter.

- Eat avocados, olives, mayonnaise, creamy salad dressings, olive oil, coconut and MCT oil, coconut milk, macadamia nuts, pili nuts, and other nuts, grass-fed butter, ghee, full-fat cheeses, and other healthy, rich, and nourishing fats!

By making these modifications to your diet, you will experience the benefits of a whole-foods, ketogenic lifestyle.

✕ DON'T EAT	✓ EAT INSTEAD
Sugar (including processed, natural, and raw)	Eliminate all sweeteners or transition with natural noncaloric sweeteners, such as pure stevia and monk fruit
Candy	Dark chocolate
Bread and other baked goods made from wheat flour	Breads and baked goods made with almond, coconut, and flaxseed flours
Pasta	Zero-carb noodles (aka shirataki or konjac noodles)
Fruit and fruit juices	Berries only occasionally; small amounts of lemon and lime juice are acceptable
Nonfat milk	High-fat dairy, such as heavy whipping cream, and coconut milk
Fat-free yogurt	Chia pudding and full-fat plain Greek yogurt (add nuts and sweeten with stevia)
Fat-free mayonnaise with added sugar	Full-fat mayonnaise without sugar
Fat-free salad dressings with added sugar	Full-fat salad dressings without sugar
Vegetable oils for cooking	Avocado oil, coconut oil, lard, duck fat, and butter
Grains	Hemp hearts, flax seeds, chia seeds, and nuts
Legumes	Legume-free alternatives such as my Ketogenic Girl Hummus (page 147)
Potatoes and other starchy vegetables	Cauliflower and radishes (Try my Cauliflower Mash [page 224] instead of mashed potatoes!)
Beets, carrots, corn, and peas	Low-carb vegetables (see chart), including asparagus, broccoli, cabbage, and leafy greens
Processed foods	Whole, unprocessed foods

Ketogenic Diet Food Guide

Instead of this, EAT THIS		Instead of this, EAT THIS		Instead of this, EAT THIS	
Mashed potatoes	Cauliflower mash	Burger buns	Portobello buns	Vegetable oils	Butter
Bread	Cloud bread	Tortilla wraps	Lettuce wraps	Carrots & potatoes	Radishes
Rice	Cauliflower rice	Low-fat dairy	High-fat dairy	Oats & granola	Chia & hemp
Pasta	Zucchini noodles	Fruit & juice	Low-fructose berries	Corn, beets, & beans	Green veggies
Pasta	Konjac noodles	Sugary treats	Dark chocolate	Anything	Bacon

Directing Your Body to Burn Fat

There are two dominant theories of weight loss:

- the energy balance theory, which says that in order to lose weight, you must take in fewer calories than you burn
- the endocrine theory, which says that your hormones determine whether weight loss or fat storage occurs

Although both theories have merit, the ketogenic diet is based on the endocrine theory. For decades, the energy balance model has dominated the Western approach to health, yet people seldom see long-term success when they focus on calories in versus calories out. After years of ascribing to this theory of weight loss myself, only to be met with failure, I finally found success by switching to the endocrine approach. Although I do believe that energy balance (calories consumed versus calories burned) plays a small role in weight loss, I feel that hormones are by far the more important part of the equation.

If you are wondering what makes the ketogenic diet more successful than other ways of eating, it begins with internal signaling and aligning with the innate design and function of our bodies. The true power of the ketogenic diet all comes down to understanding exactly how to communicate with our bodies via the foods that we eat.

Unfortunately, we cannot just speak to our bodies outright by saying something like, "Burn all stored fat now!"

If only it were that easy. If only our bodies could say in return, "Right away, boss! Commencing fat-burning sequence!"

However, we *can* tell our bodies to burn those fat stores rather than store fat. The way we communicate that message is by eating the right foods at the right times. As Dr. Jason Fung of Intensive Dietary Management puts it, we must monitor the "what and when." Dr. Fung and his partner, Megan Ramos, who founded the Toronto-based clinic IDM, are modern pioneers in the endocrine-based treatment of diabetes and obesity, and they have successfully reversed type 2 diabetes in many people. They have done so by restoring insulin sensitivity (the body's ability to efficiently respond to glucose in the bloodstream) in insulin-resistant (when one's body is unable to respond efficiently with insulin to clear the bloodstream of sugar, leading to type 2 diabetes) patients via various ketogenic and fasting protocols that limit the release of the hormone leptin, which signals the body to store fat. He and Megan have applied the hormone theory of weight loss in their practice and are achieving astonishing and consistent results. Their work has significantly advanced and validated the therapeutic promise of the keto protocol.

> "I've been using low-carbohydrate and ketogenic diets therapeutically in the Intensive Dietary Management program for many years. Many patients improve their metabolic profiles substantially—completely naturally, without medications or surgery."
>
> —Dr. Jason Fung

I just have to post this wonderful news. I am down 70 lbs since I began my keto journey. Not only do I look and feel better, but I am off all my meds, including insulin and metformin for type 2 diabetes. This is the most amazing way to live, and I sing Vanessa's and keto's praises wherever I go. Oh, and I turned 60 this year. Don't let anyone ever tell you it's too late.

—Leslee P.

The food we eat sends important signals to our bodies regarding energy storage and use. A ketogenic diet mimics the effects of fasting by creating a state of nutritional ketosis, which suppresses appetite very effectively. When we shift into nutritional ketosis by restricting carbs, consuming moderate amounts of protein, and increasing our intake of healthy fats, we no longer experience blood sugar spikes; instead, our blood sugar remains stable because we are being fueled more by ketones from the breakdown of fats and less by blood glucose.

Once you are in ketosis, the ketones circulating from broken-down fats effectively suppress appetite by appropriately signaling satiety hormones. Scientists have learned that ketones promote leptin, the hormone that makes you feel full, while suppressing ghrelin, the hormone that makes you feel hungry. A properly working endocrine system with efficiently produced leptin can lead to better metabolic performance; enhance brain function; improve mental acuity, clarity, and memory; and even positively regulate moods.

Initially, leptin binds to proteins in the blood. When leptin reaches the brain, it travels across the "blood-brain barrier" and eventually binds to leptin receptors in the hypothalamus, telling your brain that it is time to stop eating.

Your fat cells release leptin into circulation after you eat, and leptin is an effective regulator of food intake. The ketogenic diet also generates ketones, which directly provide a readily usable energy source. Because your body does not need additional food energy, it secretes leptin to suppress cravings. The opposite occurs on a high-carb diet, which suppresses leptin and revs up appetite-stimulating ghrelin.

When leptin circulating in your body makes you feel full, you stop eating; this allows the insulin in your body to do its job of clearing sugar from your bloodstream and pushing it into your cells to use for energy. Once your blood sugar has been lowered, your body stops producing insulin, which tells your body to burn stored energy. As long as insulin is being produced, your body will continue to use the energy from your food instead of the energy that has been stored as fat. The absence of circulating insulin forces your body to access that stored energy, first in the form of glycogen stored in your liver and muscle tissues. Once the glycogen has been burned, your body resorts to burning its deeper stores (fat tissue) for energy. On a ketogenic diet, the amount of food sugars in the form of carbohydrates is limited. Fullness is generated rapidly from eating satiating meals comprised of nourishing fats and adequate protein. When you feel full and you are restricting carbs, or you fast between meals, your pancreas stops secreting insulin to clear glucose from your bloodstream, which tells your body that it is now time to burn stored fat for energy.

You might think that weight loss is driven by portion control—and you would be right. What is so beautiful about the ketogenic diet is that much of your "portion control" comes naturally. Nourishing fats and proteins are satiating and naturally make you feel full. You feel full because of the restored presence of leptin (the fullness hormone) and the reduced stimulation of ghrelin (the hunger hormone). When we eat delicious and flavorful food, we feel full quickly, and the thought of eating past fullness or grazing loses its appeal. However, on a high-carb, low-fat diet, it's easy to eat an entire bag of popcorn, followed by a large container of yogurt or ice cream. The carbs in these foods suppress the secretion of leptin and rev up your hunger hormone. They also trigger a hedonic response to carbs, which is similar to the response people have to addictive drugs. Carbs light up many of the same neural reward pathways that other addictive substances do.

It is possible to gain fat weight on a ketogenic diet if you do not abide by the recommended macronutrient distribution of 80 percent fat, 15 percent protein, and 5 percent carbohydrates. Most people need to keep their daily total carb intake at or below 20 grams. In addition, be sure to observe what I refer to as the "protein threshold," which is the amount of protein that meets but does not exceed your calorie expenditure to be turned into glucose via gluconeogenesis. Carbs and protein are easy to overeat because they can trigger hormonal responses and activate reward circuits in the brain. Fat, however, is a different story. Of the three macronutrients, fat stimulates insulin release the least. It is difficult to overeat fat because it is so nutrient dense and leaves a more sustained "mouthfeel" on the tongue. If you can drink several glasses of fruit juice or eat several bowls of cereal, try eating five or six eggs, several avocados, and an entire bowl of whipped cream. Even the thought of it makes me feel full!

Because fat is very dense, some high-fat, adequate-protein, and low-carb meals that appear "average" in size can add up to a whole day's worth of calories. One-half cup of nuts or chia seeds, for example, can easily provide two to three meals' worth of energy. When portioning your meals, make sure that they are abundant in healthy fats because they will satiate you and help you get into nutritional ketosis by limiting blood sugar spikes and therefore insulin secretion. As a general rule, each of your meals should be based on a high-quality monounsaturated fat (such as extra-virgin olive oil, avocado, or macadamia nut oil) or saturated fat (such as red meat, butter, coconut oil, or MCT oil). Pair this good fat with a high-quality protein, such as grass-fed and organic meat, eggs, and seafood. Carbs should come last in the form of nutrient-dense greens, which are high in fiber. Insoluble fiber (fiber that cannot be broken down and absorbed by the digestive system) nourishes the gut, and reduces inflammation while cleaning the gut lining as it passes through the intestinal tract.

Proper keto meals, such as the recipes that appear in this book, allow you to feel full. When you aren't snacking between meals, insulin production is halted and nutritional ketosis is turned on, which uses your body's fat stores and the fat from your diet as its main source of energy. Essentially, you become fat-fueled and therefore can reap the many benefits of a ketogenic lifestyle!

Ancestral Diet Logic

When we consume sugar, whether it is processed or natural (such as the sugar in fruit or honey), it signals to our bodies to store fat for survival. Food has not always been readily available throughout our history. That meant when our ancestors came across plant-based sugars (berries or grains, for instance), they needed to consume as much of them as possible and store the energy by converting the excess sugar into fat so that it was available for future use when other energy sources weren't available. Bears do the same thing when preparing for winter. They consume as much of the abundant grasses and berries as they can in summer, build up large fat reserves, and then live off those fat stores during the winter months when they are hibernating in their dens and food is scarce. Just like bears, human survival initially depended on the body's ability to store energy for use when energy sources were not available; access to food was never guaranteed. Just like the bodies of bears, our bodies are very good at making and storing fat!

Our bodies are designed to store this energy for when it is needed, so it makes sense that our bodies would allow us to do so without the discomfort of feeling overly full. That means our bodies switch off leptin production when we consume sugar and carbs, which allows us to consume as much as we can without feeling uncomfortable.

When we eat carbohydrates such as sugar, fruit, vegetables, grains, starches, and so on, these foods tell our bodies that we are in storage mode—storing away for "winter" to survive future food scarcity. When the glucose from our food reaches the bloodstream, the pancreas releases insulin, which chases the glucose from the bloodstream; the glucose is stored in the cells for future use. The body will not burn stored fat when it is being told to store and generate more fat.

Often, people are alarmed to learn that natural sugars, such as fruit and honey, should be restricted on a ketogenic diet because they've always believed these natural sugars to be healthy. However, that teaspoon of honey in a cup of tea tells your body to store fat instead of burn it. That banana or handful of grapes tells your body that you've come across a rare source of energy and you must pack in as much as possible. Your body switches off fullness hormone signals and generates intense cravings. Your body wants you to eat as much as possible in order to stay alive later when this food source isn't available. Unfortunately for many of us, these food sources are always abundant, which means that our bodies continue to store the energy as fat even though we don't need it. The keto diet triggers our bodies to burn stored energy, which is possible because we aren't processing glucose from our food and thus our bodies aren't producing insulin. When we don't eat between meals, our bodies get a rest from circulating glucose and therefore insulin. The absence of insulin tells our bodies that it's time to burn stored energy until our next meal.

Our Bodies Were Designed to Be Either Sugar Burners or Fat Burners

Why is the ketogenic diet so effective? We first must explore the roles of glucose and fat in our bodies. Our bodies tend to be fueled by a primary and a secondary fuel. Our default fuel is glucose, and our bodies are mostly adapted to using glucose, with fat being a secondary fuel source. *Glucose* comes from the Greek word *glukus*, meaning "sweet." In a typical "healthy" diet, where carbohydrates and protein are consumed in high amounts and fat is severely restricted, glucose is the body's dominant source of energy, which occurs through the breakdown of the carbohydrates, starches, and proteins via glycolysis which is then taken up after digestion into the intestines. Glucose is then released into the bloodstream and subsequently stored in the liver and muscles in the form of glycogen. Because we are so adept at utilizing and prioritizing glucose synthesis for fuel, and our diets are predominantly high in carbs, our bodies default to using glucose as a primary energy source.

Most of us, however, have never been presented with the option of choosing sugar or fat as our dominant fuel source. Given the choice, would you rather be fueled by your own body fat or by glucose broken down from the food you eat? Because fat is considerably less appealing to deal with and a heck of a lot more visible on the body than sugar, I know which one I would choose (and have chosen by adopting the keto diet!). Also, our ability to store glucose when we take in more fuel than we need is limited to how much the liver can store in the form of glycogen (about 2,000 calories being the upper limit for the average person). As you might have noticed, our ability to store fat on our bodies is virtually unlimited.

Prior to going keto, I never knew that we had the potential to be fueled by fat, let alone as a primary fuel. I had been trained to believe that energy is measured in calories, and that when it comes to diet, a calorie is a calorie, regardless of whether it comes from fat, protein, or carbohydrate. I also believed that I needed to limit my calorie intake for weight loss, and that the easiest way to do so was to stick to lower-calorie foods, such as carbohydrates and protein, each of which contain 4 calories per gram. Fat, on the other hand, contains 9 calories per gram.

From the outset, the calories-in-versus-calories-out equation appears to be logical, which is part of the reason (aside from constant reinforcement) why it has endured. Your body fat percentage, which is an important

Today is my day 28 in round 2 [of the 28-day challenge]. I am officially down 25 pounds. It is so nice to fit into my clothes with ease. Yesterday, I even got to wear a dress I hadn't worn for 5 years. Amazing and I feel great! Thanks, Vanessa.

—Jacqueline B.

marker for long-term health, is a representation of your energy balance, just like your bank account is a representation of your funds balance. When it comes to your bank account, you want a positive balance; when it comes to your body, however, you generally want a neutral to negative balance of fat to lean mass. If you expend more calories than you take in, you will have a negative energy balance and lose weight. The best way to do so, we are told, is to lower calorie intake and increase energy expenditure. This notion is so ingrained in us that in the past, to question it would have seemed ludicrous. Fortunately, however, the endocrine theory of weight loss has resurged thanks to interest in the ketogenic diet, calling into question the energy balance theory of weight loss. Keto has become a powerful, disruptive force to outdated diet and nutrition beliefs, and it has been buoyed to new heights by the sheer numbers of people experiencing incredible weight loss and other health benefits. In short, keto has ignited hope.

My basic premise in this book is to explore the basis for why the ketogenic diet is so advantageous from an evolutionary standpoint and why it is so powerful for halting and reversing metabolic damage that underpins many modern diseases. Through this exploration, I hope to contribute to an expanding dialogue of what defines optimal nutrition for human beings in terms of overall health, performance, and disease prevention.

Although high-carb, low-fat diets are often vilified by proponents of low-carb eating, my objective is to acknowledge that carbs are a necessary part of our diet, but we must carefully regulate the kinds and amounts of carbs that we eat. In a balanced approach to eating, all three macronutrients have their place, with more emphasis on the most nutrient dense components and less on those with the least nutritional value. More importantly, I believe that being fueled primarily by fat—and thereby ketones—is much better aligned with optional functioning and health than being fueled primarily by glucose.

In the following pages, I will delve deeper into how our bodies can be fueled by stored fat rather than glucose and how to get our bodies into nutritional ketosis. When in nutritional ketosis, our bodies break down accumulated fat, and we experience many incredible benefits, such as

- easy and rapid weight loss
- increased and much more consistent energy
- mental clarity and sharpness
- satisfaction from delicious and flavorful healthy fats
- an end to food fixation because the body is being adequately nourished
- consistent calm moods
- autophagy (see page 59)

- relief from inflammation
- disease prevention and the potential to reverse diseases previously thought to be irreversible

Modern Diets Make Us All Sugar Burners

People often ask me how restricting carbs results in a balanced diet. What is so wrong with a balanced intake of healthy foods? To many, the concept of restricting grains, fruit, and some vegetables—all of which we've told are part of a "healthy" diet—sounds outlandish and extreme. My response is to ask how can we even begin to have a discussion about the concept of a "balanced" diet when more than 80 percent of the foods in the supermarket have sugar added to them? That leaves only 20 percent of foods that don't contain added sugar. Navigating the grocery store for optimal nutrition when the odds are so stacked against us is challenging. There are hidden sugars in everything, and they are taking on more and more deceptive names (see the illustration showing *sixty* different names for sugar!). How can we be expected to have balance? Even health-food stores, which do have tons of great options, offer a similar ratio of foods with added sugar, although they may take on more natural-sounding names, such as agave syrup or evaporated cane juice. Is it any surprise that modern dietary options ensure everyone will be a sugar burner?

60 DIFFERENT NAMES FOR SUGAR

Agave nectar	Coconut sugar	Golden sugar	Panela
Barbados sugar	Corn sweetener	Grape sugar	Panocha
Barley malt	Corn syrup	High-fructose corn syrup	Powdered sugar
Beet sugar	Corn syrup solids	Honey	Rice bran syrup
Blackstrap molasses	Crystalline fructose	Icing sugar	Rice syrup
Brown rice syrup	Date sugar	Invert sugar	Sorghum
Brown sugar	Demerara sugar	Lactose	Sorghum syrup
Buttered sugar	Dextran	Malt syrup	Sucrose
Buttered syrup	Diastatic malt	Maltodextrin	Sugar
Cane juice	Diatase	Maltose	Syrup
Cane juice crystals	Ethyl maltol	Maple syrup	Tapioca syrup
Cane sugar	Evaporated cane juice	Molasses syrup	Treacle
Caramel	Fructose	Muscovado sugar	Turbinado sugar
Carob syrup	Fruit juice concentrate	Oat syrup	Yellow sugar
Caster sugar	Galactose	Organic raw sugar	

The "everything in moderation" adage cannot be applied in our modern age of convenience foods because the majority of these foods only minimally nourish our bodies and can also include processing by-products that can be toxic substances that actively contribute to epidemics of disease, including obesity, diabetes, heart disease, fatty liver disease, type 2 diabetes, cancer, and Alzheimer's (now increasingly being referred to as type 3 diabetes). The ketogenic diet is a whole-foods approach that reverses this added sugar ratio of 80/20.

For starters, our diets need to maximize the ratio of positive nutrition to negative nutrition. What I refer to as "positive-nutrition foods" are foods that contribute to and enhance our health, while negative-nutrition foods do the opposite. Many foods have both positive and negative qualities. My approach to a ketogenic diet is based on maximizing positive nutrition by choosing real, whole, unprocessed foods over food products that have been processed, refined, or modified from their original forms in a lab or factory. We need to limit foods and "food-like products" that have been engineered to overstimulate our taste buds and lead to addiction.

Carbs have more negative than positive nutrition. For example, we can look at fatty liver disease, which is a serious health issue. In French, "fatty liver" is *foie gras*. Foie gras—fatty goose liver—is a rich culinary delicacy that is made by force-feeding grains to geese. Pig farmers also fatten their hogs by feeding them grains and limiting their physical movement. If dietary fat is the main contributor to body fat, then why are geese and other farm animals being fed carbohydrates? If eating fat makes us fat, wouldn't feeding the animals fat be a much more efficient way to fatten them up? Farmers know that carbs are the best way to fatten animals. The same thing happens in humans when we overeat carbohydrates: we get fatter.

A proper ketogenic diet is primarily composed of whole foods, which are foods that have been grown, harvested, or caught. You can recognize a whole food by the number of ingredients listed; it should consist of only one ingredient—that food. A package of chicken should contain only chicken, not a bunch of chemicals and added sugars. (To my horror, I have actually seen packaged chicken with sugar added to it being sold in grocery stores in the United States.) From farm to table, that food should be food that anyone in the world would recognize as nourishment.

My approach to keto is sensible and practical. People often think the keto diet is extreme because low-fat proponents have been making alarming claims for decades about the negative effects of saturated fats. However, I believe the true danger is found in diets that include copious amounts of sugar and are high in carbs and protein but low in fat. According to the USDA, the average American consumes between 150 and 170 pounds of refined sugar per year. (These numbers would be higher if unrefined sugars were included, too.) People living in Canada, the United Kingdom, Australia, and other Westernized countries are not far behind.

Day 28: lost 16.1 pounds and feeling great! For those wondering . . . I did not do formal exercise at all. This [Ketogenic Girl] eating plan is all I did. Took 3 days off plan this past weekend and still managed to eat ketogenically. Extending the first round of challenge until Thursday. Keto love to y'all!

— Toya J.

We need only look at the current state of health in the U.S. to see the results of several decades of going over a cliff when it comes to the overconsumption of carbs and protein and the elimination of fats. In many parts of Europe and Asia, people have not entirely embraced that dietary philosophy. People in the Mediterranean, for example, embrace whole-food fats and use olive oil, full-fat cheeses, and olives in their cooking, and in France people drench their food in butter. What is known as the "French paradox"—how can French people can eat so much rich food and still stay slim?—also applies to the Thai people, who eat a great deal of saturated fat, including coconut oil and coconut milk. Little did we know that they were taking advantage of all the fat-burning MCTs in coconut! (See page 76 for more on MCTs and their role in a ketogenic diet.)

We have been a fat-phobic, fat-deprived society for some time. Our great-grandparents were not deprived of healthy dietary fats, which came almost entirely from whole-food sources. You can see it in many ancient cultures still in existence today, such as the Masai and the Inuit, who primarily rely on an animal meats and/or dairy, which is consistent with our ancestral diets, without any processed carbohydrates and meeting the definition a ketogenic diet. They have been observed to have low rates of the diseases that we battle. They don't have access to processed foods and refined sugars that are readily available in modern urban environments.

When we are surrounded by easy, powerful fuel sources like the "rocket fuel" of refined sugars, we default to consuming sugars. However, in their absence, we consume mostly high-quality proteins and healthy fats, and we become fat burners rather than sugar burners. Because our modern diet is based on the high-carb model, people who try a keto diet often find that staying under 20 grams of total carbs is a challenge at first.

Hunger versus Appetite

There's a big difference between hunger and appetite. How do you know which of them you are experiencing?

Appetite is a habitual craving for food that is not related to hunger. Hunger is a physiological impulse to eat triggered by the body's requirements for food. Appetite is a perceived desire for food that is usually triggered by things like commercials (food marketers invest millions in research to make us "crave" the foods they are selling). When we see a billboard with appetizing food on it, our primal instincts to eat are triggered because those instincts are designed to keep us alive, which is why appetite is generated. The sight of favorite foods at parties or other events can also generate appetite and cravings. Once carbs hit your system, they can trigger your brain to experience intense cravings for more. In multiple trials and studies, sugar has been proven to have addictive properties, and the reasoning goes back to our ancestral makeup.

Hunger is a real instinct that is tied to survival. Our bodies tell us they're hungry and need energy. When you are a primary glucose burner, the experience of both hunger and appetite are common due to the spikes and crashes of glucose that generate constant cravings. Add a "calories in versus calories out" deprivation diet to this, and you have a recipe for disaster between feeling deprived and experiencing cravings, which can overwhelm a commitment to avoid overeating.

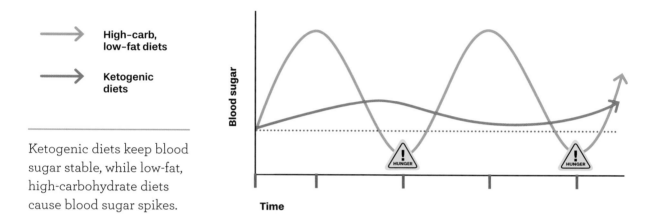

High-carb, low-fat diets

Ketogenic diets

Blood sugar

Time

Ketogenic diets keep blood sugar stable, while low-fat, high-carbohydrate diets cause blood sugar spikes.

Today marks my 4 months in the 28-day challenge group. I have enjoyed every day and learned so much about the keto lifestyle and my body. I went from 165 lbs to 125 lbs. I feel energetic and at peace. I find that when I consume lots of good fats my body feels amazing. So please don't be scared of the fat, embrace it. It's your friend! My non-scale victories are going from a size 10 to a size 6. The scale doesn't say it all. My other victories are the great energy and no hunger and great mood. Want to thank Vanessa for the prompt response to questions and support. Also this group has been awesome. Meals are delicious and easy to follow. I've been part of many different groups but they have always failed me. It seemed when you purchased the program the support and promises were no longer there. Not this program. Vanessa has kept to her word and is available every step of the way. Looking forward to my next 28 days.

—Luisa G.

As previously discussed, the keto diet is made up of positive-nutrition foods, satiating fats, and an adequate amount of protein, while restricting carbohydrates. Fat is the least insulin-stimulating hormone of those three macronutrients. Fat is the densest of the macronutrients, coming in at 9 calories per gram, which is more than double the 4 calories in a gram of protein or carbohydrate. It also makes us feel full and satisfied longer so we don't feel deprived and succumb to cravings and appetite triggered by enticing advertisements or commercials.

What Is Nutritional Ketosis?

On a ketogenic diet, we opt for positive-nutrition foods with the highest nutrition and the lowest carbohydrate content. Why do we limit carbohydrates? Because when we nourish our bodies along these guidelines, our bodies can naturally enter what is called *nutritional ketosis*.

Nutritional ketosis is a state in which the body is depleted of glucose (sugar) as a form of fuel and instead breaks down stored fat into ketone bodies and glycerol for fuel. Body fat cells contain fatty acids, and the process whereby the body breaks them down is known as *lipolysis*. When the body undergoes lipolysis, the fatty acids are released from the fat cells into the bloodstream. The liver produces ketone bodies from fatty acids, and those ketone bodies take the forms of three types of water-soluble molecules—beta-hydroxybutyrate, acetoacetate, and acetone—and a unit of glycerol. These molecules are converted to acetyl-CoA (a molecule with the primary function in energy production during metabolism) and eventually oxidized in the cell mitochondria (mitochondria are a powerhouse organelle located in the cell, breaking down nutrients and creating rich energy for the cell) for energy. They also pass through the blood-brain barrier (a membrane separating circulating blood from the brain) and are converted to energy by being used to turn acetyl-CoA into long-chain fatty acids (an acid with a long chain of carbon atoms). The heart prefers to be fueled by fatty acids and in nutritional ketosis can effectively use ketones, just like the brain. The brain's fueling from ketones will go up to about 70 percent as a primary fuel source, but it will always need some glucose as a secondary form of fuel, as the body always has a primary and a secondary fuel—either primarily glucose and secondarily fat or vice versa. That glucose can be obtained from glycerol by breaking down stored fatty acids into ketones and glycerol.

Both the brain and the muscles can utilize ketones, and the brain may prefer ketones in some cases. The ketones from omega-3 fatty acids, as well as MCT oil, have been shown to reduce cognitive deterioration in the brain and greatly aid with degenerative conditions. "Patients with memory impairment showed significant improvement in memory after receiving oral supplementation with MCTs that produced higher ketone levels in the blood," reported one study (M. A. Reger et al., "Effects of Beta-Hydroxybutyrate on Cognition in Memory-Impaired Adults," *Neurobiology of Aging* 25, no. 3 [2004]: 311–4). Another research team found that "Higher plasma levels of ketones like ß-hydroxybutyrate were directly correlated with higher performance in memory scores during this study" (Arun Swaminathan and Gregory A. Jicha, "Nutrition and Prevention of Alzheimer's Dementia," *Frontiers in Aging Neuroscience* 6 [2014]: 282).

The body depletes its glycogen stores about seventy-two hours after no more glucose or other food has been introduced, or from a few days to a week after carbohydrate restriction starts, depending on the extent of the restriction. The body will go into nutritional ketosis only when there is no available glucose for fuel. When glucose is present, the body will always opt to use it over fat because it can absorb and use glucose much more quickly than fat. For example, when you eat an apple, your body uses those sugars rapidly as they are quickly broken down into simple sugars via digestion, eventually releases them into your bloodstream, and then pushes them into your cells for use by the hormone insulin.

When you use fat for fuel, on the other hand, your body requires more time and energy for glycolysis, and the immediate fuel from breaking down sugars is replaced by a lengthier process of breaking down fat into ketones for fuel, so the immediate impact of glucose is not experienced. It's like using the existing electricity in your home versus a portable generator. When you need to power an appliance, are you going to use the power available from a plug on your wall or the portable generator? You will use the generator only when access to the electrical current is unavailable. Your body operates on the same principle. Just like a portable generator, it has backup stores of energy in the form of fat. It will burn and mobilize fat only when it needs to, not when the quicker glucose option is readily available.

When your body breaks down fat into ketone bodies, those ketone bodies pass the blood-brain barrier, move into the brain, and replace glucose as an energy source. As discussed, the body can be fueled by either glucose or fat. Carbohydrates such as bread, potatoes, wheat, pasta, fruit, and vegetables are made up of multiple sugars that are rapidly converted to simple sugar, or glucose. Because carbs are so easily assimilated, they provide near instant fuel because they don't require the more prolonged digestion and absorption of protein and fats. Carb burning results in energy highs and subsequent energy crashes, in contrast with the more stable and slow release of energy provided by healthy fats.

Fat is a denser form of energy, providing 9 calories of energy per gram versus 4 calories per gram from carbohydrate or protein. Its energy density makes it the ideal form of storage. Just like those vacuum-sealed bags that used to be advertised on television, you could stuff nine whole sweaters into the vacuum-sealed bag versus just four sweaters in a regular bag without vacuuming out the air!

The body first stores remaining glucose in the form of glycogen after our energy needs have been met in the liver. However, the body has limited storage space for glycogen, and when we continue eating past our energy needs and our glycogen storage space, the body gets creative and starts converting all that excess glucose to fatty acids (aka a vacuum-sealed bag). Our bodies can fit a lot more glucose into fatty acids, which are a dense form of energy, and it can store them all over your body! It will just keep making those dense globules of energy as fat as long as energy consumed exceeds energy required. The bodies of our ancestors would not have stored much energy as fat because food security was never a guarantee, and food was scarcer than it is in the Western world today. If our ancestors had eaten in excess of their energy needs, they still would have likely entered nutritional ketosis relatively soon afterward, as they did not have access to convenience foods or processed foods or designer lattes keeping their livers full of glycogen at all times as we do today. If they had stored any body fat, once in ketosis they would have burned that fat when food was unavailable.

In modern times, nutritional ketosis is rarely reached. The amount of leisure time we have has grown considerably, as has the abundance of and access to food, especially energy-dense carb-loaded foods. Our windows for eating have grown, too. Whereas our ancestors ate when they could secure food, we often eat throughout the day, from the time we wake up until the time we go to sleep. This constant supply of food means that we never need to access our stored energy. Instead, these energy stores are kept and grow as we continue to eat more of the wrong foods.

Being in a state of nutritional ketosis is nothing new; it has been around as long as humans have been around. Before the rise of modern agriculture, which provided food security in the forms of cultivated rice and maize, humans existed mostly as nomadic hunter-gatherers. In Neolithic times, humans spent most of their days hunting animals and foraging for wild plants and berries. Around 12,000 BCE, many humans gave up a nomadic existence for a settled existence. As humans began to domesticate animals and formalize the planting and harvesting of foods, surpluses started to develop for the first time in history. Farmers optimized production by choosing crops that had the best returns on investment, including wheat. Over time, wheat was modified to maximize yield and seed endurance.

Most planted and harvested foods are grains and carbohydrates. For the first time in human history, we started to have surpluses of carbohydrates at our disposal rather than relying primarily on wild meats and limited amounts of gathered plants, grains, and berries. A diet composed of wild

I hit my weight goal!!! Woot woot!! 135.0 lbs today!!!! :) I started the keto lifestyle July 4 at 178 lbs. 43lbs! I have gone from a size 14 to a size 6. I have to admit Christmas was very tempting to go off! But luckily my spouse was very supportive and told me I had come too far to go off now. That was what I needed to hear and stay strictly keto. I don't usually have cravings. Thanks to all of you and your support and to Vanessa Spina!! Keto on, my friends!!

—Stacey C.

animal meats with limited foraged berries and plant foods would have qualified as a ketogenic diet, which means we thrived for thousands of years in nutritional ketosis with regular fasting incorporated due to food scarcity.

It is said that sugar was introduced into Western diets in 1099 in England. At that time, sugar cost about $100 per kilogram in today's prices; it started out as a luxury "spice." As trade between the West and East grew, so did the importation of sugar. In the fifteenth century, sugar was being refined in Venice and was taken by Christopher Columbus to the New World. Sugarcane grew well in North and Central America thanks to the favorable climate.

Sugar remained a luxury for the English upper class into the eighteenth century. It was known as "white gold" because the margins on its sale were so high. Because of its profitability, the government taxed sugar heavily, and it was not until 1874 that the sugar tax was dissolved, leading to prices that were affordable for the general population.

The cost of producing sugar continued to decline with the introduction of beet sugar. Today's sugar industry is dominated by beet sugar, sugarcane, and corn syrup, or maltodextrin. Global consumption of sugar has reached more than 100 million tons per year, with heavy government subsidies supporting low sugar prices.

It is quite a reversal for this once-rare luxury "spice" to be so commonplace today that it is added to 80 percent or more of today's supermarket foods. This transformation occurred over the last forty years. Many studies have demonstrated the addictive properties of sugar, so it is not surprising to see that it has come to dominate our modern food supply. If adding sugar to a food that a company is selling makes that food addictive and sell well, then to *not* add it puts the company at a disadvantage in the marketplace.

In studies of mice, sugar has been shown to be more addictive than cocaine, one of the most addictive drugs in existence. Is sugar a drug? We think of it as a food, and when it takes the form of fructose and is blended with other nutrients, we think of it as healthy. What defines a drug versus a food? A drug alters behavior and generates dependence. I believe that sugar falls into this same category. In many situations, sugar's addictive properties make it a hazard for people dealing with illnesses like diabetes and obesity.

The Effects of Being a Sugar Burner in a Sugar and Processed Food–Filled World

Prior to going keto, I had a great deal of affection for sugar and carbs. Both had been there to comfort me whenever I needed them. Sugar provided instant relief in the form of a glucose rush that made me feel like everything was going to be okay. Because I grew up as a child of the fat-phobic, high-carb nutritional paradigm, I consumed a lot of fruit, juice, "healthy" whole grains, reduced-fat milk, potatoes, rice, and corn, and sometimes even daily candy or soda. As long as fat wasn't in the picture, I believed I was eating a healthy diet.

You might find this description of my typical day alarming, or you might find it all too familiar.

You're probably well versed in the high-carb, low-fat paradigm. It extols the virtues of carbohydrates while underlining the dangers of dietary fats, presenting itself as a "balanced" diet. In my opinion, nothing could be further from balanced in terms of adequate and optimal nourishment. I would even go so far as to call this paradigm extreme because it names fat as the culprit behind the rising incidence of heart disease and therefore virtually eliminates it from the equation. Nonfat yogurt, fat-free salad dressings, and other foods are presented as the epitome of a healthy, "balanced" diet. The "ideal plate" recommended by the USDA is high-carb, typically high-protein, and low-fat. By definition, this approach to eating cannot be referred to as balanced, especially when fat, which is essential for the proper functioning of our bodies, has been eliminated.

Having healthy blood that is free of excess sugar and fat is one of the best ways to ensure that our bodies function optimally, prevent disease, and prolong life. It has been said that if you live in the West, you are likely to die from heart disease, cancer, or dementia, such as Alzheimer's. We all live in fear of these conditions, and many of us have lost loved ones or seen them suffer from the ravages of disease and from uncomfortable procedures used to treat them.

The Energy Balance Model versus the Endocrine Model

We have been sold the false notion that caloric intake is not affected by the form in which those calories are taken in. We're told that a calorie is a calorie, regardless of its composition.

A calorie is *not* a calorie—just like the fuels with which we power our cars are not all the same. If you fill up your diesel-run car with ethanol, for example, you might get interesting results. Just like cars, our bodies require specific forms of fuel—namely glucose and fat. Many people don't know that there is more than one fuel source that can be dominant, and we can decide which one we want our bodies to use as a primary fuel. And being fueled primarily by fat instead of glucose can drastically improve our health and prevent disease!

Contrary to what we've been led to believe, we don't need to exercise more and eat less to burn fat and lose weight. It's a little-known fact that weight loss comes from proper hormone function, not from calorie restriction or exercise. Our hormones control our body's set weight, as well as how hungry we are and whether we are in energy-storage or fat-burning mode.

The human body has evolved to store fat diligently to keep us alive in times of food scarcity. In modern times, though, food scarcity is rare for most of us; we have food all around us. We're even encouraged to eat constantly to "speed up our metabolism" as if eating *more* would somehow make us slimmer. It runs completely counter to logic, yet we've accepted these notions. Meanwhile, our society is facing soaring rates of obesity, diabetes, and heart disease. The key fact that we have been missing is not just *what* we should be eating, but also the *timing* of our meals. We need to make sure that we eat to satiety at mealtimes and then fast between meals, just as our ancestors would have, rather than "grazing," "nursing" (as I call sipping on sweetened beverages), or snacking between meals.

Insulin is a hormone that performs important functions in the body; among them, it regulates body weight. Most diets that center on consuming less food at each meal, grazing to speed up metabolism, and moving more don't work in the long term. The body's set weight stays the same because it was "set" by the overstimulation of insulin from the low-fat, high-carb way of eating that most of us have been following since the 1970s, when Ancel Keys declared that dietary fat was the cause of rising heart disease. Keys's work propelled our society to replace fat with unlimited carbs and sugars.

So what happens when you cut calories and exercise more? Your body adjusts by lowering its energy expenditure, slowing your metabolism and shutting off certain less-critical functions to conserve energy and keep you alive in case of a prolonged food shortage. You feel depleted and tired because your body is shutting off nonessential functions to sustain you. Now you're feeling worse, but you believe that you need to exercise despite your low energy. You might lose a few pounds at first, but once your body lowers its energy expenditure by slowing your metabolism, you will gain it all back, or you will live in a constant state of deprivation without seeing the weight loss you want.

Our ancestors ate meals to fullness and then fasted between meals. Today, with snacks between breakfast and lunch, lunch and dinner, and after dinner, our bodies never get a break, which means that our hormones never get a break. Although there are dozens of hormones in the body related to energy management, insulin is the most important hormone in the fat-loss equation. Insulin is released whenever we eat; it pushes glucose into our cells and liver to be used for energy. It is also an effective fat-storage trigger when it is released on a continuous basis. It functions so well that we are all naturally adept at storing fat despite our best efforts to the contrary!

When we are grazing and "nursing" all day, insulin is released constantly to clear the bloodstream of sugar and push that sugar into the cells. If glucose is excessive and therefore cannot all be cleared from the bloodstream, it is extremely detrimental to the body and to overall health. An excess of glucose in the blood turns into concentrated forms of energy known as triglycerides or lipids (fats) in the blood. The bloodstream always needs to be cleared of any circulating glucose or triglycerides or these can cause congestion and blockages. Depending on the location of the blockage, these blood lipids can lead to heart disease, stroke, and deep vein thrombosis. Contrary to popular belief, fats in the bloodstream are not caused by the consumption of fat but more so by the overconsumption of carbohydrates.

Because fats in the bloodstream are dangerous, insulin clearly has an extremely important role. Consequently, when insulin is present and clearing glucose, it tells the body to store all that energy. We cannot both store and burn energy (fat) at the same time. We are either in fat-burning mode or in fat-storing mode, and it is the balance between these two states that regulates our daily average and the health of our blood and bodies.

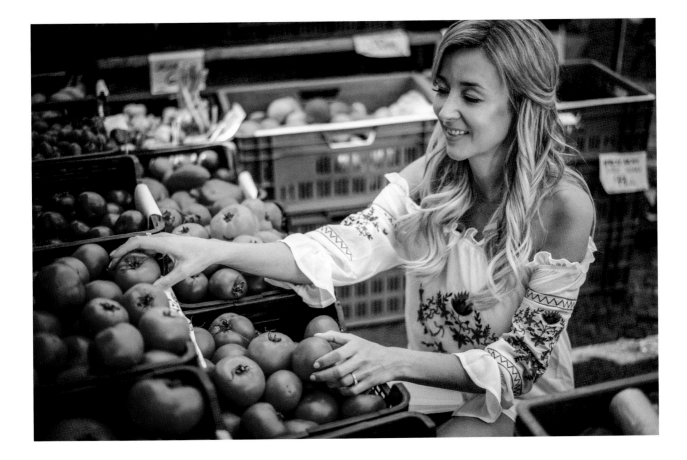

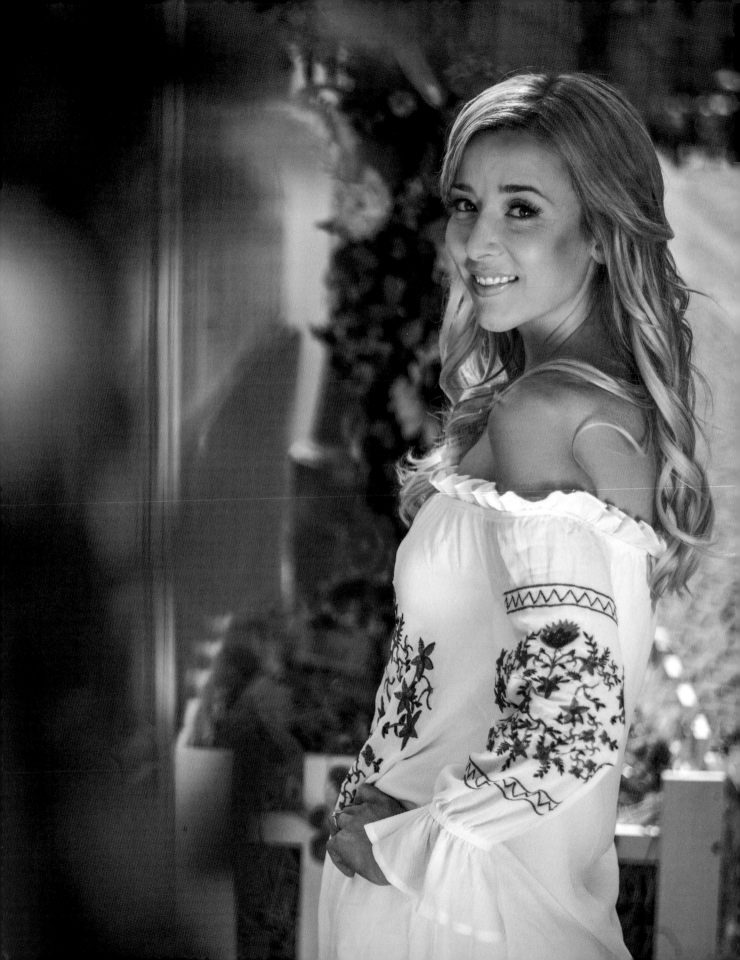

Chapter 2
Exercise and Weight Loss

We've all been told that there is only one way to lose weight: eat less and exercise more. Everyone "knows" that this is how you shed pounds: You eat fewer calories than you burn in a day. You avoid "fattening" foods. You eat a lot of salads, whole grains, and fruit. Like lab rats on hamster wheels, we run and run on the treadmill, sweating for those endorphin highs. I remember a study published in *Time* magazine about ten years ago that asked why obesity rates are soaring given that exercise and gym activity have been steadily rising for decades. If exercise is what makes us "burn" stored fat, why is obesity rising?

It takes a lot of willpower to run in place for 30 minutes or more—going nowhere—in a gym facility or at home! Running in place, just for the purpose of "burning calories," must be one of the most insane things we do in our modern age. As reported in the *Time* study, one of the core findings behind why obesity was rising in tandem with exercise was the "compensation factor," whereby exercise gives people a license to reward themselves. Most of the participants in the study ended up splurging on reward treats on the days they worked out, such as sugary smoothies or a muffin with their latte. The math is simple: burn 250 calories jogging or doing hard cardio at the gym and then eat a 400-calorie muffin, and you are now 150 calories worse off than if you had not exercised at all! The *Time* study was one of the first studies I read that made me start to question the role of exercise in burning fat. As it turns out, *Time* magazine and I were both on the right path.

I was determined to lose weight via both diet and exercise despite this insightful study. As my exercise obsession persisted, I came across more information upholding the premise that exercise might not help us burn fat, might be detrimental to our health, and might even prevent us from losing weight. It took me years to embrace this conclusion. However, I started following the keto protocol and cut out my daily self-inflicted suffering of running to nowhere because I realized that I was only doing it for that sense of burning fat and the endorphin rewards near the end. Runner's high is a real thing, indeed. However, the body's release of endorphins is not a survival reward. Instead, these endorphins mask the pain that our joints and limbs suffer after prolonged running. Steady-state cardio, such as running, jogging, elliptical training, and spinning, is now being uncovered as one of the most detrimental forms of movement for the body. It does more harm than good.

Exercise for the sole purpose of burning calories also requires willpower. It takes willpower to do things we don't enjoy. I was addicted to cardio for many years, unable to go a day without running on a treadmill for up to two hours at a time. I exercised every day because I thought it would help me burn fat (it didn't) and make me smaller (I just got larger). Instead, all that exercise revved up my appetite and depleted my energy. It also interfered with social engagements. I ran so much and so frequently that I tweaked my knee and did damage that I know will cause suffering in my later years. However, I thought that if I didn't exercise intensely, I would gain weight. Exercise should be a reward for the body, in my opinion, not a punishment.

I have worked with well over 2,000 people to date who have followed my meal plan programs, and the majority of them have lost weight with relative ease, without any scheduled form of strenuous exercise.

Exercise stresses our bodies. A little bit of stress, such as from strength training, can be good for us because stressing our muscles helps build muscle. However, much of the exercise we do for health puts *too much* stress on our bodies. This includes strenuous steady-state cardio. According to conventional modern medicine, health is about eating less fat and moving your body more. Because of this, many of us spend hours in the gym, working the treadmill or stair machine like it is our job, believing that if we sweat enough, we will attain the body weight and health of our dreams. Unfortunately, all this punishing exercise not only depletes willpower but also generates a lot of cortisol in the body, which can cause blood glucose to spike and keep you out of nutritional ketosis. Stress is the number-one enemy to healing, slowing and preventing proper repair. On a keto diet, the main focus is on restoring optimal function, not depleting our bodies with strenuous exercise.

Also, weight loss can be sabotaged because the willpower strenuous exercise can rob you of the willpower you need to stick to a keto diet. After working out, many people reward themselves with smoothies, muffins, or other treats; working out becomes a license to indulge because the treat has been "earned" through the burning of calories.

Think of your willpower reserve as being measured in a finite number of units. For the sake of this example, let's say we all have ten willpower units to use each day. We spend our willpower units in many various ways. We might use one unit for each of the following activities: getting out of bed when the alarm clock goes off earlier than we'd like, another unit for providing loving patience to a spouse or children, and another unit for getting to work and accomplishing our daily tasks. Add a visit to the gym, which can easily use up any remaining willpower for the day, leaving no units for the most important task of all when it comes to weight loss: controlling what we eat and don't eat (using willpower).

Doing strenuous cardio exercise for ninety minutes used most of my ten willpower units, if not more. Because I had depleted my daily allowance, I didn't have any willpower left when it mattered most for weight loss—to stop eating when I felt full or to avoid late-night snacking while relaxing and watching television. Simply put, I had no willpower left to control myself against the addictive effect of carbs.

This depletion of willpower is why I now embrace and recommend good-feeling movement. When I started exploring these concepts, I asked myself what I love most. The answer was walking and listening to audio books and podcasts while taking in beautiful views. So I started walking for pure enjoyment. I have always enjoyed weight training, too, but I always placed punishing cardio ahead of weight training in terms of importance. Now I enjoy sculpting my body with resistance training. I also switched to yoga, which always feels like a reward for my body and my mind. I also enjoy the occasional bike ride or spontaneous tennis match.

When you shift the purpose of exercise from weight loss to rewarding, good-feeling movement, you discover how incredible it is to be in your own skin. Ask yourself right now—what kind of movement do you most love to do? What activities bring you joy from being in your body?

Many people are under the impression that I don't believe in exercise because I often state that my programs do not *require* exercise for weight loss. On the contrary, I think exercise is phenomenal for health. However, I emphasize good-feeling movement that puts you in a great state of mind, along with resistance-based exercise that enhances your body composition. I cannot say enough good things about moving your body— but my golden rule is that exercise should be a reward, not a punishment. When you feel good, inhabiting and moving your body is a delicious experience. So I am far from being against exercise.

If you love to run, keto will fuel you like never before. Your liver can store only about 2,000 calories in the form of energy—but the average fat-burner has access to 40,000 calories of energy in the form of stored fat.

Movement should be a celebration of health and feel like a delicious reward for the body, mind, and soul; it should never feel bad or punishing. Because we want to reduce stress as much as possible on our path to healing and weight loss, it is key to practice good-feeling movement that is not overly strenuous. Walking, cycling, weight training, and playing sports, such as volleyball or tennis, are great ways to move and can lower stress. And yoga provides healthy movement, while its focus on controlled breathing is excellent for relieving stress.

I'm almost finished with round 2 [of the 28-day challenge]—feeling great. Have lost close to 26 pounds and lots of inches!! I've adapted to this way of eating, even on vacation! THANK YOU, Vanessa Spina!

—Lori C.

Ketosis: Receiving Proper Nutrition for Optimal Health

As I have covered, a ketogenic diet is generally defined as being high-fat, moderate-protein, and low-carbohydrate. It is called *ketogenic* because when properly followed, it puts your body in a state known as *nutritional ketosis*, in which your primary fuel is fat rather than glucose, which becomes a secondary fuel. Your body breaks down both stored fat and the fat you consume into ketone bodies, which fuel your body.

Although glucose is the body's default fuel and is the fuel that powers most people today, I believe that being primarily glucose-fueled is not aligned with optimal health, and that being fueled by fat and ketones is much better aligned with optional health.

When we look at our current model of "healthy" eating, the other controversial aspect of the ketogenic diet is its shunning of most fruits and many vegetables and its embracing of healthy fat. We have been programmed to believe that vegetables and fruits are the epitome of healthy nourishment, and that fat is the worst food we can eat. "Vegetables and fruits" are always grouped together, even though fruits are high in fructose and vegetables provide tons of vitamins and nutrients without fructose. We choose to eat large amounts of fruit and avoid fat without realizing that this high-carb, low-fat combination has the following ill effects:

- Our essential nutrient needs are not met.

- We are left feeling deprived.

- Food fixation is heightened.

- Our livers are overburdened by the fructose that they must store, which can lead to the development of nonalcoholic fatty liver disease (NAFLD).

In my opinion, the current food pyramid or MyPlate model needs to be turned on its head, with healthy fats rather than high-carb foods such as fruit, bread, pasta, and "healthy" whole grains making up the largest component.

I am feeling so good about this hourglass. I now measure 2 sizes smaller than I ever have, I was once 30 lbs lighter but a diet soda and carb eating mess. I love my shape, I love the way my skin is tightening, I love that I'm not counting every calorie in fear and working out 7 days a week. I am living a healthy life with a healthy routine and seeing such gorgeous changes in my body.

Just weighed in today, another 5 lbs down, 28 in total now. Keto on, girls!

—Chantel C.

Ketogenic Food List

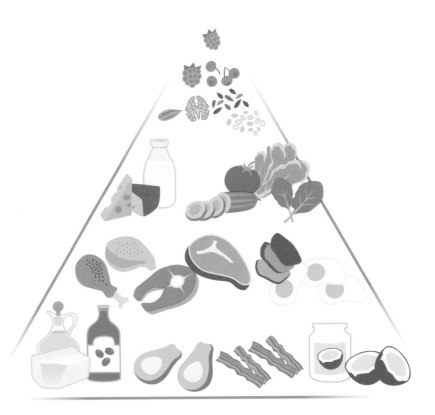

We increase our intake of healthy fat because

- Fat makes us fuller longer and satiates us, so we require less carbohydrate and protein.

- Fat is the macronutrient that stimulates insulin the least.

- Because healthy fat, such as coconut oil, is so dense, it has some thermogenic qualities, meaning that it requires quite a bit of energy to break down. This breakdown revs the metabolism.

Restricting glucose via limiting carbs, moderating protein, and increasing the intake of healthy fats compels the body to seek an alternative fuel source. Lucky for us, our bodies are just as adept at burning fat as they are at storing it.

What the stereotypical view of a diet high in saturated fat looks like . . .

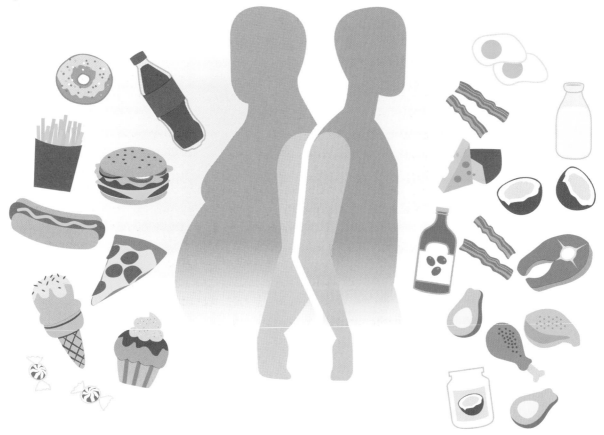

. . . and what a diet high in saturated fat actually looks like.

Following a ketogenic diet also turns you into a fat burner through natural fasting between meals (you're already being fueled from ketones just as though you were fasting). As long as you are not "grazing" or "nursing" sweetened beverages all day, your body will be in a fasted state outside of mealtimes. Many people believe that "grazing" will speed up their metabolism. However, what it actually does is prevent your body from accessing stored energy.

Keto allows fasting to occur naturally because you feel full and your body's satiety signals are restored. In today's society that is built on convenience, the notion of choosing to go without food is beyond most people. Opting to forgo food for any length of time is so counter to the way our society operates that the mere mention of it shocks people. I love how low-carb blogger and author Jimmy Moore refers to it as "the other F word." He says you could call it the other, *other* F word after "fat." Our way of life has developed to a point that the only time we are not consuming food is usually in our sleep.

If you are like so many people, you drink or eat within an hour of waking and have your last bite to eat or gulp of a drink within an hour of sleeping. Consumption is a pervasive part of the day, along with food fixation. Most people eat three "square meals" per day, and a day would not be complete without periodic snacks between those three meals, as well as sweetened (caloric or noncaloric) beverages—most of which qualify as meals when you consider their calorie contents and their effects on the body.

Because carb-heavy diets lack essential fats and nutrients, they result in us never feeling fully satisfied, and we become fixated on food. The body is craving nutrients, and instead of giving our bodies those nutrients, many people continue to eat carbs. However, when we give our bodies the full quota of essential nutrients, we can experience food peace, being liberated from the thought of food. For people who have lived most of their lives overfed and undernourished or experienced any kind of disordered eating, food peace is a novel concept. But it is a real thing! Prior to going keto, I experienced only brief glimpses of food peace. Those glimpses came right after overly indulgent holiday meals when I felt so stuffed that I was ready to assume the fetal position. Otherwise, I was so fixated on food that I was always looking forward to my next meal and what form it might take—even while eating my current meal.

When you begin to properly nourish your body with real foods and all the essential fatty acids and amino acids it needs, the focus on food gradually dissipates. You begin to reframe food in terms of its original purpose: as fuel for your body. Our energy should be released from fixating on food to focusing on the many more constructive aspects of life. We should be eating to live, not living to eat. Beyond what we are going to eat next, there are so many more rewarding aspects of life in which we should invest our energy and time.

When the body is being fed by ketones, the script is flipped as food fixation is reduced through proper nutrition and fasting naturally occurs. You might have heard that when people fast for long periods, their hunger dissipates. I remember hearing this and thinking that the absence of hunger must be a survival tool. I now realize that the real reason hunger disappears is because the body is not hungry when it can rely on its own plentiful stored energy. Your body can readily access virtually unlimited stores of energy packed away all over the body when you have converted to being a fat burner through long-term keto adaptation (aka becoming fat-adapted). Once you are fat-adapted, you don't experience hunger, which is a signal to eat food for survival. We rarely experience true hunger today, but we regularly experience appetite.

When your body can draw on an abundance of stored energy, it does not need to send hunger signals, which is why the sensation of hunger dissipates quickly when fasting. Fasting is the voluntary election to forgo feeding on energy from external sources. However, just because you are fasting does not mean you are going without nourishment. On the contrary, your body has access to its stored energy. An average person with no visible fat has access to about 40,000 calories' worth of energy. Just imagine how many stored calories are available to someone who has a small amount of visible fat, let alone someone with dozens or even hundreds of pounds of body fat. One pound of fat equals 3,500 calories—enough to fuel a person for about two days.

Natural fasting between meals or for dedicated fasting hours or days during the week is the antithesis of the culture of nonstop consumption that has generated widespread insulin resistance. The fact that it occurs naturally on a keto diet shows how satisfied the body is by real, whole-food nutrition.

How Keto Differs from Other Low-Carb Diets (Paleo, Banting, LCHF, JERF, and Atkins)

Keto and other low-carb diets limit carbohydrate intake and encourage the consumption of healthy fats. The Paleo (short for Paleolithic) diet is built on many of the same principles: emphasizing a variety of whole foods, modeling an ancestral way of eating, and avoiding processed foods. Modeling an ancestral diet calls for consuming foods that would have been hunted or gathered in Paleolithic times—which is where the Paleo diet gets its name. The whole-foods model dictates a focus on foods that have been grown, raised, or produced in natural environments. Organic foods grown without the use of pesticides and chemicals are encouraged, as are sustainable and humane farming practices for farm-raised animals.

The Paleo diet is based on balance and variety. Many keto meals can also be categorized as Paleo. Paleo and keto share whole foods as well as ancestral diet principles. For many people, a Paleo diet is very effective. For people with more metabolic resistance, however, further restriction of carbohydrates is required. Keto differs from Paleo in its level of carb restriction.

The following table compares the keto and Paleo diets.

Food	Paleo	Keto
Wheat	No	No
Gluten	No	No
Grains such as quinoa	Not encouraged	No
Legumes (beans, lentils, and peanuts)	No	No
Starches (plantains, potatoes, squash)	Yes	No
Soy, tempeh, tofu	Not encouraged	No
Meat and eggs	Yes	Yes
Dairy	Not encouraged	High-fat dairy is acceptable
Vegetables	Yes	Yes, except for high-sugar veggies such as beets, carrots, and sweet peas
Fruit	Yes	No, except for the lowest-carb fruits in some cases
Unrefined natural sweeteners (agave, dates, honey, maple syrup)	Yes	No
Artificial sweeteners (ace-k, aspartame, sucralose)	No	No
Natural sweeteners (stevia)	Yes	Yes
Low-carb sweeteners (erythritol, xylitol)	Not encouraged	Yes

I am happy to announce I have reached my number one goal that I set out for when I started this [Ketogenic Girl] plan in mid January!!! I truly never believed I could achieve my goal and thought it was farfetched. I am down 67.6 pounds!!! I started at 242.2 and thought it would be a dream to achieve 175! I achieved and beat it!! 174.6 this morning!!! Just goes to show you never give up!!! My new goal is 150!!! I've got this!! Thank you so much, Vanessa, for this plan, and thank you to my sister Bethany, who without telling me about this plan and asking me to take this journey with her I could not have achieved these goals!!!! Keto on!!!

—Eryn W.

Both Paleo and keto restrict:

- Wheat and gluten

- Legumes (beans, lentils, and peanuts)

- Grains such as corn and quinoa

Keto and Paleo differ in the following ways:

- **Natural sweeteners:** Dates, honey, maple syrup, and other natural sweeteners are generally okay on a Paleo diet but not on a keto diet. Most natural sweeteners are identical to table sugar on a molecular level; in fact, some, such as agave syrup, are worse.

- **Starches:** All starches are restricted on a keto diet, but many are allowed on a Paleo diet, including white potatoes, sweet potatoes, yams, squash, taro, and plantains.

- **Vegetables:** Keto restricts higher-sugar vegetables such as beets, carrots, and sweet peas. Paleo does not restrict these foods.

- **Fruit:** On a Paleo diet, both fresh and dried fruits are allowed. On a keto diet, only the lowest-fructose fruits and some berries are allowed; avocados, blackberries, cranberries, raspberries, and rhubarb are generally okay. However, many people who do strict keto do not consume these fruits on a regular basis. Some avoid them until their blood sugar has normalized and is consistently low due to restored insulin sensitivity.

Keto is a low-carb, high-fat diet with a moderated protein intake. Paleo does not abide by these specific macronutrient distributions; on a Paleo diet, carb intake tends to be high to normal, as do intakes of protein and fat. Some people require higher amounts of carbohydrates than a typical keto diet provides; see page 65 for more on "carb-up" days and how they might help.

Banting, LCHF, and JERF

William Banting was an English undertaker who came to fame after trying a low-carbohydrate diet to deal with weight gain. He had so much success that in 1863, he published a pamphlet called "Letter on Corpulence, addressed to the Public." In this letter, Banting details his struggle to lose weight via diets and exercise programs and outlines how he started a mostly ketogenic diet of meats, greens, fruits, and very dry wine while avoiding sugar, starches, beer, milk, and more. It was so popular that it was picked up by a British publisher. Interestingly, Banting was a distant relative of Sir Frederick Banting, who was one of the discovers of insulin. Banting's legacy lives on today, although much of this low-carb knowledge has been lost for the past few decades, and we are only now reconnecting with it.

I am officially down 32 pounds as of this morning and I'm about to take Ruckus, our Jack Russell pup, out for her first–ever 2k run! I asked [my husband] to take my photo to see what 32 lbs off me looks like, and I was pleasantly surprised!! So much love for this program!! Vanessa Spina, we love you!

—Lyndsay M.

The term "Banting" also refers to a low-carb, high-fat protocol based on whole foods that was popularized in England and South Africa. LCHF (Low Carb High Fat) and JERF (Just Eat Real Food) are similar to Banting and are very popular in Sweden.

The Atkins Diet

The Atkins Diet is known for being low-carb and, to an extent, high-fat. However, when I first read *Dr. Atkins' Diet Revolution* in about 2002 and tried it myself, I did not understand that protein was to be moderated as well. Also, I did not understand the emphasis on moderating protein or testing for ketones. Atkins is known for being low-carb and includes fats, closer to a 60 percent ratio. However, the ketogenic diet is known for being high-fat, closer to 70 and 80 percent or higher and moderate in protein as well as low in carbs.

These diets are all based on carbohydrate restriction. However, what differentiates the ketogenic diet is its emphasis on moderating protein to a specific macronutrient percentage, and for the testing and tracking of ketones.

Who Should Not Follow a Ketogenic Diet

The ketogenic diet is not for everyone. Before beginning a ketogenic diet, it is strongly recommended that you undergo a health screening to rule out any undiagnosed conditions or contraindications with your health or medications. Keto might not be appropriate or ideal for:

- People with any stage of kidney disease or preexisting liver, pancreatic, or kidney issues or conditions. Keto could complicate and severely stress the pancreas, liver, or kidneys in people suffering from rare conditions such as muscular dystrophy and gallbladder disease.

- People with blood sugar issues such as hypoglycemia or type 1 diabetes. It might or might not be appropriate for people with type 2 diabetes; however, type 2 diabetics will require medical supervision while on keto.

- Women who are pregnant or nursing or who have gestational diabetes.

- Anyone suffering from or recovered from an eating disorder.

- People who have been experiencing adverse symptoms for a prolonged period, including poor circulation, numbness in extremities, and hair loss; these symptoms could indicate undiagnosed thyroid issues that are not being supported by a carb-restrictive diet, and more carbohydrates might be required.

There are some additional considerations, such as that you might need to adjust your medications while on this diet. If you are considering keto, it is important to speak with your physician or endocrinologist, especially if you have any kind of medical condition. If you are new to low-carb eating and to keto, it is important to decrease your carbohydrates gradually in order to avoid hypoglycemia (low blood sugar).

Easing Your Transition to Keto

Because your body loses a lot of water and sodium on a ketogenic diet, it's important to maintain your electrolyte levels on a ketogenic diet by both upping your sodium intake. With regard to sodium, opt for a high-quality source, such as Himalayan sea salt or Celtic sea salt. I like to add these salts to bone broth, meals, or even glasses of water. If your body is healthy and well-functioning, it will regulate the appropriate amount of potassium to retain based on how much sodium you ingest.

If you experience lethargy, muscle cramping, or twitching while on keto, these are usually indicators that your sodium intake needs to be increased and your electrolytes need to be increased. Magnesium is also safe to supplement with. Taking potassium supplements, however, is never recommended. Discuss your supplementation regimen with your physician.

When it comes to water, more is not always better on keto. Maintaining a consistent water intake, without overdoing it is important. Too much water can dilute your electrolytes. It's important to get at least one half fluid ounces per pound of body weight as a minimum per day as recommended by the NIH. I also recommend the urine color guide (page 90) for clues on your level of hydration. The best indicator is always thirst, just as hunger is the best indicator we need to eat. It's crucial to listen to your body, and see your physician if you have a condition that causes underlying electrolyte imbalances before considering a ketogenic diet.

The Incredible Benefits of a Ketogenic Diet

The ketogenic diet is an effective way to optimize health and vitality. It is also being recognized as a powerful healing protocol, demonstrating the potential for treating and in some cases reversing chronic inflammation, insulin resistance, obesity, and much more. The latest science is presenting the incredible benefits of ketones as well as highlighting the key role that healthy fats, as well as dietary cholesterol, plays for proper brain function.

A ketogenic diet has amazing benefits, such as:

- Easy and rapid weight loss

- Increased energy

- Mental clarity (no more brain fog!)

- Consistent, calm moods

- Satisfaction from eating delicious and flavorful high-fat foods

- Food peace (freedom from food fixation)

- Restored insulin sensitivity

- Anti-aging (generated via autophagy clearing cellular debris, restored metabolic health from enhanced insulin sensitivity, detoxification, loss of visceral fat, disease prevention, and more)

- Therapeutic applications for diseases or conditions, such as epilepsy, lupus, ulcerative colitis, PCOS (polycystic ovarian syndrome), obesity, insulin resistance or type 2 diabetes, Alzheimer's (increasingly referred to as type 3 diabetes), high blood pressure, stroke, heart disease, cancer, autism, migraines, adrenal fatigue, and much more!

- Disease prevention

With all these benefits, keto is clearly a powerful protocol. And if disease prevention, mental clarity, increased energy, or easy weight loss don't convince you, how about the fact that keto is anti-aging? A keto diet provides fat-soluble vitamins such as vitamin E, as well as boosts human growth hormone during fasting. Also, whole foods provide antioxidants. We tend to age at the speed of our insulin sensitivity and metabolic health. Having persistently high blood sugar is one of the worst things for our health and long-term wellness. A keto diet restores insulin sensitivity; this diet keeps us looking and feeling young!

Why does a keto diet do all this? Here are some of the main reasons:

- It represents a return to diet that is centered on real, whole foods and avoids processed foods and sugars.

- It restores insulin sensitivity by lowering carbohydrate intake and restricting all forms of sugar, including white sugar, fruit sugar (fructose), milk sugar (lactose), and "natural" sugars such as honey and maple syrup. These natural sugars are identical to processed sugar when it comes to their effects on our bodies. Consuming sugar is known to disrupt blood sugar, interfere with hormone function and intracellular communication, and feed tumors.

- Fasting between meals allows your body to take a rest from insulin. It also allows your body to undergo autophagy, whereby it "eats" old, dying cells. Through autophagy, your body consumes excess skin left over from rapid weight loss and even consumes growths, such as benign tumors and cysts.

Just wanted to share my success so far because I've never lost this kind of weight before. Or stuck to anything!! It is officially six weeks into this program and I am down 25 pounds!!!! That is even with loosely following the program while my mom was in town for a week!! Thank you, thank you, thank you, Vanessa Spina!!!

—Kimberly F.

- IGF-1 and human growth hormone are stimulated by fasting, and on a ketogenic diet, you will naturally fast between meals and sometimes through regular mealtimes because your body is fully nourished and does not need additional food.

- A keto diet provides your body with essential fatty acids and amino acids, as well as the fat-soluble vitamins A, D, E, and K and B vitamins from high-quality proteins. It also feeds your beneficial gut bacteria with cruciferous veggies, fermented prebiotic foods (foods that promote the growth of beneficial gut bacteria), and probiotics.

- It removes inflammatory foods such as wheat, soy, peanuts, and in some cases dairy; it allows your body to reduce chronic pain and inflammation and to focus on healing.

- It allows for proper hormone balance and function. Diets that are high in carbs and contain soy are highly estrogenic, which can interfere with hormone function. High-carb diets can cause excess testosterone, and excess soy can generate too much estrogen.

- It makes weight loss natural and easy because your body becomes a fat burner and accesses stored fat for energy rather than relying on glucose.

- It greatly enhances the health of your blood. Excessive glucose consumption often leads to a fatty liver and fatty blood. The body needs to clear excess sugar in the blood, and when the liver and cells are full, it turns that excess blood glucose into fat, a more concentrated form of energy. This leads to high triglycerides, which in turn generate high blood pressure because the blood has an increasingly difficult time circulating. Poor circulation can also result. As we age, healthy circulation is one of the most important contributors to good health. Once the body is depleted of excess sugar, it can clear the bloodstream of these blood lipids.

- It provides your body with plenty of medium-chain triglycerides (MCTs), which promote brain health and ketone production. Breast milk is full of MCTs—and is ketogenic—to provide babies with the highest-quality fats and proteins for their rapidly developing cells.

There are many more reasons why keto does what it does. I've simply listed some of the main reasons why keto is so powerful for healing and for managing and preventing disease. Our bodies are restored to a healthy equilibrium when we get out of the way of their brilliant healing genius, in which more than a hundred trillion cells work hard to keep us alive and in optimal health. When you injure yourself, you can watch your body go to work, with inflammation fending off bacteria and repairing wounds. However, when we constantly eat unhealthy foods or are exposed to environmental toxins, inflammation is ever-present. When we put only nutrient-rich foods in our bodies and steer clear of those toxins, on the other hand, we will heal rapidly.

So happy I took the plunge with this awesome Challenge! 28 days done, feeling great, and so thankful for being able to lose 27 lbs total! Thank you, Vanessa Spina!!! Love this program.

—Lisa C.

The Latest Science Supporting Low-Carb Diets

According to investigative journalist Nina Teicholz, author of *The Big Fat Surprise: Why Butter, Meat and Cheese Belong in a Healthy Diet*, there is a vast amount of evidence—more than seventy-four randomized and controlled trials—proving that low-carb diets are safe and highly effective for treating obesity, diabetes, and heart disease. Low-carb diets also are proven to dramatically improve health. More and more studies are being released, including a study published in the *Lancet*, titled "Associations of fats and carbohydrate intake with cardiovascular disease and mortality in 18 countries from five continents (PURE): a prospective cohort study." As reported in the *New York Times*, the researchers tracked more than 135,000 participants and found that "High carbohydrate intake is associated with a higher risk of mortality, and high fat intake with a lower risk." (Nicholas Bakalar, "New study favors fat over carbs," *New York Times*, September 8, 2017. Accessed via www.nytimes.com/2017/09/08/well/new-study-favors-fat-over-carbs.html?mcubz=3.)

According to another recent study, saturated fat does not cause heart disease. (Aseem Malhotra, Rita F. Redberg, and Pascal Meier, "Saturated fat does not clog the arteries: coronary heart disease is a chronic inflammatory condition, the risk of which can be effectively reduced from healthy lifestyle interventions," *British Journal of Sports Medicine* 51, no. 15 (2017), http://bjsm.bmj.com/content/51/15/1111.) As reported in a widely read story by CBC News, "The belief that saturated fat in foods such as butter, cheese and meat clogs arteries is 'just plain wrong.'" According to the authors of the study, instead of meat and dairy, people should eat a Mediterranean-style high-fat diet, reduce carbohydrate intake, take brisk daily walks, and keep stress to a minimum. (CBC News, "Pass the butter: cutting saturated fat does not reduce heart disease risk, cardiologists say," posted April 25, 2017, www.cbc.ca/news/health/pass-the-butter-cutting-saturated-fat-does-not-reduce-heart-disease-risk-cardiologists-say-1.4085453.)

It is beyond the scope of this book to compile and present them here, but many books, including *The Big Fat Surprise*, cover this subject in much greater detail.

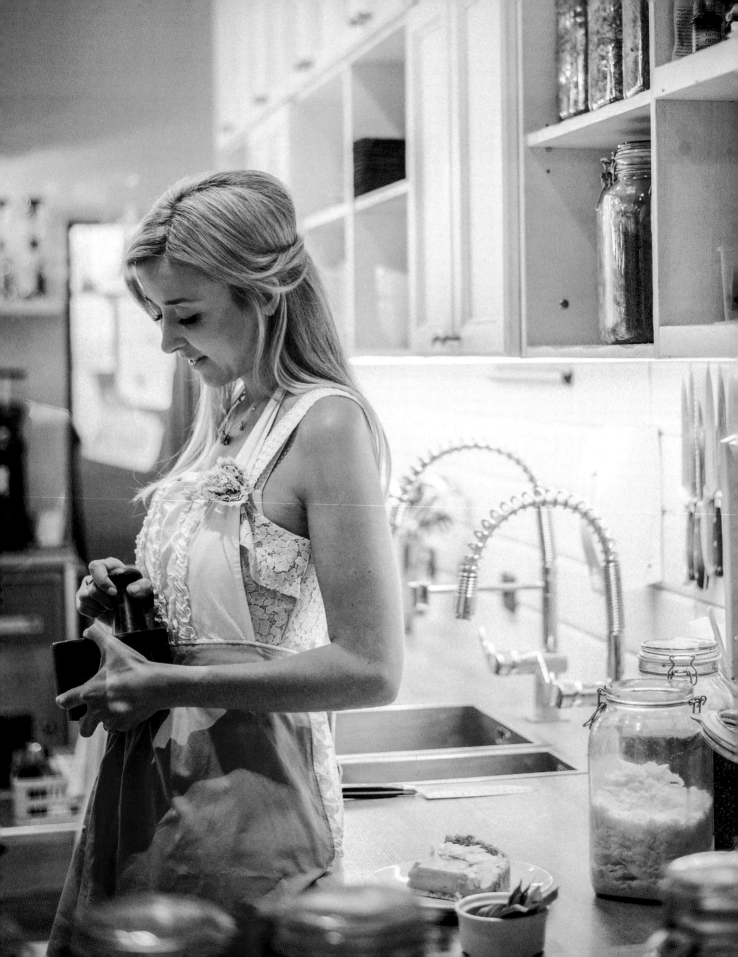

Chapter 3

Following Keto

In this chapter, I will cover exactly what following keto means and how to do it, breaking down the concepts into simple guidelines so that you can get started on this way of life.

Macros: 80/15/5 Fat, Protein, and Carbohydrate

My approach to a keto diet is based on a therapeutic application whereby the macronutrients of each meal are broken down into an 80/15/5 percent distribution. What does this mean? It means that in a day's worth of eating, approximately 80 percent of your total calories should come from healthy fats, 15 percent should come from quality proteins, and 5 percent should come from carbohydrates. This macronutrient, or "macro," distribution is what makes a ketogenic diet high-fat, adequate-protein, and low-carb.

At first glance, 80 percent fat might seem shockingly high, especially when we have been conditioned to eat low-fat diets. The distribution of fat is so high because 1 gram of fat has 9 calories—more than twice the number of calories in 1 gram of protein or carbohydrate, each of which has 4 calories per gram. Because fat is very energy-dense, having it account for 80 percent of your diet is easy because it doesn't represent that much food. For example, 1 tablespoon of oil or butter contains 100 calories, whereas 100 calories of salad greens is a whopping 4 to 5 cups.

For example, If we were to apply the 80/15/5 rule to someone on an 1,600-calorie-per-day diet, then we end up with the following:

- 1,200 calories from fat, or 133 grams of fat
- 320 calories from protein, or 80 grams of protein
- 80 calories from carbohydrate, or 20 grams of carbohydrate

In the example above, I have provided an illustration of how the 80/15/5 percent macronutrient breakdown might look like. It is not necessary to consume 133 grams of healthy fats per day, however; the critical part to get into ketosis is to restrict total carbohydrates to 20 grams or less, and to moderate protein as well. For many of the people I work with, this will get their bodies into a state of nutritional ketosis, whereby they begin producing ketones from the breakdown of stored energy in the form of body fat. For some individuals, the threshold to get into nutritional ketosis is much higher than 20 total grams, and levels of protein will range as well. You can see that in this example there are 70 grams of protein, which may be less than what the average person is used to consuming, but if it is sourced from high quality proteins, this amount of can well provide all the essential amino acids required by the body for optimal nutrition.

The easiest way to figure out what percentage of each macronutrient you are getting is to use a tracking program that allows you to keep a daily food diary and calculates the macronutrient percentages for you. I use a couple of different food-tracking apps and online sites, including MyFitnessPal. The app allows you to enter food nutrient data by scanning bar codes on food packaging. When you are first getting started, I recommend scanning bar codes because you need the data to be as accurate as possible. After tracking your food for a while—especially if you are like most people and tend to repeat the same rotation of meals—you will only need to track when you are trying new foods or when you are traveling.

A side benefit of tracking your food—with an app or in a journal—is that it keeps you accountable. Making a deal with yourself to track everything you eat will make you think twice about having an extra portion. You can also add a friend who's doing keto to your food app account and share your daily totals; doing so brings a fantastic sense of accountability.

If the idea of tracking all your food seems overwhelming, I suggest starting with 21 keto meals—seven breakfasts, seven lunches, and seven dinners. You can use the meal plans in this book (see page 367) and on my website, www.ketogenicgirl.com, or you can choose your own meals that fit the keto profile. Repeat those meals so you don't need to track everything you eat. You can repeat these 21 meals each week for a month, or you can pick your favorite days and repeat them without needing to do any tracking whatsoever!

Adjusting the Keto Diet to Your Individual Needs

Although the 80/15/5 guideline works for most people on a ketogenic diet, you can modify it to accommodate your health conditions. In some ways, keto is an all-in approach to nutrition; however, it's not necessarily going to be successful for everyone. (See page 57 for details on who should not follow a keto diet.) The only way to really know if it is for you is to try it out, for yourself and see how you feel and if you enjoy the lifestyle and the results that you achieve (with your doctor's approval). For some people, it is better to just "lean in" to keto—follow a whole-foods diet and eliminate sugar and processed foods. If you do these things, you will be moving in the right direction, and you will be ahead of the game healthwise. Even if you don't go all-in with keto, making just a few positive, keto-related changes is better than doing nothing at all.

For more information about modifying keto for special health conditions, see Chapter 5.

I am happy to say today I reached a mini goal of mine. Down 40 lbs!!! Thank you so much for the support and a huge thank you to Vanessa!!!

—Marybeth D.

Net Carbs versus Total Carbs

Net carbs are total carbs minus fiber. So, if you've eaten 40 grams of carbs and 20 grams of those carbs were in the form of fiber, your net carbs would be 20 grams. This net carbs approach is widely used among those doing keto. It was popularized by Michael R. Eades and Mary Dan Eades in their book *Protein Power: The High-Protein/Low Carbohydrate Way to Lose Weight, Feel Fit, and Boost Your Health—In Just Weeks!*

The net carbs approach is based on the idea that the fiber you eat negates part of the carbs you eat, as some fiber is insoluble and is not digested. In my opinion, however, fiber does not make carbohydrates "disappear" whether you digest them or not. Although *Protein Power* is a wonderful and important book and the net carbs concept may work for many people, I find that it is often not strict enough. Many of the clients I work with require a stricter approach, so I work with total carbs instead. Tracking fiber intake is important because fiber is great for the gut microbiome (see page 82). For this reason, I have included both total carb and fiber counts for the recipes in this book. However, I believe that you will be much more successful at getting into nutritional ketosis if you focus on total carbs. If you subtract the fiber, more often than not you are going to eat too many carbs to get into and stay in ketosis. This is a mistake that I see people make too often, and as a result they struggle to get into ketosis and do not see the results they want to see.

Carbing Up

Some people require higher amounts of carbohydrates because of their specific weight training regimens or thyroid-related conditions or other issues, or can follow a keto diet by doing "carb-up" days. If you are interested in following a keto diet but feel that you need greater amounts of carbs to fuel your workouts, or if you are not seeing improvements in your overall condition, I suggest doing one carb-up day each week. On a carb-up day, eat two to three times the normal amount of carbs. Using our earlier example of a 1,600-calorie daily diet, you would eat between 40 and 60 grams of carbs on a carb-up day instead of only 20 grams. Get your extra carbs mostly from green vegetables that are high in vitamin C, such as kale and mixed lettuces. You can add some berries or eat large salads with keto dressings. There are a few recipes in this book that fit this description, such as the Caesar, Cobb, and Niçoise salads.

How to Know Whether You're in Ketosis: Testing Your Blood Sugar and Ketone Levels

One thing that sets the ketogenic diet apart from other diets is that we can use the latest technology to give us feedback on how we're doing.

Ketones take three forms—acetone on your breath, acetoacetate in your urine, and beta-hydroxybutyrate in your blood—and therefore can be measured via the breath, urine, and blood. Many people start with urine test strips when first dipping their toes into keto, which are great because the strips change color when ketones are present. The breath meter works in a similar way. I have used both urine test strips and breath meters. Both indicate the presence of ketones, but they are not particularly accurate, and they do not tell you your exact ketone level or your blood sugar reading. In my opinion, the blood sugar reading is even more important than the ketone reading. For these reasons, I recommend blood testing if you are serious about getting into nutritional ketosis and experiencing its incredible benefits.

Some people might find the idea of pricking your finger to test your blood sugar and ketones bizarre or over the top for someone who does not have diabetes—not to mention that having a fear of needles is a very real thing! After all, diabetics test their blood with glucometers out of necessity, and as a matter of life and death in many cases. However, knowing that the technology exists (and at our fingertips, no less!), there is no reason not to avail ourselves of these useful devices even if we are testing not for life and death but to optimize our nutrition and health. Persistently high blood sugar in a healthy person can lead to diabetes, among other conditions, such as elevated triglycerides, which can lead to stroke and heart disease. Gone are the days when you had to depend on a doctor to get a blood sugar or ketone reading; now you can do it in the privacy of your own home.

Does going keto means a lifetime of pricking your finger? Not at all. You'll do most of your testing when you first start the keto diet. Once you get the hang of it, you will only need to test occasionally, such as when you are introducing a new food or are traveling and want to make sure that you stay in ketosis.

What You Need

The most important tool to ensure that you are not consuming too much glucose is a glucometer that also measures ketones. This device can test blood sugar, blood ketones, or both. I recommend the Abbott Precision

I hit my goal! Woohoo, finally! I'm down 25 pounds since the middle of April. The best part is my physical health and mental health are healthy again, and that's priceless! Thanks for the easy plan and great coaching, Vanessa!

—Rhonda G.

Xtra or the Abbott Freestyle Neo. You will also need lancets (I use 28- or 30-gauge), which are micro needles that you insert into the lancing device. The lancing device typically comes with the glucometer, along with some lancets to start with. Finally, you will need both glucose test strips and ketone test strips. You can start with just glucose test strips if you like; however, I recommend getting ketone test strips as well.

In a state of nutritional ketosis, blood sugar and ketones are inversely correlated. In other words, as blood sugar goes down, ketones go up because your body is fueling itself with them. As long as your fasting blood sugar is below 90 mg/dL or 5.0 mmol/L and your blood ketones are between 1.0 and 3.0 mmol/L, your brain is being fueled by ketones and burning fatty acids, which means you are burning fat!

In my opinion, testing your fasting blood sugar when you wake up is essential to your success. You can use your results as a barometer to gauge whether you stayed within the carb and protein thresholds to remain in nutritional ketosis. There is no need to test at any other time of day if you test in the morning, fasted, and keep a record of your results. Hitting at or below 90 mg/dL or 5.0 mmol/L is the strongest indicator that your previous day's food choices fell within the prescribed parameters.

How to Test Your Blood Sugar and Ketones

Following are the steps for testing your blood sugar:

1. Purchase a glucometer, lancets, blood glucose test strips, and ketone test strips. The Freestyle brand of test strips is compatible with the meters by Abbott mentioned above.

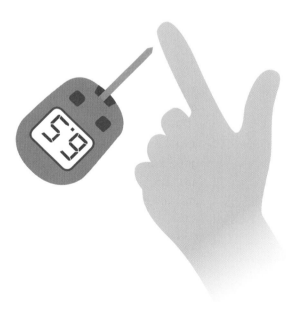

2. Watch a video on how to test yourself (I have a couple on my YouTube channel, Ketogenic Girl).

3. Test your fasting blood sugar and ketones in the morning when you first wake up. Here's the general procedure:

   a. Have the glucometer ready and standing by.

   b. Load the lancing device with a lancet by removing the cap from the lancing device, inserting the lancet, and pushing it down until it clicks into place. Then twist off the top section to reveal the micro needle. Replace the cap on the lancing device.

   c. Prepare the glucose and ketone test strips by removing them from the packaging. If they are the Abbott Freestyle brand, the glucose test strip will be blue in a blue foil packet and the ketone test strip will be purple in a purple foil packet.

   d. Pull the bottom of the lancet away from it; it should pull away like a rubber band and snap back. Place the lancing device against the side of your finger and then push the button in the center to release the needle. It will make a very fine prick, and a small droplet of blood will form.

   e. Insert the glucose test strip with the black-and-white-coded end into the machine. Dip the other end of the strip (the small white absorbent part) into the droplet, using a very small amount for the glucose test strip; save a larger amount for the ketone test strip. It should take about 5 seconds to get the blood glucose reading. Remove the glucose test strip from the device and insert the black-and-white-coded end of the ketone test strip into the machine. Make sure that you have a small to medium-sized droplet of blood; if you don't put enough blood on the test strip, it will read "Error."

4. Keep a log of your blood sugar and ketone readings.

I just wanted to comment on Vanessa's program. Took me a while to buy unfamiliar items. So I started late around early Feb. so for the 28-day program and lost about 22 pounds. This is results for a 56-year-old.... Great results, Vanessa! You were a godsend to me and others. I'm starting to want more variety now, and looking forward to your cookbook.

—Maryann M.

Testing Summary

MACHINE: Glucometer — I like the Abbott Precision Xtra

TEST STRIPS: Glucose test strips and ketone test strips

LANCETS: 30-gauge lancets

NUMBERS:

Fasting blood sugar below 90 mg/dl or 5.0 mmol/L

Ketones between 1.0 and 3.0 mmol/L

Interpreting the Results

Ideally, your blood glucose should be 5.0 mmol/L (90 mg/dL) or below; ketone levels between 1.0 and 3.0 mmol/L are ideal for burning fat. A reading of 0.5 mmol/L is defined as the start of nutritional ketosis, and 1.0 mmol/L is the optimal ketone zone marker.

When you are in nutritional ketosis, you have measurable ketones that are breaking down fats into ketone bodies and glycerol.

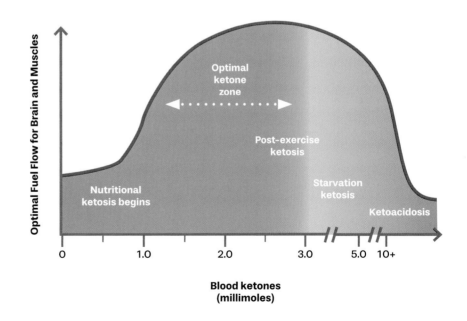

Chart adapted from the book *The Art and Science of Low Carbohydrate Performance* by Jeff S. Volek and Stephen D. Phinney

In the past, knowing whether you were doing the right things when it came to dieting and weight loss involved a lot of guesswork. You would read a diet book, put the concepts into practice, and then weigh yourself once (or a few times) a week, hoping that each time you hopped on the scale, you would see a lower number staring back at you. In the old way of dieting—high-carb, high-protein, low-fat, "exercise more and consume fewer calories, but eat more often to have a faster metabolism"—we often saw some initial success from lowering or controlling calorie intake and exercising excessively. After a while, however, despite our best efforts, we stopped seeing results. Traditional dieting is somewhat like looking for something in a dark room. Try as you might, you can't seem to locate it.

A ketogenic diet, on the other hand, is like turning on the lights in that room, putting an end to your fumbling around in the dark. If you are measuring your ketones and blood sugar, you get immediate feedback, which means you know definitively whether your efforts have been successful. Your ketone readings will tell you whether your body is breaking down fat into ketone bodies. Your blood sugar readings will tell you how efficiently your body is clearing out blood sugar after you eat, how responsive your cells are to insulin, which foods overwhelm your system, and which foods support and heal your body.

Each of our bodies behaves differently, so the only way to know for sure whether you are reaching nutritional ketosis is to test your blood. I commonly hear people say that they are not seeing the weight loss and energy gain that they wanted to see. Inevitably, when I ask them what their ketone and blood sugar readings are, they tell me that they are using breath or urine tests. While they are detecting the presence of ketones, they are not seeing specific amounts, and they aren't testing blood sugar at all! Another common scenario is that someone will have ketones in the 1.0 to 3.0 range, but their waking fasted blood sugar will still be above 90 (or even 100). What this usually means is that ketones are present, but they are coming from the breakdown of dietary fats and not stored body fat. Their bodies have not yet fully healed, and they are not in a state of nutritional ketosis because their blood sugar is still too high for their bodies to be burning fat as a primary fuel and glucose as a secondary fuel. Rather, the reverse is still occurring.

When glucose is available, your body will always default to using glucose as its primary fuel source because it is so powerful. It is similar to having access to a sports car to take you from point A to point B every day; there are other modes of travel, but the sports car is faster and more efficient. If someone else is using that car, however, you will need to choose another option, such as your bicycle. It takes a bit more work to get out the bike and inflate the tires, and it takes more energy to pedal the bike than to press the gas pedal of the sports car. The bike is slower than the sports car, too, but the exercise is good for your body, and it's fun to be outside moving under your own power. Ketones are an incredible source of energy, and the brain and body love to be fueled by ketones. However, if any glucose is available, the body is programmed to rely on glucose as its primary fuel source, leaving stored body fat as a secondary or backup energy source to be accessed only when glucose is not present.

Remarkably, testing your blood sugar can also help you identify food intolerances and potential allergies. If you are intolerant of or allergic to, say, coconut, your blood sugar might be consistently higher than normal. I have had clients who were consistently getting high blood sugar readings even though they were following my program to the letter. It tuned out that they had an intolerance to coconut, and when they removed coconut from their diets, their blood sugar went back to the normal range for people who are in nutritional ketosis. Food allergies can cause cortisol to be released due to inflammatory responses, leading to higher blood glucose readings, which can normalize when the problematic food is removed from the diet. You can learn so much about your body and how sensitive or resistant you are to insulin through testing.

Testing yourself keeps you off the scale. If you are following a ketogenic diet for weight loss, I believe in weighing once a week, on the same day, at the same time. It's important not to get overly wrapped up in the day-to-day changes because your weight can fluctuate by as much as 6 pounds based on your electrolyte balance and water retention (or lack thereof). I believe in testing because it keeps us accountable for our food choices without the obsession that the scale can bring. I believe in focusing on and celebrating non-scale victories, such as feeling comfortable in looser-fitting clothing and the sense of freedom that comes about when food fixation falls away. Growing confidence, increased energy, better sleep, less medication, and greater overall health and wellness are all non-scale victories. However, we cannot truly achieve progress unless we are measuring the results.

Following a ketogenic diet involves tracking food intake, which keeps you honest. When you know you have a daily target to hit—80 percent fat, 15 percent protein, and 5 percent carbohydrate—and you are tracking the food you eat, you might think twice about indulging in carbs or excess protein. You'll be motivated when you see the results moving in the right direction—blood sugar decreasing and ketones increasing. Testing yourself has many benefits that I believe far outweigh any mental barriers regarding the momentary pain involved. Having the health of your dreams

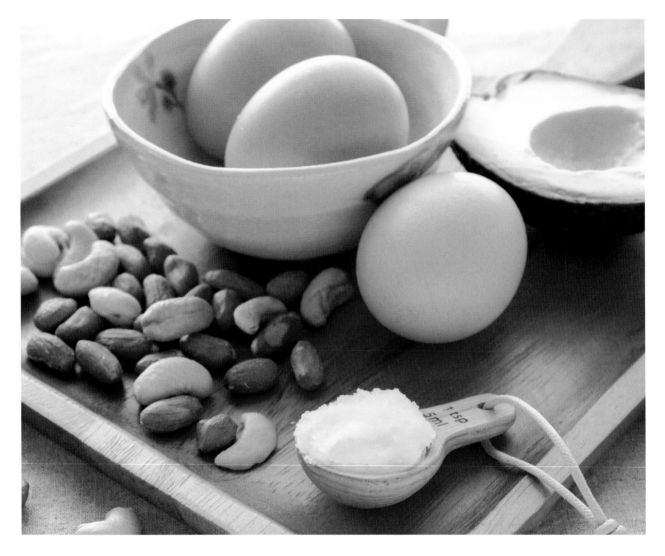

is worth the minuscule finger prick required to test your ketone and blood sugar levels. Of course, you absolutely can follow a ketogenic diet without using a glucometer. And if you are getting the results that you want without testing your blood glucose and/or ketones, then more power to you. However, if you want to get those results with the least amount of time and guesswork, the feedback from blood sugar and ketone testing is truly invaluable. Testing has been a major key to my success and that of the thousands of clients with whom I have personally worked to unlock the power of keto.

A Health Revolution

I believe that this is just the beginning of medical technology in the home. I have read that Google is working on contact lenses that can measure blood sugar. A time is coming when we'll be able to take our blood or urine samples to a local pharmacy for interpretation. These technologies will enable us to take further responsibility for our own health and wellness.

However, a persistent disconnect between health and food is not being addressed in medical training. I attended a health conference in London at which a speaker asked the physicians in the audience what kind of nutritional training they received (if any). The answers ranged from a few hours to a half-day at the most. Why aren't doctors receiving more nutritional training when we literally become what we eat, and nutrition is one of the most important aspects of health? Why does the modern approach to medicine persist in subjugating the relevance of food and nutrition for weight loss, diabetes, and obesity while recommending increased exercise and eating less? This is especially frustrating when eating less and exercising more do not yield positive results. Why do doctors recommend drugs and surgery to manage these health conditions rather than starting with balanced nutrition?

Encouragingly, due to the increasing number of studies being released on the importance of diet in treating and preventing disease, a growing number of health practitioners are learning about the power of reducing sugar consumption. Also, more medical professionals are learning that all calories are not considered equal, the types of calories we eat are vitally important, and the quality of the nourishment we receive is of unparalleled importance. In my opinion, food and nutrition should be the first aspect of treatment when it comes to addressing many health conditions that have been proven to be treatable—and reversed completely—with dietary changes. Unfortunately, telling a patient to eat more whole foods is not a protocol that generates any revenue, but prescribing an expensive medication does. The incentive to prescribe natural cures to ailments is nonexistent. I have a great deal of respect for the vast number of dedicated physicians in the world; I don't know where we would be without them. However, it is time for a change on a grand scale, and the health revolution begins with individuals taking responsibility and advocating for their own health and well-being.

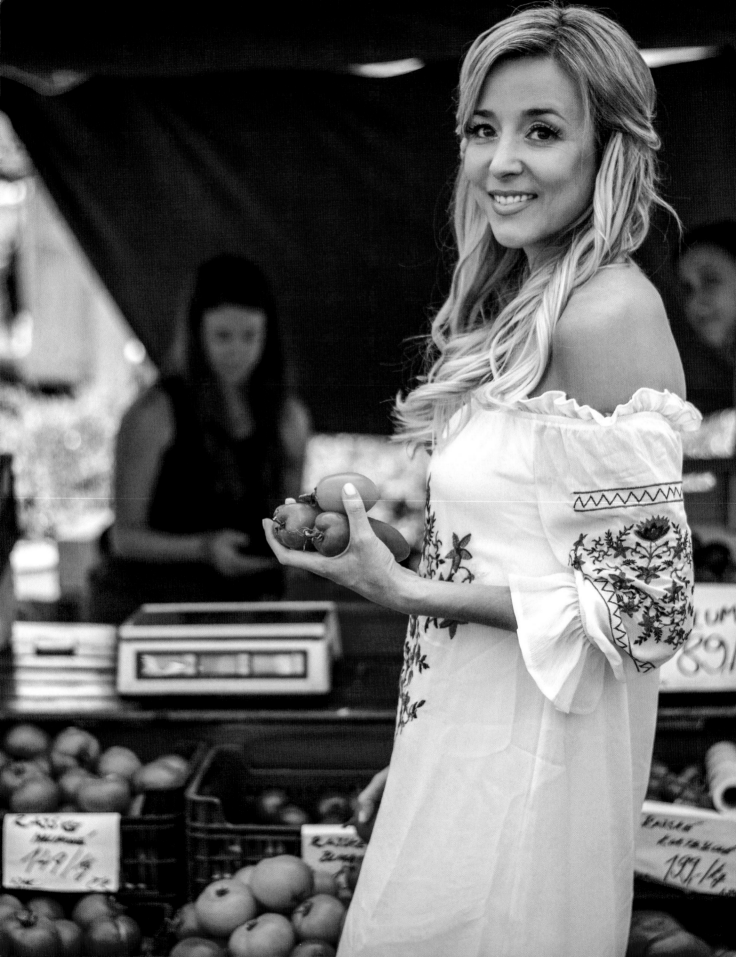

Chapter 4

Beyond Macros:
The Essentials of a Healthy Diet

Our bodies require essential amino acids and essential fatty acids, and they depend on us to deliver these necessary nutrients via the food we eat. Although some people consider the ketogenic diet a fad diet, I believe high–carb, low–fat diets that deprive the body of essential nutrients and fat–soluble vitamins while constantly flooding it with glucose are much more compromising to health.

Essential nutrients are nutrients that our bodies are unable to generate or synthesize on their own. Essential fatty acids from fats and essential amino acids from proteins are vital to our existence, but our bodies are not able to produce them, so we must ingest them in the form of food. Unlike fats and proteins, carbohydrates are not essential. Before writing them off completely, however, you need to know that there are some high-quality carbohydrates that play an important role in our bodies.

Essential Fats

Omega-3 and Omega-6 Fatty Acids

Our bodies require the healthy fatty acids alpha-linolenic acid (an omega-3 fatty acid) and linoleic acid (an omega-6 fatty acid) to thrive. These building blocks play a significant role in the function of all cells and tissues. Deficiencies in these essential fatty acids can lead to compromised liver and kidney function, lowered immune function, slowed or halted growth, dry skin, and depression. Getting the necessary fatty acids is extremely beneficial for overall health and can:

- Reduce the incidence of heart disease
- Provide relief from issues related to inflammation, such as ulcerative colitis and joint pain
- Prevent heart disease and stroke
- Decrease breast cancer risk

We need to consume both omega-3 and omega-6 fats, but in the correct proportions. In the standard American diet, we typically see ratios of omega-6 to omega-3 fats of 10:1 or even 20:1. Omega-3 fatty acids lower triglycerides (blood fats), help alleviate chronic inflammation; reduce symptoms of depression, asthma, and ADHD; assist with baby development; and lower cholesterol. Because omega-6 competes with omega-3 in the body, too much omega-6 prevents omega-3 fats from being utilized. To keep the body from relying too much on omega-6 fatty acids and therefore not utilizing omega-3 fatty acids, a better target ratio for omega-6 to omega-3 fats, in my opinion, is 2:1 or even 1:1.

Therefore, it is important to seek out foods that supply significant amounts of omega-3 fatty acids and make them a regular part of your ketogenic diet. Some of the richest sources of omega-3 fats include:

Caviar or fish roe	Oysters
Chia seeds and chia seed oil	Pumpkin seeds and pumpkin oil
Cod liver oil	Salmon and salmon oil
Flax seeds and flaxseed oil	Sardines
Anchovies	Spinach
Herring	Walnuts and walnut oil
Mackerel	

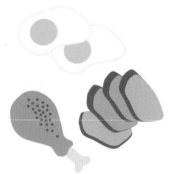

Here are some additional sources of omega-3:

Almonds	Eggs
Beef	Pine nuts
Chicken	Pork
Dairy products	Sesame seeds

Medium-Chain Triglycerides (MCTs)

Medium-chain triglycerides, or MCTs (also known as medium-chain fatty acids, or MCFAs), are highly beneficial for health and for generating ketones. They are quickly broken down and absorbed by the brain and body, so they provide us with a lot of energy. Unlike other fats, MCTs go straight to the liver, where they can be used for fuel or turned into ketone bodies.

MCTs are known for boosting fat loss. Because they are absorbed rapidly, the body is not likely to store them. They increase levels of leptin and other hormones, which reduce appetite and generate a feeling of fullness. MCTs can also help you get into and stay in nutritional ketosis.

MCTs are also known for strengthening the immune system. They are naturally present in human breast milk, which is ketogenic, and which is why baby formula is sometimes made with coconut oil or MCT oil. (MCT oil is similar to coconut oil but has six times the concentration of MCTs; it is used in several of the recipes in this book.)

Most dietary fats are made up of long-chain fatty acids (LCFAs) containing 13 to 21 carbon atoms or short-chain fatty acids (SCFAs) containing fewer than 6 carbon atoms. MCTs fall in the middle and contain 6 to 12 carbon atoms. The main MCFAs are:

C6: caproic acid

C8: caprylic acid

C10: capric acid

C12: lauric acid

Some of the top sources of MCTs are:

MCT oil (mostly caprylic acid or capric acid)

Coconut oil (mostly lauric acid)

Full-fat dairy products

Fat–Soluble Vitamins

Consuming healthy fats provides the hardworking cells in our bodies with the fatty acids they need to perform myriad functions to keep us in good shape. These healthy fats also furnish the important fat-soluble vitamins A, D, E, and K:

- **Vitamin A** is known for its vision-boosting properties and plays a key role in maintaining eyesight, as well as boosting immunity and supporting cell and hair growth, reproductive function, and fetal development.

- **Vitamin D** is essential for overall health, a strong immune system, and the regulation of circulating phosphorous and calcium, which are critical for bone growth and maintenance. Many people living in North America have vitamin D deficiencies.

- **Vitamin E** is an important antioxidant that prevents free radical damage and supports skin health, as well as prevents the risk of blood clots by acting as a blood thinner.

- **Vitamin K** is needed for blood clotting, bone health, and avoiding calcification in the blood vessels, which is critical for reducing heart disease risk. Vitamin K has also been shown to be associated with lowered cancer risk.

Once our bodies are getting their fill of these essential fatty acids and fat-soluble vitamins, plus essential amino acids (see the next page) and B vitamins, they are well nourished and can operate optimally!

Essential Proteins

Many health and fitness proponents focus on the *amount* of protein we should consume per day to meet our nutritional needs. In my opinion, there is too much of a focus on quantity. Protein *quality* is just as important as, if not more important than, the amount consumed. For this reason, a ketogenic diet emphasizes protein quality over quantity and focuses on moderating protein intake.

Protein quality is determined by how well a food satisfies our nutritional requirements by providing essential amino acids, which are the building blocks of our cells. There are nine essential amino acids: histidine, isoleucine, leucine, lysine, methionine, phenylalanine, threonine, tryptophan, and valine. Six other amino acids are conditionally essential, and five that can easily be synthesized in the body are considered not essential.

As long as your body is receiving essential amino acids from high-quality proteins, there is no need to overconsume protein, whether you are following a regular diet or a muscle-gaining or bodybuilding regimen. The right range for protein depends on your activity level; however, meeting your body's amino acid requirement is the most important factor in optimizing your ketogenic diet.

Some of the highest-quality proteins that best deliver the essential and conditionally essential amino acids also happen to be some of the central foods consumed as part of a ketogenic diet, including:

Eggs	Chicken
Cheese	Nuts
Fish	Seeds
Beef	Nut and seed butters

> *It happened! I crossed over into the 130s this morning. 139.5 is a 20–pound loss from where I started. . . . My goal jeans were a size 6. I have them on today and had to add a belt. Just tried on a pair of size 4 jeans I've kept for years and they are completely wearable now. Keto on!*
>
> —Lana W.

The Role of Healthy Carbs

For the average healthy person, there is no such thing as an essential carbohydrate. The human body does not require carbohydrate in the same way that it requires essential fatty acids and essential amino acids. We need much smaller quantities of carbohydrate than we have been advised to consume in recent decades. We also need to consider their type and form, because not all vegetables, fruits, and grains are created equal.

For years, the notion that fruits and vegetables are the epitome of a healthy diet has been drilled into us. However, it's important to understand the nutrient-to-sugar balance in plant foods. We want to consume those that are the most nutrient-dense and the lowest in sugar. The following sections lay out the best and worst choices.

Grains

It's true that grains are not completely devoid of nutrients. However, in modern agriculture, grains are significantly processed and, more importantly, modified so that they are almost unrecognizable as compared to their ancient forms. The initial cultivation of grains propelled human society forward by providing a readily accessible and inexpensive food staple. However, grains today are so devoid of nutritional value that they need to have nutrients added to them. In direct contrast, you have high-quality proteins, fats, and vegetables that are nutrient-dense and therefore do not require fortification. Plus, today's processed and modified grains trigger inflammatory reactions in growing numbers of people and are the source of widespread gluten intolerance and more serious conditions, such as Crohn's disease. For these reasons, grains can be considered nutrient-negative, as their drawbacks outweigh any beneficial contributions they might make to our diets. In formulating a diet based on optimal nutrition, grains have no place, in my opinion. Therefore, the ketogenic diet completely eliminates grains.

Vegetables

Vegetables are known as *complex carbohydrates* because they contain fiber and vitamins as well as sugars. However, many vegetables contain just as much sugar as fruit! Some of the highest-carb vegetables are potatoes and sweet potatoes (which are also classified nutritionally as starches) and corn (which is also classified nutritionally as a grain and a fruit). Starches have higher concentrations of sugars chained together than other vegetables, and for this reason they have a stronger effect on blood sugar than nonstarchy veggies. Many other vegetables that we think of as healthy are also very high in sugar. Beets, for example, are used to make beet sugar, and beet juice is often used to make candy because it adds a vibrant pink color as well as sweetness.

Shockingly (to me, anyway), carrots contain a lot of sugar. For years, I relied on carrots because I believed that I was doing good for my body and my diet. Then I got into using a juicer to mix carrots with apples. I drank this juice every morning for months because I thought it was healthy, but the reality was that I was jolting my system with a sugar overload by ingesting several carrots and apples at once without any fiber to slow their absorption.

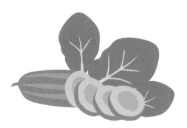

So, even when it comes to vegetables, it's critical to make smart choices. Some of the other highest-sugar *(nutrient-negative)* vegetables (some of which are also nutritionally classified as grains and starches) include:

Beets	Potatoes
Carrots	Squash (especially butternut squash and acorn squash)
Corn	Sweet potatoes
Peas	
Plantains	

The following vegetables should become your go-to selections because they are low in carbs, low in sugar, and high in fiber; in other words, they are *nutrient-positive*:

All cruciferous vegetables, including broccoli, cauliflower, and green and red cabbage	Lettuce (all varieties)
Avocados	Mushrooms
Asparagus	Mustard greens
Alfalfa sprouts	Mung bean sprouts
Arugula (rocket)	Okra
Bell peppers (mainly green)	Onions (green onions are ideal because they are the lowest in carbs; the carbs in yellow and red onions can add up quickly, so it's good to limit our intake)
Bamboo shoots	
Bean sprouts	
Celeriac	Radishes
Celery	Shallots
Cucumbers	Spinach
Collard greens	Summer squash
Dandelion greens	Swiss chard
Eggplant	String beans
Escarole	Turnip greens
Endive	Tomatoes
Garlic	Watercress
Kale	Zucchini
Leeks	

As a general rule, lettuces and greens tend to be quite low in carbs and high in nutrients, making them excellent choices! This is especially true because they tend to be eaten raw and therefore contain live enzymes, which make it easier for our bodies to digest and assimilate them.

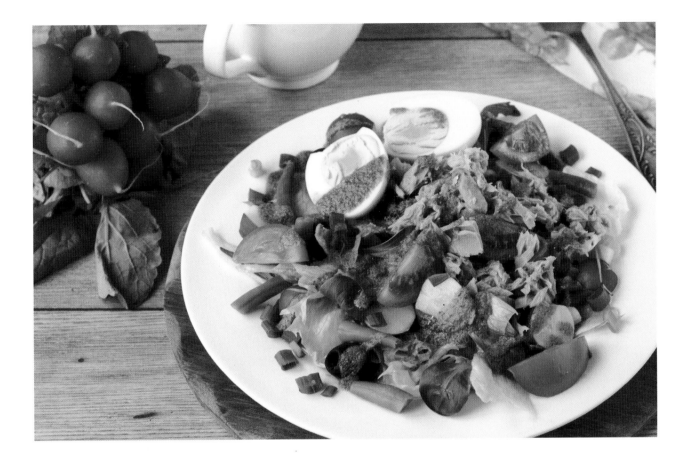

A Warning About Salads

We need to unlearn much of what we have been told regarding what is healthy when it comes to food. Take salads, for example, which are often treated as a "free" food. Contrary to what we have been trained to believe, salads with fat-free dressings are not the holy grail of health (and neither is juicing). A pile of zero-calorie lettuce makes almost anything appear healthy—even if it is full of sugar from the fat-free dressing! Tossing in some dried fruits or other sugar-loaded ingredients makes the situation even worse. Salads can be great choices on a ketogenic diet, but we need to be smart about how we put them together. As a rule, base your salads on low-carb vegetables and avoid adding dried fruits or croutons. See pages 164 to 179 for some excellent keto salad recipes.

These low-sugar, nutrient-dense, and nutrient-positive vegetables have an unparalleled ability to feed and support the friendly bacteria in the gut, known as the microbiome. The microbiome performs essential functions such as producing neurotransmitters (including serotonin, which helps us feel happy and calm) and keeping "bad" bacteria (think *Candida*) at bay. The microbiome weighs about 2 pounds and is made up of trillions of cells. Because of its size and function, it is under consideration for being reclassified as an organ; it is a vital organ indeed! For more on this topic, check out Dr. David Perlmutter's book *Brain Maker: The Power of Gut Microbes to Heal and Protect Your Brain–for Life*.

Fruit

Fructose is one of the most health-compromising sugars in existence. Many studies are now pointing to the dangers of fructose consumption. Due to the liver's inability to process fructose like it does sucrose, in many cases fructose is stored as fat, irrespective of caloric intake. This can overload the liver with fat and lead directly to the development of nonalcoholic fatty liver disease (NAFLD), which is a precursor to type 2 diabetes.

In many ways, pure fructose is worse for the body than table sugar, which is a combination of sucrose and fructose. Another pitfall of fructose is that because we think of refined white sugar as being bad for us, many of us attempt to moderate our consumption of it—for example, we use restraint when adding sugar to coffee or tea. However, because we have been taught that fruit is a healthy food that we should consume daily, we assume that fructose must also be good for us. Because it is given the health halo associated with fruit, we don't hold back when consuming it. Similarly, we have no issues with juicing fruit or adding fructose to our food as a sweetener. Fructose is now packaged in stores as a "healthy" alternative to table sugar. Yes, fruits are full of healthy antioxidants and vitamins, but so are vegetables. For the most part, vegetables give us all the same nutrients, but without the sugars.

That being said, *some* fruit is allowed on a ketogenic diet, provided that it is consumed in moderate amounts. Here's some information to help you make the best choices.

The following fruits have a very high fructose content (they are *nutrient negative*):

Apples	Melons
Apricots	Nectarines
Bananas	Oranges
Cherries	Papaya
Figs	Peaches
Grapefruit	Pears
Grapes	Plums
Guava	Pomegranates
Kiwi	Tangerines
Kumquat	Any dried fruit, such as dates, raisins, and prunes
Lychee	
Mango	

The following fruits have a medium to low overall sugar content:

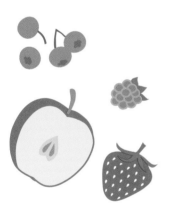

- Blueberries
- Strawberries

The following fruits have the lowest overall sugar content (they are *nutrient positive*), so they are the best choices for a ketogenic diet:

- Blackberries
- Cranberries
- Lemons
- Limes
- Raspberries
- Rhubarb

I started this challenge in August 2016 with a goal to be able to reduce the amount of medications I take every day. I recognized that my ill health was directly related to the choices I had been making. [As of] yesterday I officially have lost 50 lbs. My doctor has reduced my blood pressure pills from 50 mg a day to 12.5 mg a day and my potassium pills from 4 pills a day to 2 pills a day. I have gone from size 16 pants to comfortably wearing size 4 pants. I have gone from a 2XL top to a L top (and from an E cup to a DD). I am very excited by these positive changes and am hopeful that when I lose the remaining 15 lbs I will be able to completely stop both the aforementioned medications. I have gained a sense of freedom and clarity. I have more energy than I have had for the past two years. I love this program! Thank you to this whole group and especially Vanessa for helping me to become the best me possible.

—Doreen M.

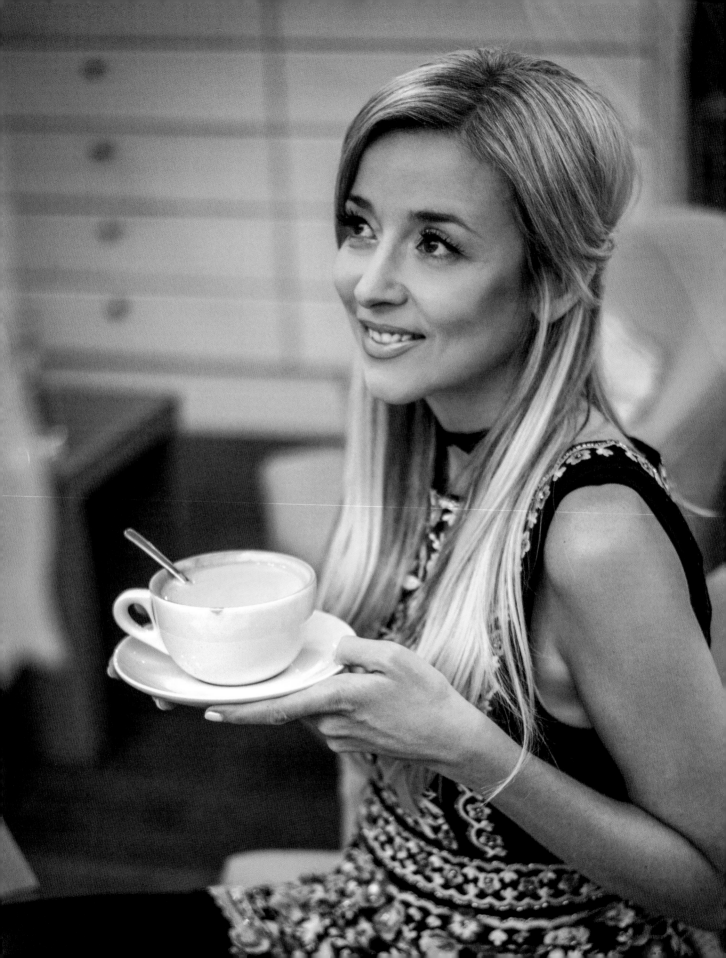

Chapter 5

Hot Topics

I love to answer people's burning questions about keto, and some topics come up more often than others. In this chapter, I cover some of the hot topics I see that I think warrant additional attention.

What's the Difference Between Nutritional Ketosis and Ketoacidosis?

People sometimes confuse the ketogenic diet with *ketoacidosis*, an extremely rare, life-threatening complication that can arise in people with diabetes. Ketoacidosis and nutritional ketosis are not connected in any way other than that both involve the presence of ketones. Ketoacidosis occurs when the body lacks insulin and blood sugar cannot be pushed from the cells; the result is high blood sugar and extremely high ketones. Typically, ketoacidosis involves ketone levels of at least 20 mmol/L and blood sugar readings of 240 mg/dl or higher.

Healthy people whose pancreases can produce insulin are not at risk for ketoacidosis. If you do not have diabetes or rare kidney or pancreas issues and you are following a ketogenic diet for the purpose of achieving nutritional ketosis, your ketone and blood sugar levels are always going to be inversely correlated: as ketones go up, blood sugar goes down. Ideally, you want your blood ketones to be between 1.0 and 3.0 mmol/L and your blood sugar to be at 90 mg/dl or below. Some people enter ketosis at 0.5 mmol/L.

After a period of fasting, ketones can go above 3.0. The highest ketones I've had during a fast were 8.0, but my blood glucose was very low—in the 56 to 70 range—as my body was being fueled almost entirely by fat. Sometimes eating large quantities of fat can push your ketones higher. If I eat a lot of cream cheese, for example, my ketones can go all the way up to 6.0. Going above 3.0 does not generate any additional benefits, however. For more information on nutritional ketosis, see page 39.

Bodybuilding and Keto

If you love to lift weights, you might discover that the keto diet is incredible for fueling your body in the gym. Many people find that some of their best workouts come during fasting, with or without a supplemental dose of branched-chain amino acids (BCAAs). Eating keto is generally muscle sparing because when you are in ketosis, your body burns fat, not muscle. Keto also mimics the effects of fasting, which can produce human growth hormone, or IGF-1, which boosts muscle building.

A ketogenic diet optimizes nutrition. You will need to play around with your protein intake to determine how much protein is ideal for you and to establish your protein threshold for when you enter or leave nutritional ketosis.

Ketone Supplements

Ketone supplements (also known as exogenous ketones) have been growing in popularity in recent years along with the popularity of the ketogenic diet itself since researchers discovered that ketones could be ingested and then utilized by the body. Rather than having their bodies generate ketones from the breakdown of dietary or stored fats, some people consume them instead. Ketone supplements take various forms, including drinks that can be added to water and food products, and generally come as packaged, prepared foods. Many people claim that ketone supplements help them get into ketosis without needing to follow a ketogenic diet, or that they boost the effects of following a ketogenic diet.

I am excited about the leading-edge scientific applications and discoveries in the field of ketone supplements. This science could help millions of people who are unable to get into nutritional ketosis via diet alone experience the therapeutic benefits of an intake of ketones to be used as energy for the brain and body. I am optimistic about the power of exogenous ketones for people who cannot make their own.

That being said, I don't believe in magic pills. My approach is based on nutritional ketosis, which, as the name implies, is ketosis derived from the food we eat. The body is programmed to make ketones just like it grows nails, heals wounds, and performs many other essential functions. Ketosis requires a mindful approach to eating and living, and there are no easy outs.

Counting Calories

Many people think that counting calories is not important when following keto, or that the *type* of calories being consumed is more important than the *number* of calories being consumed. The amount of food you eat is a factor, of course. However, what is much more important for weight loss and maintenance is how much of the food you eat is readily absorbed and processed by your body with a minimal release of the hormone insulin to clear your bloodstream during and after digestion, and how often this process occurs.

If you are eating only 1,000 calories a day but are eating a high-carb diet centered around low-fat foods such as bagels with fat-free cream cheese, coffee with sugar-free sweetener and nonfat milk, fruit and fruit juices, and smoothies, those 1,000 calories could be spread throughout the day. This prevents your body from benefitting, as you are continuously stimulating insulin, which prevents your body from burning fat. We want real, sustained weight loss from optimally functioning hormones, not temporary weight loss from caloric restriction that does nothing to restore proper hormone function and health.

Cheat Days and Carb-Loading

Many people have a hard time with the idea of giving up high-carbohydrate diets. For one, we learn to eat bulk, and we get used to eating large amounts of salads, vegetables, fruit, low-fat dairy such as yogurt, and the like. The average person on a high-carb diet consumes six to eight meals a day (including beverages that supply as much energy as a meal). Because we are constantly thinking about our next meal, food fixation can develop.

When you start a ketogenic regimen, one of the adjustments you need to make is to your portion sizes, as high-fat food is much denser than high-carb, low-fat food. This is where the importance of macronutrient allocation comes in. However, portion control also happens naturally on keto; healthy fats and high-quality proteins are much more satisfying than carbohydrates because they nourish the body and provide essential fatty acids, essential amino acids, and power-packed ketones from the fat stored on your body. They are a longer- and cleaner-burning fuel.

Make no mistake, sugar and carbohydrates are extremely addictive. Studies have shown that lab rats will forgo cocaine for sugar! It is an incredibly addictive substance and provides instantaneous high energy (and subsequent crashes). Sugar also creates dependence, which is met with a large number of side effects from withdrawal.

If you are picturing white crystals, then you might think your diet doesn't contain a lot of sugar. However, when you think about carbs as a whole, you will realize that sugar makes its way into our diets in many forms, from baby carrots to bagels. Carbs include everything from the flavoring syrup you use in your coffee to the grapes or apple that you enjoy as a mid-afternoon snack.

Many diets are based on low-carb principles but also include "cheat days," "high-carb" days (on which you would "carb-load"), or even "carb nights." Several years ago I followed a program in which I ate low-carb during the week and then had the option to have a cheat day when I could eat whatever I wanted. I ended up eating a lot of carbs on this single day because they were so restricted during the rest of the week. I have two main issues with this mindset: one, it can lead to bingeing, and two, it can interfere with insulin sensitivity. Let's dig into each of those issues in a little more depth.

Bingeing

First, cheat days can cause food fixation and lead to an unhealthy food-related behavior known as bingeing. For anyone who has a history with bingeing behavior, a cheat day is a binge with permission. You are used to dealing with food fixation when you eat a high-carb diet that fails to supply essential fatty acids and fat-soluble vitamins. Severely restricting carbohydrate intake for most of the week until a specific day only heightens food fixation because you cannot help but think about this magical day coming our way. How could you *not* obsess about the coming food free-for-all?

So, until that cheat day, you fixate on your favorite cereals, packaged treats, bread, candy, pizza, and more. However, after what often ends up being a decadent and overindulgent day, you wake up the next day feeling sick and remorseful with a sugar hangover, and you want nothing more than to return to your disciplined ways that make you feel so good.

Insulin Resistance

The second issue I have with cheat days is that spiking your blood sugar with a binge full of sugary and carb-loaded foods reverses all the effort you've put into healing insulin resistance and restoring insulin sensitivity (see page 21). When you eat a high-carb, low-fat diet, insulin suppresses the release of leptin, your satiety hormone, which means that you never really feel full, even when your stomach is full. This is partly why ketogenic diets are so effective. On keto, you fill up on fat, which is the macronutrient that stimulates the production of insulin the least, and the resulting release of leptin makes you feel full easily. Leptin gives your body a break from insulin, making you more insulin sensitive.

Real whole nutritional food! . . . I've been following Ketogenic Girl for over a year, and I've never felt better! My overall health has improved greatly, I have more energy, and my mental clarity is amazing. It is more than just a weight-loss program, it is a complete health overhaul program that Vanessa personally walks you through. Her recipes are extremely easy, elegant, and so satisfying and filling. There are many keto sites and programs popping up, but none compares to Ketogenic Girl. She is the real deal! I've lost two pant sizes and many, many other non-scale victories and health gains, such as decreasing my medication by half! And the food is so good!!

—Lisa R.

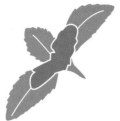

Natural and Artificial Sweeteners

Avoid artificial sweeteners at all costs. Recent studies have found that sucralose—one of the most common artificial sweeteners—can devastate the healthy bacteria in the gut, which is responsible for many important functions in the body. Aspartame, another common artificial sweetener, is also a neurotoxin and compromises brain health. Diet soda is very deceptive; a can of artificially sweetened soda can spike glucose even higher than a soda containing sugar and can kick you out of ketosis for several days.

Ideally, a ketogenic diet should be centered on whole foods without additives. In the beginning, I relied on natural sweeteners to help me make the transition away from sugar and artificial sweeteners; this strategy was especially helpful for getting me off a sweetened beverage that I used to drink throughout the day. However, I now eat mostly satiating real foods with a very limited amount of sweetener. If I do use sweetener, it tends to be in an occasional sugar-free dessert sweetened with stevia. Because I believe that ridding ourselves of cravings for sweet tastes is an important part of the keto lifestyle, the recipes in this book are mostly savory, though I do include a few sweet desserts especially for those of you who are still working on changing your habits.

Some people have a cephalic response to both artificial and natural sweeteners, in which insulin secretion is triggered when the tongue tastes sweetness; this prepares blood sugar to rise. The cephalic response can end up causing blood sugar to *drop* as insulin clears the bloodstream of glucose. It can then spike cortisol and cause the adrenals to mobilize stored glucose and raise blood sugar. This process can lead to cravings, irritability, and other symptoms. Because both natural and artificial sweeteners can lower blood sugar, they are not recommended for everyone. Speak with your doctor about consuming sweeteners if you take blood sugar medication or insulin.

Hydration

On a keto diet, hydration is a key to weight loss, healing, and simply feeling your best. Many people (myself included) find it challenging to drink enough water throughout the day, but doing so is even *more* important on a keto diet. Ketone bodies can be acidic in the body, and we need to support our livers with ample hydration to assist them in processing those ketones. Additionally, the kidneys release a lot of water when carbs are no longer eaten, so it is important to replenish that water, and to maintain electrolytes with added sodium in many cases.

The following chart shows you how to use the color of your urine to determine whether you are properly hydrated. If your urine is a pale yellow, you are well hydrated. If it is a darker yellow, you are okay, but you need to drink more water for optimal hydration.

Urine can take on a variety of colors. It typically ranges from a deep amber or honey color to a pale straw color, with many golden-hued variations in between. The color of your urine can tell you a lot about your body. Here's a chart of urine colors and what they indicate.

No Color (Transparent)
You're drinking a lot of water. You may want to cut back.

Pale Straw Colored
You're normal, healthy, and well hydrated.

Transparent Yellow
You're normal.

Dark Yellow
You're normal, but drink some water soon.

Amber or Honey Colored
Your body isn't getting enough water. Drink some water now!

Supplements

I believe in getting the nutrients we need from whole-food sources. Many supplements are not needed on a keto diet as they are on high-carb, low-fat diets that do not supply the essential fatty acids or essential amino acids that our bodies require. As always, it is important to speak with your healthcare provider about the appropriateness of following a ketogenic diet given your individual health situation and about any supplements you are considering. That being said, I have found the following supplements to be generally supportive for people who are following a ketogenic diet. See your healthcare provider or nutritionist for specific recommendations based on your unique needs.

- **Omega-3 fatty acids:** As previously discussed, to maximize our health, we need to ensure that we balance the ratio of omega-3 to omega-6, which is often skewed way too far toward omega-6 in our modern diet. This becomes even more important on a ketogenic diet because we are consuming a lot of fat. Opting for rich food sources of omega-3 fatty acids, such as wild-caught fish, walnuts, flax seeds, and chia seeds, is recommended over taking supplements; however, additional supplementation may be beneficial.

- **Vitamin C:** Vitamin C is an important antioxidant for neutralizing free radicals. In some cases, it can be lacking on a ketogenic diet, as the consumption of fruit is limited; however, there are abundant food sources to meet the need for vitamin C, including lemons, limes, bell peppers, and leafy green vegetables such as kale and broccoli.

- **Probiotics, such as high-quality *Bifidobacteria:*** Probiotics are essential for the friendly bacteria in the gut to thrive. In my opinion, probiotics are the most important supplement to take, whether or not you eat a ketogenic diet. The gut microbiome is an important factor for digestion, regularity, assimilation of vital nutrients, and keeping the gut flora in great health, and it is essential for supporting proper neurotransmitter production in the gut.

- **Biotin, prenatal vitamins, and collagen for healthy hair and nails:** With the hormone fluctuations and other changes that can occur on a keto diet, a lot of detoxification takes place. Symptoms of detoxing can include hair loss and dry skin, as the skin is the body's largest detoxification organ and pathway. Biotin, prenatal vitamins, and collagen have been shown to assist with these symptoms in some people.

- **Magnesium:** Most people are lacking in magnesium, as modern agricultural practices have depleted our soil and the foods that grow in that soil of nutrients. Magnesium is important for regulating levels of calcium, potassium, and sodium in the body and can help calm nerves, alleviate anxiety, improve sleep, soothe muscle aches, and even aid in digestion and constipation. On a keto diet, supplementing with magnesium can be highly beneficial. See your physician, healthcare provider, or nutritionist for specific recommendations based on your individual needs.

- **Electrolytes (sodium):** The body loses a lot of water and sodium on a keto diet, so it is important to supplement with high-quality sodium, such as Himalayan salt or mineral-rich sea salt. The body will then regulate its critical sodium-to-potassium balance on its own, so there is no need to supplement with potassium (self-directed supplementation with potassium is dangerous and *never* recommended; it should be done only under the care of a physician).

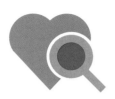

Keto for Special Health Conditions

Many people come to the ketogenic diet because of persistent health conditions that they have not found success in alleviating or treating with traditional healthcare approaches. Their quests lead them to keto for one main reason: success is loud! People who have succeeded in treating their conditions share their experiences, and good news travels fast. The commonality among all these issues is hormones, and the keto diet has the potential ability to rebalance and regulate hormones. Although I am not qualified to discuss the medical aspects behind these conditions, I wanted to mention some of the empirical evidence that I have observed through the stories shared by members of my coaching program, the 28-Day Ketogenic Girl Challenge, which has had more than 2,300 members to date whom I have personally worked with through their participation. Many of them have experienced significant health benefits through their own applications of keto or my program.

Thyroid Issues, Infertility, and PCOS

Many of the women I coach through my programs suffer from conditions that are related to the endocrine system, whereby there is a hormone function connection, including thyroid conditions, infertility, and PCOS (polycystic ovary syndrome)—and many of them have experienced the tremendous benefits of keto. Women often tell me that following a ketogenic diet enabled them to become pregnant after many years of trying. It has been wonderful to see several women announce pregnancies in our online coaching group for the 28-Day Ketogenic Girl Challenge in the past couple of years.

One possible explanation for these women's increased fertility is that high-carb diets interfere with hormone function. One theory is that high-carb diets can cause the body to generate a lot of testosterone or androgen, an excess of which could lead to improper hormone balance. High-carb diets can do so by a) generating too much insulin, which can lead to androgen production, b) generating excess testosterone, and c) generating too much estrogen.

We have already established that eating high amounts of carbohydrates can generate too much insulin. Many popular high-carb foods, including dried fruits, beans, chickpeas, peas, tempeh, tofu, alfalfa sprouts, cereals (including flax in some cases), and soy milk, are estrogenic and contain high levels of concentrated sugars. An energy bar containing dried fruit or a visit to a salad bar, which features a lot of the aforementioned foods, is commonly thought of as a "healthy" meal. These foods not only mimic the effects of estrogen in the body but also spike glucose and insulin, creating an imbalance in normal balanced hormone production.

In addition, high-carbohydrate diets tend to be more processed, and modern food products contain a lot of soy, which is estrogenic when absorbed by the body (which means that it acts similarly to estrogen in the body). The plastics frequently used in product packaging also contribute to excessive estrogen leaching into our foods and beverages from plastic containers. Alcohol is estrogenic as well.

Most people who eat high-carb diets have some degree of insulin resistance. If you have excess body fat, then you may have insulin resistance and built-up metabolic dysregulation from years of (unintentional) abuse to your bloodstream. As previously discussed, 80 percent of supermarket foods contain added sugars. Their sugar content spikes insulin, potentially leading to androgen creation. The processes used to create them (the refinement and addition of chemicals) and the estrogenic compounds found in their packaging can also generate persistently elevated blood sugar levels. Elevated blood sugar can prevent individuals from experiencing weight loss or proper hormone function.

On a so-called "healthy" low-fat, high-protein, and high-carb diet, blood sugar is raised by many other factors in addition to carbohydrates, including adrenaline and cortisol from stress, processed foods, chemical additives, allergenic foods, environmental toxins, and excess dietary protein. Insulin must singlehandedly combat all these triggers without any backup. It is the only hormone that has the ability to remove glucose from the bloodstream for use by and storage in cells. The human body is incredibly adaptive, and we have adapted to these continuous blood sugar stimulants and triggers to keep us alive. When you first begin the keto diet, your body goes through some healing—maybe a little, maybe a lot. By healing, I am referring to a return to a state of homeostasis wherein the body is functioning optimally, the way it was designed to function, without compromise in the form of chronic pain, impaired metabolism, infertility, excess weight, impaired insulin sensitivity, or disease. Healing is not an overnight process; however, the ketogenic diet has shown real promise in relieving symptoms of a compromised endocrine system because it is based on restoring hormonal homeostasis in the body.

Thyroid Function and Keto

The thyroid gland is located in the neck, just below the larynx, and has two lobes. It main function is to take iodine from food sources and convert it to two thyroid hormones: thyroxine (T4) and triiodothyronine (T3). The thyroid cells absorb iodine and combine it with the amino acid tyrosine to generate T4 and T3, which are then released into the bloodstream to be transported throughout the body, where they control the metabolism (the conversion of calories from food and oxygen into energy to fuel the body). All cells in the body depend on the thyroid hormones T3 and T4

UNBELIEVABLE!! 9 weeks [on the Ketogenic Girl Challenge] . . . 20 lbs GONE!!! Happy dance!!!

—Rhonda W.

to regulate the conversion and production of energy via the metabolism. Thyroid production in the body is managed by the pituitary gland, which in turn is regulated by the hypothalamus, both of which are located in the brain (source: endocrineweb.com).

With regard specifically to women and hormones, female hormone function can be affected by eating high-carb, low-fat diets and experiencing too much stress from modern lifestyles, leading to high levels of cortisol, for example, which throws the body's hormones off-balance. We see women's hormone function being more and more disrupted via the epidemic levels of thyroid issues known as either underactive (hypothyroid) or overactive (hyperthyroid). In the case of underactive thyroid, the thyroid gland does not produce enough thyroid hormone. Symptoms can include fatigue, weakness, weight gain or increased difficulty with weight loss, coarse or dry hair and rough skin, hair loss, cold intolerance, muscle cramps, and more. Symptoms of overactive thyroid or hyperthyroidism can include nervousness, anxiety, irritability, mood swings, trouble sleeping, weakness, chronic tiredness, swelling in the neck, palpitations, and more. Many women seek medical treatment to alleviate symptoms, which can include prescription medication or surgically invasive treatments to obliterate the thyroid. However, some women have experienced a reduction in symptoms after following a ketogenic diet, which is exciting to see.

Hashimoto's thyroiditis is an autoimmune condition in which the immune system attacks the thyroid. In some cases, it can lead to hypothyroidism, as the ability of the thyroid gland to generate thyroid hormone becomes compromised.

Graves' disease, on the other hand, is an autoimmune disorder whereby the thyroid gland produces *too much* thyroid hormone, which is a common cause of hyperthyroidism.

If you have thyroid or hormone issues and are interested in trying the ketogenic diet, it is best to transition into ketosis gradually; otherwise, you might see disruptions in your monthly cycle or experience hypoglycemic (low blood sugar) reactions. This applies to either hypothyroidism or hyperthyroidism. Some women might also need to do what is known as "carbohydrate cycling" or "carb-up" days while on keto, such as eating a higher amount of carbs once per week in order to stabilize the conversion of the thyroid hormone T3. See page 65 for more on carb-ups.

Many women are estrogen-dominant due to the amount of processed, soy-based foods we consume. Estrogen levels will drop when we begin eating a whole foods–based diet. The body will adapt to having lower levels of estrogen coming in through the diet. Excessive amounts of estrogen in the body can interfere with proper thyroid function as the thyroid is connected to sex hormones and adrenal function.

The thyroid gland manages metabolism and growth. Proper thyroid function combats lethargy, fatigue, depression, constipation, and

Finished my first 28 days yesterday [and] starting round 2 today!! Vanessa, thank you so much for this program. It was clear, it had amazing recipes, and your online support and everyone's help has given me what I needed to be successful on this way of eating!! I am happy to report I am down 24.1 pounds!!!!!! In just 28 days!!! But even more is how great I feel. I sleep better (no medication!!), I have a ton of energy, my headaches are gone, and I am in a great mood all the time!!!! Thank you, thank you!!! Here is to the next 28 days!!!!

—Marcie C.

more. It has been stated that 80 percent of women in North America have undiagnosed thyroid issues. Women who have hypothyroid, thyroidectomies, hyperthyroid, or PCOS have seen incredible success on my strict keto program.

Thyroid, Iodine, and Keto

Unless you have autoimmune Hashimoto's (in which case you must avoid iodine at all costs), you need iodine. It is essential for a properly functioning thyroid. The keto diet can provide a lot of iodine and is another reason it can be highly beneficial to the thyroid. Dried seaweed is one of the best sources of iodine; 7 grams of seaweed contains 4,500 micrograms of iodine, which is about thirty times the recommended daily intake. Other rich food sources of iodine include iodized sea salt, Himalayan sea salt, cod, baked turkey, boiled eggs, canned tuna, high-fat Greek yogurt, cheddar cheese, lobster, green beans, and cranberries. Iodine supplements are available as well. Speak with your healthcare provider if you are considering iodine supplementation.

For more on thyroid conditions, I recommend the work of Dr. Amy Myers and the Myers Way Protocol.

Fertility

Ketogenic diets can go a long way toward restoring hormone balance and can be excellent for fertility. The changes on keto are so dramatic, I have even seen menopausal women get their cycle again! However, the effects vary considerably from woman to woman. My clients' monthly cycles often lengthen in the first few months of a ketogenic diet and then gradually return to twenty-eight– to thirty-three–day cycles. Estrogen can be stored in fat, so when you first lose weight on keto, more estrogen is released into your body, which can affect your cycle. I have seen cycles lengthen to thirty-four to forty or more days. As the body's pH changes from becoming a fat burner, changes occur throughout the body. Delays and changes in cycle length are typical when starting a ketogenic diet and usually persist for a few months. These changes then regulate themselves once the body adapts to nutritional ketosis.

PCOS and Weight Loss

PCOS (polycystic ovarian syndrome) is a condition in which a woman's sex hormone levels are out of balance, which can cause the growth of ovarian cysts (benign masses on the ovaries) and can compromise fertility, disrupt the menstrual cycle, and even affect cardiac function. According to the U.S. Department of Health & Human Services, between 1 and 10 and 1 and 20 women of childbearing age have PCOS, up to 5 million women in the United States. Symptoms can include infertility, excessive hair growth or hair loss, decreased breast growth, deepening of the voice, acne, and weight gain, potentially leading to depression and an inability to lose weight (source: healthline.com).

The cause is unknown; however, it is theorized that women who have PCOS are overproducing the hormone androgen, which can interfere with ovulation. The connection to keto with regard to androgen overproduction is that excess insulin, triggered by high-carb diets, may be the cause of this androgen overproduction. It is theorized that drastically limiting carbohydrate intake can reduce the production of androgen.

Dozens of women on my program have thyroid issues, PCOS, and insulin resistance or are in menopause and have struggled to lose weight. They tell me that my Ketogenic Girl 28-Day Challenge is the first thing that has worked for them to heal and lose weight. To learn more about the challenge, go to www.ketogenicgirl.com.

Cholesterol

According to Dr. Adam Nally, an obesity specialist and leading proponent of low-carb diets, one of the fastest ways to reduce your cholesterol levels is to cut your carbohydrate intake. The most common reaction people have when they hear about keto is fearing high cholesterol levels. However, when speaking about heart disease, stroke, and other health risks, it is important to examine triglycerides first.

Persistent high blood sugar is one of the greatest health risks our society is facing today. The body converts the excess blood sugar that it cannot clear to blood lipids (fats), which are denser forms of circulating glucose. These blood fats are called triglycerides, and their presence in the bloodstream puts us at risk for blockages. Most people understand that having high triglycerides is bad for us but have been led to believe that the cause is dietary fat, not realizing how significantly excess sugars contribute to the problem.

Cholesterol also has a bad reputation, but it is a vital substance that plays a role in maintaining sex hormones (testosterone and estrogen) and synthesizing vitamin D while being essential to cell membranes and the production of bile. It is needed for hormone generation and facilitates intracellular communication.

The liver makes about three-quarters or more of the cholesterol needed by the body. Most of the cholesterol in our bodies does not come from the consumption of cholesterol, just as blood fats do not come from the consumption of dietary fats. Our bodies convert excess glucose in the bloodstream into a denser form of energy (or fat) to deal with and lower high glucose levels. Consistently high blood sugar can cause many health issues, so it is converted to triglycerides in the blood to manage it and to avoid blockages.

Cholesterol levels and the consumption of dietary fat have been on the decline since the 1970s, yet heart disease remains the number-one killer in the Western world. Rates of heart disease, diabetes, and obesity are higher than ever. Cardiovascular disease and total mortality are reduced when carb intake is decreased, and overall cardiovascular health improves when we add healthy fats to our diets. According to Nina Teicholz, an investigative journalist and author of *The Big Fat Surprise: Why Butter, Meat and Cheese Belong in a Healthy Diet*, a study that will reveal that saturated fats do not cause heart disease has been conducted by the former president of the American Heart Association, Dr. Salim Yusuf. I expect more of these studies to reveal the immense and powerful benefits of consuming healthy fats and the important role of cholesterol.

A major, groundbreaking study done at McMaster University in Canada following 135,000 adults was just published in *The Lancet*, demonstrating that low-fat diets are linked to higher death rates and could raise the risk of early death by almost one-quarter. People who reduced their consumption of fats such as butter, cheese, and meats lived far shorter lives than their counterparts who enjoyed high-fat diets, contrary to the mainstream health advice we are repeatedly given. The participants in the study who ate the most carbohydrates in addition to eating low-fat faced a nearly 30 percent higher risk of early death. Eating high levels of all fats reduced the mortality rate by up to 23 percent! In reaction to this study, *Time* Magazine proclaimed, "The Low-Fat vs. Low-Carb Diet Debate Has a New Answer!" (http://time.com/4919448/low-fat-v-low-carb-diets/).

Another recently published article in the CBC News showed that ketogenic diets are effective for weight loss and health, are safe, and reduce cholesterol, triglycerides, and more. "The present study shows the beneficial effects of a long-term ketogenic diet. It significantly reduced the body weight and body mass index of the patients. Furthermore, it decreased the level of triglycerides, LDL cholesterol and blood glucose, and increased the level of HDL cholesterol. Administering a ketogenic diet for a relatively longer period did not produce any significant side effects in the patients. Therefore, the present study confirms that it is safe to use a ketogenic diet. These results indicate that the administration of a ketogenic diet for a relatively long period is safe. Further studies elucidating the molecular mechanisms of a ketogenic diet are in progress in our laboratory" (Hussain M. Dashti et al., "Long-term effects of a ketogenic diet in obese patients," *Experimental & Clinical Cardiology* 9, no. 3 [2004]: 200–205).

Major non–scale victory to report! I was diagnosed with PCOS a little over a year ago after rapid weight gain when I quit my birth control. I gained 45 lbs in 4 months after my husband and I started trying having a baby. I eliminated gluten, dairy, soy, and sugar from my diet, which helped me stop gaining but did nothing to help me lose. 11 months later, after 16 months of trying to get pregnant and still not losing weight, I started the 28–day challenge. It was the first thing that has worked for me! Happy to say I'm down 26 lbs and earlier this week I got the greatest little surprise! Expecting a little one December 26! I KNOW the keto diet played a role in me finally conceiving. Thanks, Vanessa!

—Jaime M.

Potential Side Effects of Keto

The main side effects that I see in people on a keto diet originate from a lack of dietary sodium because of the loss of electrolytes that occurs on a low-carb diet. Increasing your sodium intake can assist with low energy, muscle cramping, headaches, and other symptoms of the "keto flu." I like to supplement with 1 to 1¼ teaspoons of high-quality sea salt per day by adding it to my food.

Another potential side effect is brief and moderate to severe skin rashes and bruising. The body stores a lot of toxins in body fat to keep them away from our organs. Your skin is the body's biggest organ. That means when you burn fat, the skin is one of the best pathways for detoxification. You should consult your doctor with regard to the appearance of either rashes or bruising, as they could be unrelated to diet. Temporarily doing some carb cycling or "carbing up" can reduce the symptoms of rashes related to fat loss.

People beginning a keto diet sometimes experience a lack of regularity or constipation as their bodies adapt from a high-carb diet to a low-carb diet. Regularity is critical to maintain at all times, so it is beneficial to be aware of elimination habits and ensure that proper elimination is taking place. Consult with your physician or healthcare provider if you are experiencing constipation. In working with the clients who follow my program, I have found that daily supplementation with probiotics containing *Bifidobacteria* and eating fermented prebiotic foods, such as unsweetened sauerkraut, kimchi, full-fat yogurt or coconut milk yogurt, and unsweetened kombucha, can be helpful in maintaining proper and regular elimination. Additionally, making sure that your ketogenic diet contains at least 20 grams of carbohydrates daily, especially from green leafy vegetables and cruciferous vegetables such as broccoli, cauliflower, and cabbage, will optimize nourishment for healthy gut bacteria, which will support regular elimination. Bulking agents, such as psyllium husk, chia seeds in water, and flax meal, are high in omega-3 fatty acids as well as providing bulking insoluble fiber, which supports bowel function, and are excellent foods to include in a ketogenic diet.

A Last Note on Health

We've all heard the adage that people trade health for money in their youth and then trade money for health in old age. Poor health does not develop overnight; it is an accumulation of years of health-compromising choices. Going keto is a choice to love your body; it is an act of self-love. The only way to communicate with those trillions of hardworking cells that are working on your behalf is to nurture them and provide them with optimal nutrition. Feeling trapped in an unhealthy or overweight body is a recipe for self-hatred. When you are vital, full of energy, and functioning at your best, on the other hand, you can love being in your body and live life to the fullest!

Keto is a long-term lifestyle, not a short-term "diet" for quick results. When you adhere to the 80/15/5 macronutrient ratios and make use of my meal plans (see page 367, or check out the plans on www.ketogenicgirl. com), results will come quickly. In my experience, people who follow the keto diet strictly see the most success; the biggest winners are those who truly commit to this way of life. The new you that you are creating begins *right now*. The new you begins the moment you open yourself up to the possibility of finding a way of life that will work for you. Imagine a life for yourself in which the following are true:

- You have the health and body of your dreams.

- You can enjoy food and see it as your friend, not the enemy.

- You appreciate your body and relish being in it.

- You have the vitality and zest for life that you were meant to have!

You really can have your keto cake and eat it, too!

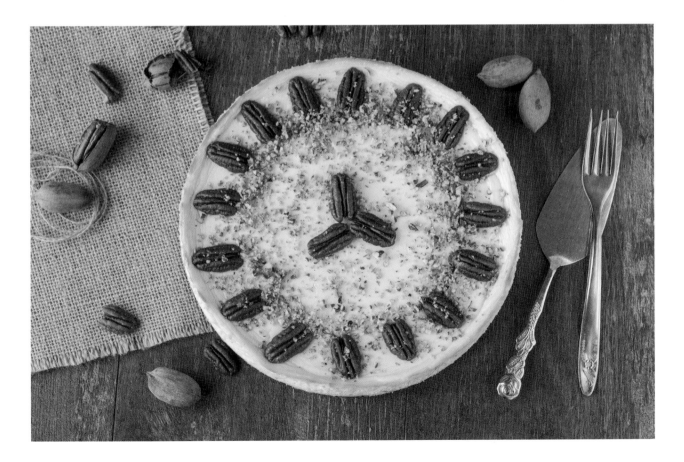

PART TWO

Recipes and Meal Plans

Chapter 6

Introduction to the Recipes

I like to call my approach to keto a sensible whole-foods lifestyle. The emphasis is on real, whole foods that are grown or caught, not packaged or canned, and undergo as little processing possible. A whole food is something that would be recognizable as food to our ancestors from a previous century. Cooking with and being fueled by whole foods is a real joy!

My approach to cooking has many influences. From the time I was young, my mother, Marilyn, instilled in me a love of cooking and entertaining. My cooking influences are French, which tends to be high in fat (except for all the wine!), and Asian, after so many years of living abroad.

My culinary range has been enhanced by the many diverse cultures in which I've had the privilege to live, including countries in Africa, Asia, and Europe. When I was growing up, my parents worked for the Canadian diplomatic service, and we lived in Beijing, China, for two postings as well as a posting in Manila in the Philippines, both of which were great bases from which to explore Southeast Asia. Getting to live in and travel around these countries exposed to me to many diverse culinary traditions.

Over the years, one of my favorite hobbies has been to take delicious meals and re-create them with all the same decadence and flavor, while also being healthy and nourishing instead of being detrimental to health. And now I am fortunate to live my passion every day by creating and sharing recipes full-time!

These recipes generally follow the 80/15/5 macronutrient distribution for the therapeutic approach to keto, while adhering to a few additional rules that I developed while working to help more than 2,000 clients effectively get into a state of nutritional ketosis. I have created flavorful ketogenic versions of many of my favorite dishes and go-to comfort foods, and these dishes can help heal the body, restore homeostasis, and burn fat.

I won't lie; I am definitely a foodie, and I am a fan of the delightful sensory experience that is food. But I also enjoy the natural health-boosting effects that proper nourishment can provide.

How Important Is It to Choose Organic Produce and Grass-Fed/Pastured Meats?

Whenever possible, choose humanely raised grass-fed and pastured meats. If you go for grass-fed and pastured meats, you can opt for fattier cuts. Because toxins are stored in animals' body fat, it's best to choose leaner cuts if you're buying conventionally raised, non-organic meats. You can then add healthy fats, such as coconut oil or mayonnaise (see page 355 for my recipe), to your meals in order to get an adequate amount of quality fat.

It is crucial to avoid meats and other products from animals that have been treated with antibiotics. When we consume those foods, the residual antibiotics ravage the friendly bacteria in our gut microbiome, which play a critical role in keeping us calm and happy by producing serotonin.

Stocking Your Keto Pantry

I try to use only readily accessible ingredients in my recipes. When going keto, however, you will probably want to stock up on some items that you might not have used before. The following is a quick roundup of the ingredients that are handy to have on hand in a ketogenic kitchen.

All the ingredients that you purchase should be free of added sugars. Many foods, such as bacon and sausage, can contain hidden sugars (see page 35 for some of the names those hidden sugars go by). Almost any ingredient that ends in "-ose" is a sugar. You can buy pork belly and slice it into bacon instead of hunting down uncured bacon, which is tougher to find, but recently I have found some brands offering uncured, unsweetened bacon. More and more of these healthier products are becoming available all the time thanks to the growing popularity of this incredible low-sugar diet!

Pantry Essentials

Unsweetened almond milk

Unsweetened cashew milk

Unsweetened coconut milk

Coconut butter

Coconut cream

Unsweetened shredded coconut

Unsweetened almond butter

Unsweetened cocoa powder

Unsweetened baking chocolate

Coconut flour

Nut flours

Shirataki (konjac) noodles

Chia seeds

Flax seeds

Flax meal

Hemp seeds

Pumpkin seeds (pepitas)

Sweeteners

Pure stevia

Erythritol

Monk fruit

Fats

Avocado oil

Coconut oil

Hazelnut oil

MCT oil

Olive oil

Walnut oil

Grass-fed butter

Ghee

Other

High-quality Himalayan or Celtic sea salt

Dried herbs

Nutritional yeast

Extracts and flavorings, such as almond extract, vanilla extract, and blueberry or raspberry flavoring

Some Notes on the Recipes

I hope the recipes in this book will convince you that eating keto can be simple, accessible, and delicious. I've modified all of my (and, I'm sure, your!) favorites so that you can have French onion soup with croutons, or Eggs Benedict, or your favorite Thai soup and still stay keto.

To better understand how I have put together the recipes and what options you have, please review the following quick notes.

Selecting Ingredients

I choose my ingredients carefully, and you should, too. Sugar pops up in unexpected places, so always check ingredient labels.

Use the following guidelines when purchasing these ingredients:

Eggs: The recipes were created using large eggs. I suggest using organic eggs as available and as your budget allows; whenever possible, buy them from a local source that you trust.

Butter: In recipes in which the butter should be specifically salted or unsalted, I indicate which you should use. If I don't specify, either type will work based on your preference. Look for grass-fed butter as available and as your budget allows.

Mayonnaise: Should be sugar-free and unsweetened, with homemade being best. (See page 355 for my Homemade Mayonnaise recipe.)

Cream cheese: Should be full-fat—at least 30% fat.

Sour cream: Should be full-fat—at least 30% fat.

Yogurt: Should be full-fat—at least 30% fat.

Almond milk: Should be unsweetened.

Beef: As your budget allows, use grass-fed and organic beef, preferably locally sourced.

Pork: As your budget allows, look for pasture-raised and organic pork, preferably locally sourced.

Chicken: As your budget allows, look for antibiotic-free, organic, free-range chicken, preferably locally sourced.

Ketchup: Should be unsweetened and sugar-free.

Balsamic vinegar: All balsamic vinegars contain a small amount of sugar from the concentrated grape must, but look for the brand that is lowest in sugar and does not contain caramel coloring.

The Use of Sweeteners

Many of the recipes in this book call for sweeteners, and they show the range of sweetener usage and preferences available. But all sweeteners are optional. Many people enjoy consuming sweetened foods, just as there are many who choose not to use any sweeteners.

The two most keto-friendly sweeteners are pure stevia and erythritol. Pure stevia is made from a plant that can be grown in your garden; it can be purchased in plant form as well as in liquid and powdered form. It is my number-one choice if I'm using a sweetener. Erythritol is a derivative of sugar and contains 4 grams of carbohydrate per teaspoon; although some people believe that it is an indigestible fiber, I count all of its carbs in my calculations.

A phenomenon known as the *cephalic response* can happen with any sweetener, including calorie-free stevia, and I believe it is more prevalent than people think. This response causes the pancreas to react to the taste of sweetener and anticipate blood sugar to rise thinking you are consuming a sugary food; the pancreas releases insulin to clear the bloodstream of sugar and push it into the cells for energy metabolism. This causes blood sugar to dip, as no sweet food has actually been ingested, which results in low blood sugar, potentially leading to cravings.

Over the years of eating whole foods on keto, my sweet tooth has shifted to more of a "savory tooth," and my palate has adjusted and normalized from its previous overstimulation from sugar and artificial sweeteners. For this reason and because I am aware of cephalic response, I have reduced my own use of sweeteners to nearly none. While I still enjoy an occasional sweet-tasting treat, especially at family events and celebrations, I have not included as many sweet recipes in this book as you'll find in some other keto cookbooks. I have found that people see the most success when they eat whole foods, and whole foods tend to be savory. I have, however, included some savory desserts and a few sweet ones. If you need sweets as you transition to keto, then by all means avail yourself of these recipes.

A Note on Net Carbs

If you have heard of *net carbs* and *total carbs*, you probably know that net carbs are the total carbs from your food diary for the day, or for a meal, with the fiber subtracted. For example, if you've eaten 40 grams of carbs but your fiber intake totals 20 grams, your net carbs would be 20 grams. The majority of people on keto use this net carbs approach, aiming to eat 20 or fewer grams of net carbs per day. My approach, however, uses *total* carbs, without subtracting fiber. In my opinion, eating carbohydrates in the form of fiber does not magically negate the effects of those carbs.

It's great to be aware of fiber, though; we want to be sure to choose carbs that are high in fiber, which is beneficial for the gut microbiome. Because consuming fiber is important, I have included fiber content in the nutrition breakdown for each recipe. That said, please remember that getting into nutritional ketosis generally requires counting total carbs; if you subtract the fiber, your total carb consumption is likely going to be too high to get you into ketosis.

Chapter 7
Breakfast

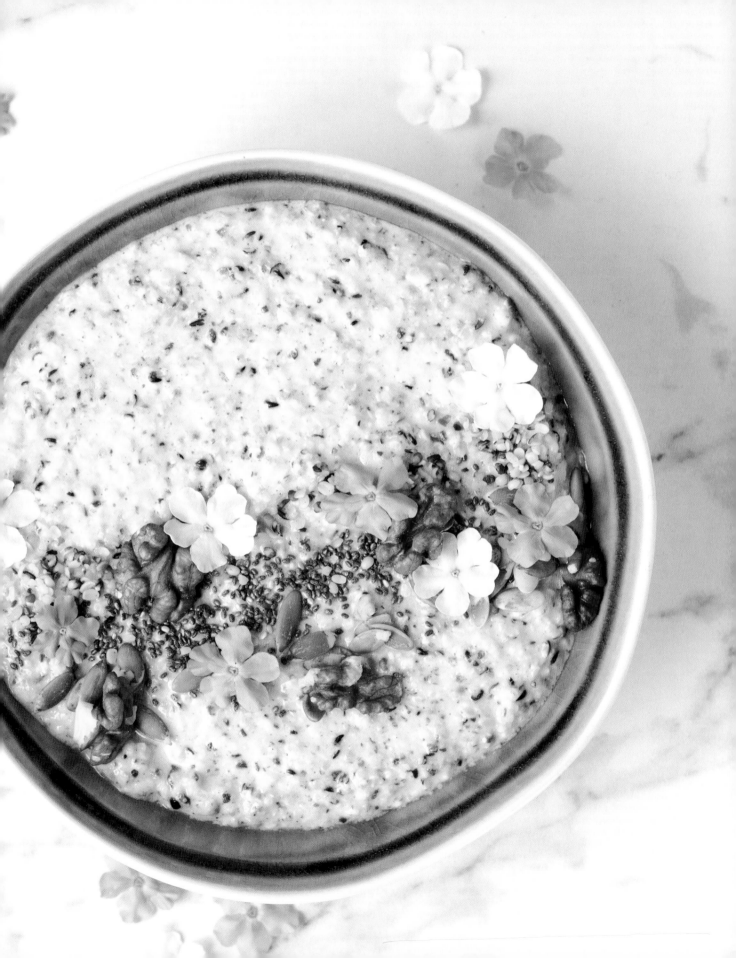

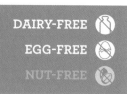

DAIRY-FREE

EGG-FREE

NUT-FREE

Avocado Smoothie

Prep Time: 10 minutes
Yield: 2 servings

Smoothies are a popular breakfast staple because they can be a big timesaver in the morning. I am not typically a proponent of smoothies on keto; I prefer that people eat whole foods. Smoothies are requested so often, however, that I created one for this cookbook!

1½ cups (1¾ ounces/50 g) fresh spinach

½ cup (1 ounce/35 g) stemmed and chopped fresh kale

1 medium-sized ripe avocado, peeled and pitted

1½ teaspoons freshly squeezed lemon juice, or to taste

1 teaspoon peeled and grated fresh ginger, or to taste

½ cup (2½ ounces/70 g) crushed ice or ice cubes

1½ cups (12 fluid ounces/340 g) almond milk

¼ cup (2 ounces/55 g) coconut cream (see note)

2 tablespoons coconut oil or MCT oil

6 or 7 drops liquid stevia, or 1 to 2 teaspoons other keto sweetener of choice

Pinch of sea salt

1 to 2 tablespoons chia seeds (optional)

1. Place all the ingredients except the chia seeds in a blender. Blend to combine.

2. Stir in the chia seeds, if using, and allow to bloom in the smoothie for about 10 minutes before serving.

3. Divide between 2 glasses and serve.

note

For the coconut cream, you can either purchase canned coconut cream or refrigerate a (13½-ounce/400-ml) can of coconut milk overnight so that the cream and water separate; drain the coconut water and scoop out the remaining coconut cream.

MACRONUTRIENTS
(per serving)

Fat	Protein	Carbs	Fiber	Energy
30.5g	3g	11.5g	6.5g	329 cal
82%	4%	14%		

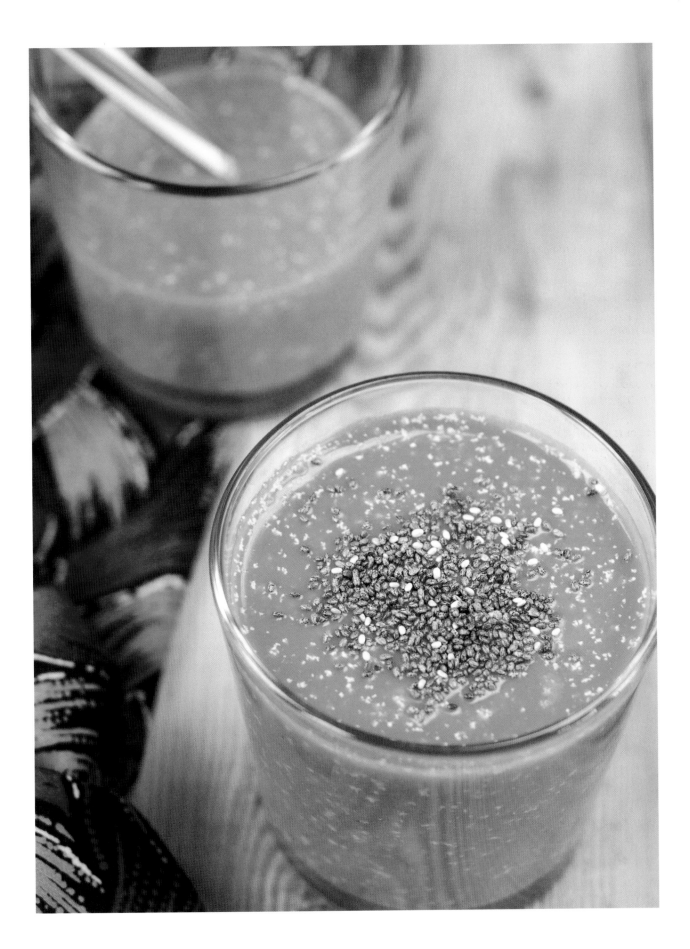

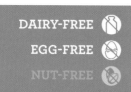

DAIRY-FREE

EGG-FREE

NUT-FREE

Omega-3
Keto Porridge

Prep Time: **5 minutes, plus time to chill overnight** | Cook Time: **4 minutes**
Yield: **1 serving**

This recipe is my keto take on Elizabeth Rider's overnight oats recipe (www.elizabethrider. com/chia-hemp-overnight-oats-recipe/). I love using this chewy overnight breakfast cereal as a tasty oatmeal substitute. Omega-3 fats are important on a regular diet, and they're especially critical on a ketogenic diet to maintain an omega-6 to omega-3 ratio of closer to 2:1 or 1:1. The average ratio is 10:1 or even 20:1, which contributes to chronic inflammation. Omega-3 fatty acid sources such as the chia seeds, walnuts, and pumpkin seeds in this porridge are wonderfully anti-inflammatory.

2 ounces (55 g) hemp hearts

1 tablespoon whole or ground raw pumpkin seeds

½ teaspoon chia seeds

⅛ teaspoon fine sea salt

½ teaspoon ground Ceylon cinnamon or regular cinnamon, divided

¼ cup (2 ounces/55 g) coconut cream (see note, page 108), room temperature

¼ cup (2 fluid ounces/60 ml) almond milk, room temperature, plus more if needed

1 teaspoon powdered stevia

2 to 4 drops liquid stevia, to taste (optional)

1 teaspoon unsweetened shredded coconut

6 walnut halves, chopped if desired

1. Combine the hemp hearts, pumpkin seeds, chia seeds, salt, and ¼ teaspoon of the cinnamon in a bowl.

2. In a separate bowl, whisk together the coconut cream and almond milk. Pour into the seed mixture and stir to combine. Set in the refrigerator to chill overnight.

3. When ready to serve, heat the porridge in a saucepan over low to medium heat for 3 to 4 minutes, until warmed through. Alternatively, heat it in the microwave for 1 minute.

4. Mix in the remaining ¼ teaspoon of cinnamon, powdered stevia, and liquid stevia (if using), adjusting the sweetness to your taste. Add more milk if a thinner consistency is desired.

5. Top with the shredded coconut and walnuts and serve.

tip

Top the porridge with some berries if you are in weight-maintenance mode rather than weight-loss mode.

MACRONUTRIENTS
(per serving)

Fat	Protein	Carbs	Fiber	Energy
54g	23g	12g	12g	594 cal
77%	15%	8%		

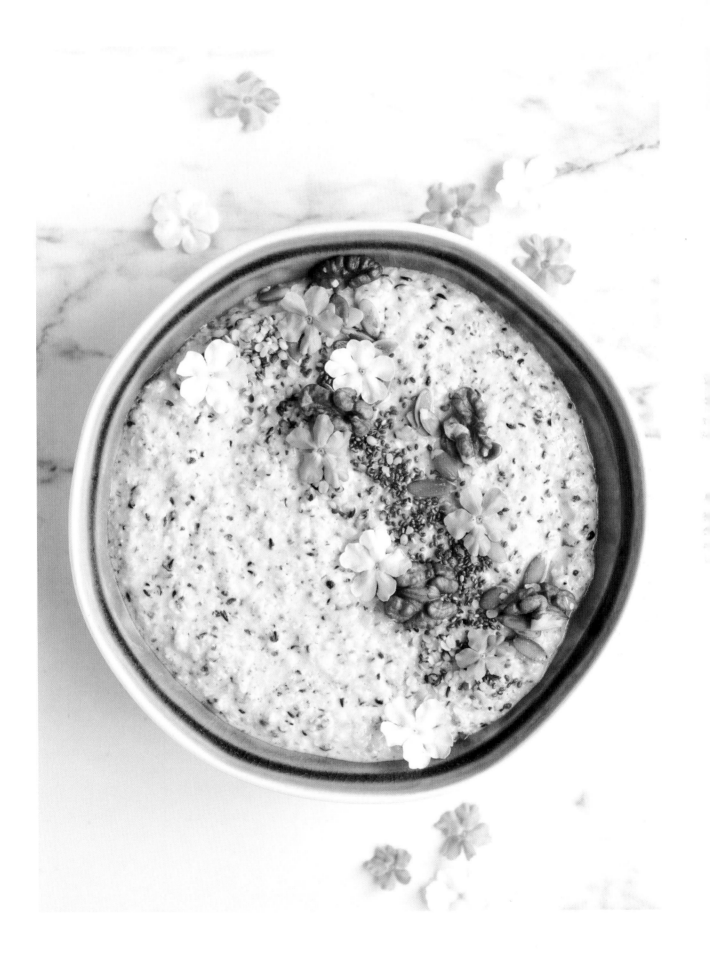

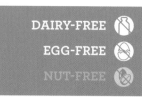

DAIRY-FREE

EGG-FREE

NUT-FREE

Omega-3
Seed and Nut Mix

Prep Time: **10 minutes**
Yield: **10 servings**

Seeds and nuts are a portable, densely nutritious food that in ancient times would be taken on long treks to provide energy. They are also a fantastic source of fiber. This energy mix is a great option to pack with you on hikes or road trips; it can also be used as a topping in other dishes.

¼ cup (2 ounces/55 g) flax seeds

¼ cup (2 ounces/55 g) raw pumpkin seeds

¼ cup (2 ounces/55 g) raw sunflower seeds

¼ cup (2 ounces/55 g) hemp hearts

¼ cup (2 ounces/55 g) raw almonds, half coarsely chopped in a food processor and half left whole

¼ cup (2 ounces/55 g) raw walnuts, finely chopped in a food processor

¼ cup (2 ounces/55 g) unsweetened coconut flakes

¼ cup (2 ounces/55 g) cacao nibs

Combine all the ingredients. Store in an airtight container in the refrigerator for up to 2 weeks.

MACRONUTRIENTS
(per serving)

Fat	Protein	Carbs	Fiber	Energy
20.4g	9.12g	7.5g	3.1g	225 cal
77%	15%	8%		

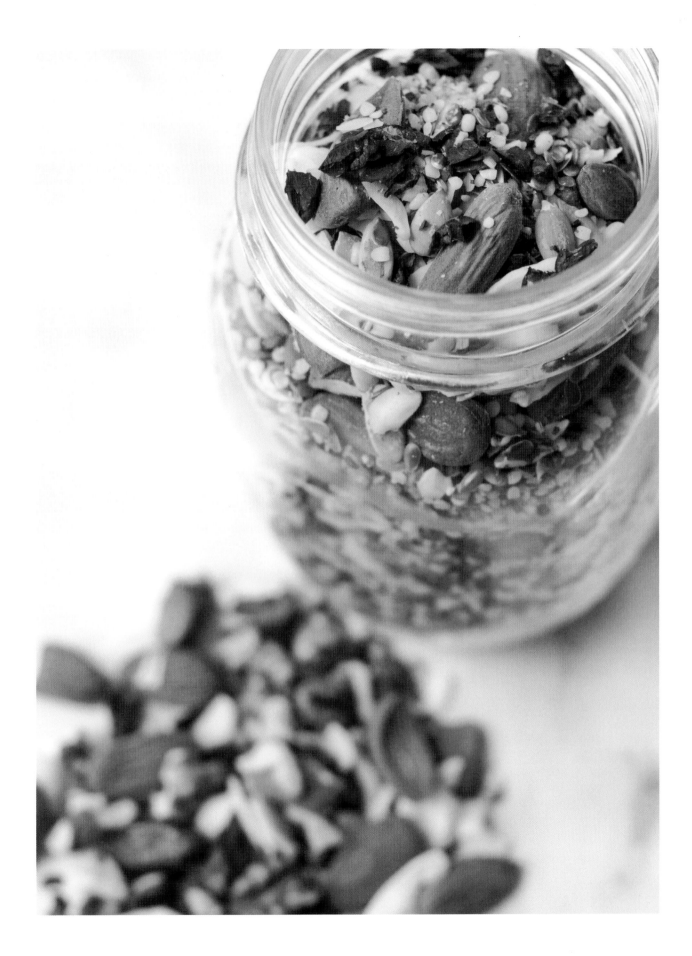

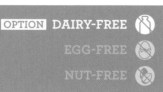

OPTION DAIRY-FREE

EGG-FREE

NUT-FREE

Omega-3 Portable
Seed and Nut Energy Bars

Prep Time: **10 minutes, plus time to cool overnight** | Cook Time: **25 minutes**
Yield: **10 bars**

This is a variation of the Dark Chocolate and Coconut Energy Bars (page 116) but is baked, so it is more portable. Use 10½ to 12½ ounces (300 to 350 grams) of your favorite seeds and nuts. I love the combination called for in this recipe because the flax seeds, walnuts, and pumpkin seeds are full of omega-3 fat, which we need all the more on a keto diet. Also, the hemp hearts are low in carbs, and the fiber is ample.

¾ cup (6 ounces/170 g) butter or coconut oil

3 tablespoons granulated stevia or erythritol

1 teaspoon vanilla extract

½ teaspoon liquid stevia

¼ teaspoon ground Ceylon cinnamon or regular cinnamon

½ cup (3 ounces/85 g) hemp hearts

¼ cup (2 ounces/55 g) raw sunflower seeds

¼ cup (2 ounces/55 g) whole or ground raw pumpkin seeds

¼ cup (2 ounces/55 g) flax seeds

¼ cup (2 ounces/55 g) raw almonds, coarsely chopped in a food processor

¼ cup (2 ounces/55 g) raw walnuts, finely chopped in a food processor

2 tablespoons unsweetened almond butter

¼ teaspoon fine sea salt

2 eggs, whisked

1. Preheat the oven to 350°F (177°C). Grease a 13 by 9-inch (33 by 23-cm) baking pan. Line the bottom of the pan with parchment paper.

2. In a medium saucepan over low heat, melt the butter. Stir in the granulated stevia, vanilla, liquid stevia, and cinnamon.

3. Remove from the heat and stir in the hemp hearts, seeds, nuts, almond butter, and salt. Add the eggs and mix well.

4. Pour the mixture into the prepared pan. Cover with another sheet of parchment paper and use your hands to press the mixture firmly into the pan.

5. Bake for 20 to 25 minutes, until lightly browned. Let cool in the pan overnight.

6. Remove from the pan and cut into 10 bars. Store in an airtight container for up to a week, or freeze for longer storage

tip

I like to grind the almonds and walnuts together so they are broken up a bit, but you can still identify what they are in the bar.

MACRONUTRIENTS
(per bar)

Fat	Protein	Carbs	Fiber	Energy
31.4g	8.9g	6.3g	3.2g	341 cal
78%	15%	7%		

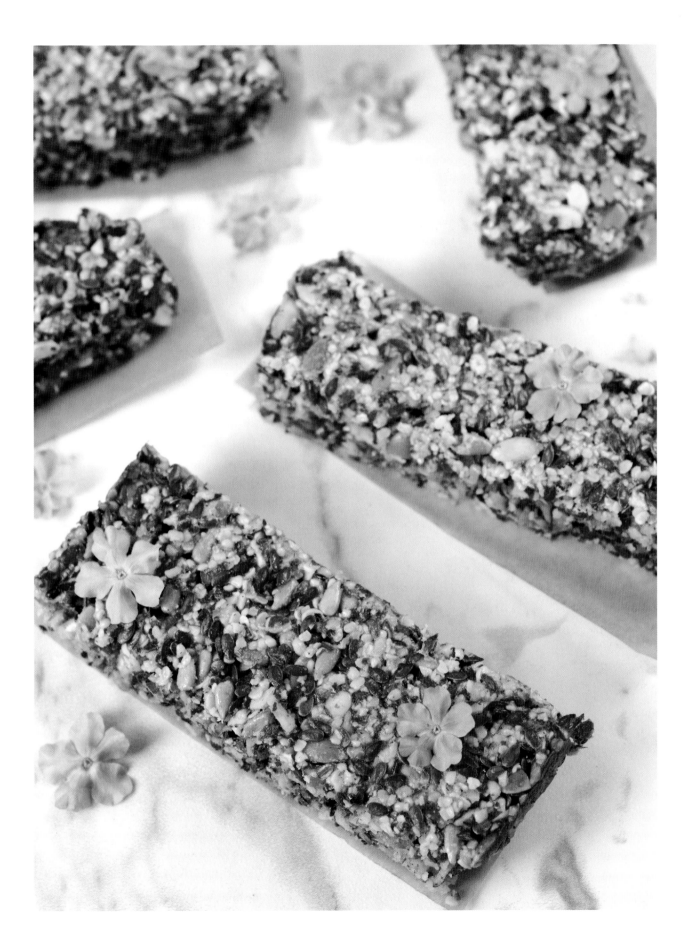

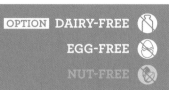

OPTION DAIRY-FREE

EGG-FREE

NUT-FREE

Dark Chocolate and Coconut
Energy Bars

Prep Time: **10 minutes, plus 1 hour to refrigerate** | Cook Time: **4 minutes**
Yield: **10 bars**

This recipe uses a seed and nut base but adds dark chocolate and coconut to make it more of a dessert bar. I love the combination of omega-3–rich flax seeds, walnuts, and pumpkin seeds, low-carb hemp hearts, and abundant fiber. This is probably the healthiest dessert on the planet! These bars need to be kept in the refrigerator or they will melt, but they can be taken on the go in a cooler with ice packs.

¾ cup (6 ounces/170 g) butter or coconut oil

3 tablespoons granulated stevia or erythritol

1 teaspoon vanilla extract

½ teaspoon liquid stevia

¼ teaspoon ground Ceylon cinnamon or regular cinnamon

½ cup (2¾ ounces/80 g) hemp hearts

¼ cup (2 ounces/55 g) flax seeds

¼ cup (2 ounces/55 g) whole or ground raw pumpkin seeds

¼ cup (2 ounces/55 g) raw almonds, coarsely chopped in a food processor

¼ cup (2 ounces/55 g) raw walnuts, finely chopped in a food processor

2 tablespoons unsweetened almond butter

2 tablespoons unsweetened shredded coconut

¼ teaspoon fine sea salt

1¾ ounces (50 g) unsweetened baking chocolate (100% cacao) or dark chocolate (99% cacao), chopped into small pieces

1. Line the bottom of a 13 by 9-inch (33 by 23-cm) pan with parchment paper.

2. In a medium pan over low heat, melt the butter. Stir in the granulated stevia, vanilla, liquid stevia, and cinnamon.

3. Remove from the heat and stir in the hemp hearts, seeds, nuts, almond butter, coconut, and salt.

4. If you prefer large chunks of chocolate in the bar, let the mixture cool in the refrigerator for 10 to 15 minutes or on the counter for about 30 minutes. When it is completely cool, gently fold in the chocolate. If you prefer a chocolate-flavored bar, add the chocolate while the mixture is still hot and stir until completely melted.

5. Pour the mixture into the prepared pan. Cover with another sheet of parchment paper and use your hands to press the mixture firmly into the pan. Place in the refrigerator to chill for 1 to 2 hours.

6. Remove from the pan and cut into 10 bars. Store in an airtight container in the refrigerator for up to 2 weeks.

tip

I like to grind the almonds and walnuts together so they are broken up a bit, but you can still identify what they are in the bar.

note

You can also make these bars without the dark chocolate. Simply omit the chocolate and skip Step 4.

MACRONUTRIENTS
(per bar, with chocolate)

Fat	Protein	Carbs	Fiber	Energy
30.6g	7.9g	7.5g	4.6g	330 cal
82%	9%	9%		

MACRONUTRIENTS
(per bar, without chocolate)

Fat	Protein	Carbs	Fiber	Energy
27.9g	7.2g	6.1g	3.8g	298 cal
80%	11%	9%		

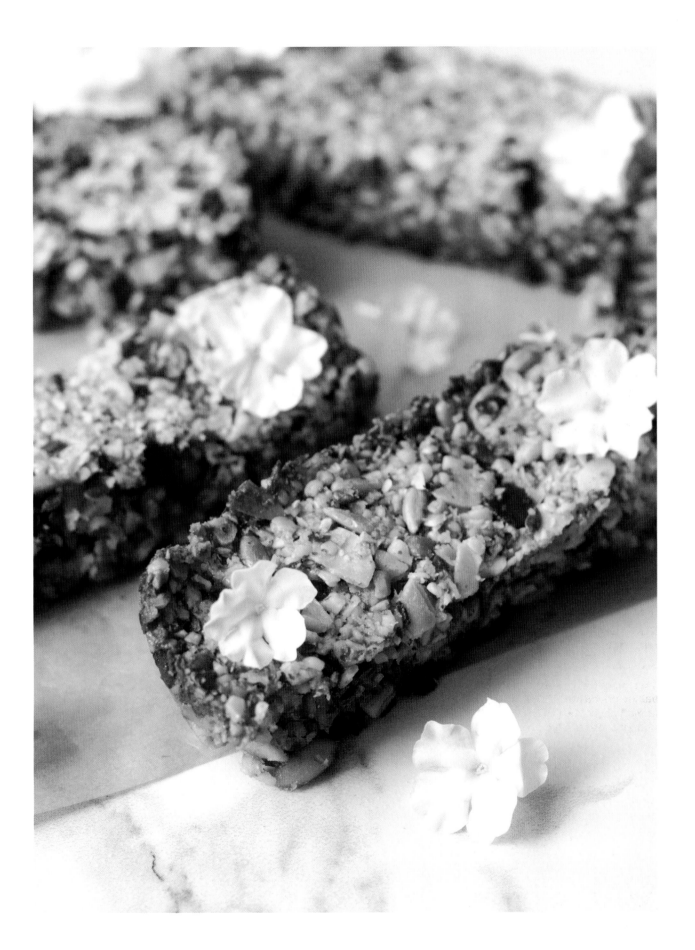

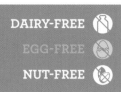

DAIRY-FREE

EGG-FREE

NUT-FREE

Avocado Bacon
Deviled Eggs

Prep Time: **15 minutes** | Cook Time: **10 minutes**
Yield: **12 egg halves (2 servings as a meal or 3 servings as a snack)**

This is one of the best portable snacks to bring with you to a party or other event. Everyone loves deviled eggs, keto or not! I have provided macronutrient information for eating them as a meal or as a fat bomb snack.

6 slices bacon

6 eggs

½ medium-sized ripe avocado

5 tablespoons (2.5 ounces/70 g) mayonnaise

½ teaspoon fine sea salt

Ground black pepper

Paprika, for garnish (optional)

1. In a skillet over medium heat, fry the bacon until slightly crispy, 3 to 5 minutes. Set aside.

2. In a small pan of water over high heat, boil the eggs for 6 minutes. Remove from the heat and immerse in cold water until cool. Drain and peel.

3. Cut each egg in half lengthwise. Place the yolks in a bowl.

4. Add the avocado to the bowl with the egg yolks. Add the mayonnaise, salt, and pepper to taste. Mash together with a fork or an immersion blender until smooth and creamy.

5. Finely chop the bacon. Add about half to the bowl of filling and mix together.

6. Fill a piping bag with the egg yolk mixture. Pipe the filling evenly into the egg white halves. Garnish with the remaining chopped bacon and paprika, if desired. Serve at room temperature or chilled.

tip

Don't have a piping bag? Fill a resealable plastic bag with the filling. Move the filling to one lower corner of the bag and snip off that corner, about ¼ inch (6 mm) from the end. Use the plastic bag as you would a piping bag to squeeze the filling into each egg white half.

MACRONUTRIENTS (6 egg halves per serving)				
Fat	Protein	Carbs	Fiber	Energy
53g	28g	4g	2g	610 cal
79%	18%	3%		

MACRONUTRIENTS (4 egg halves per serving)				
Fat	Protein	Carbs	Fiber	Energy
34g	19g	2.6g	1.6g	399 cal
78%	18%	3%		

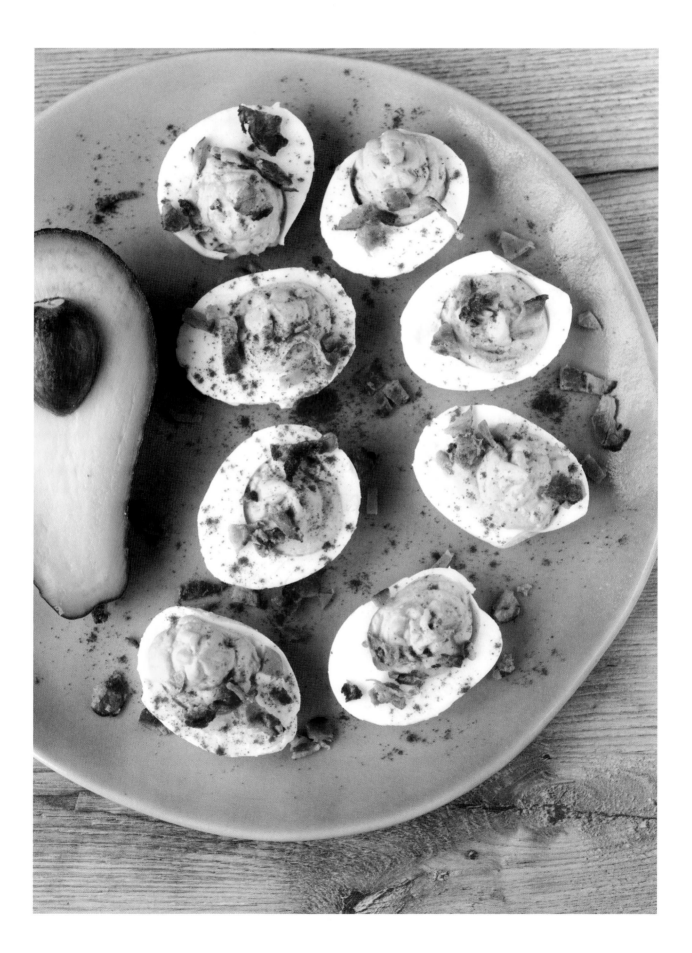

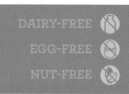

DAIRY-FREE

EGG-FREE

NUT-FREE

Baked Eggs Benedict
Casserole

Prep Time: **10 minutes** | Cook Time: **45 minutes**
Yield: **6 servings**

This delicious egg bake tastes just like eggs Benny but is easier to prepare, especially when serving guests. You may make it 24 hours ahead of time and then reheat it in the oven, covered with aluminum foil or a lid, for 15 to 20 minutes before serving. This casserole is traditionally made with English muffins; feel free to enhance this version with keto bread slices or zero-carb English muffins.

12 ounces (340 g) bacon, chopped

6 eggs

2 cups (16 fluid ounces/475 ml) almond milk

1 tablespoon finely chopped fresh chives or dill

1 tablespoon chopped fresh parsley

½ teaspoon onion powder

½ teaspoon fine sea salt

¼ teaspoon ground black pepper

¼ teaspoon paprika

1 batch Hollandaise, for serving (page 354)

Hot sauce, for serving (optional)

1. Preheat the oven to 375°F (190°C).

2. Layer the bacon in the bottom of a 9-inch (23-cm) square baking dish.

3. In a bowl, whisk together the eggs, milk, chives, parsley, onion powder, salt, pepper, and paprika.

4. Pour the egg mixture over the bacon. Cover with an ovenproof lid or aluminum foil.

5. Bake, covered, for 25 to 30 minutes. Remove the lid and bake for another 10 to 15 minutes, until a toothpick or knife inserted in the center comes out clean.

6. Remove the casserole from the oven and let cool slightly before cutting. Serve each portion drizzled with 3⅓ tablespoons of the hollandaise and a little hot sauce, if desired.

MACRONUTRIENTS
(per serving)

Fat	Protein	Carbs	Fiber	Energy
55.7g	31g	2g	0.3g	645 cal
79%	19%	2%		

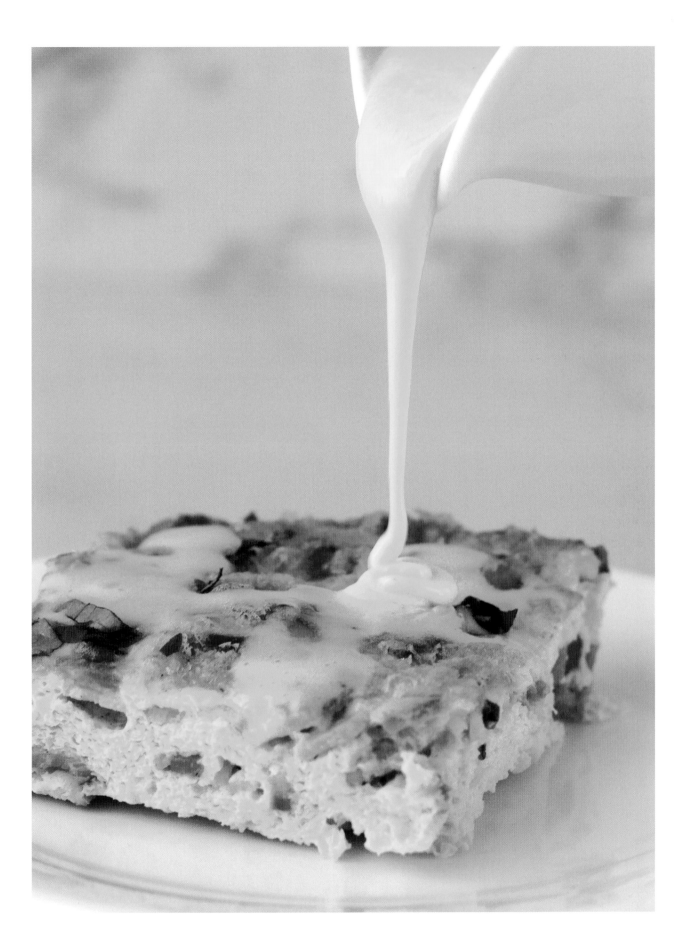

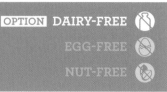

OPTION DAIRY-FREE

EGG-FREE

NUT-FREE

Breakfast Crêpes

Prep Time: **5 minutes** | Cook Time: **15 minutes**
Yield: **6 crêpes (2 per serving)**

I grew up on my mother's delicious English crêpes. They always seemed like such an indulgence with the flour, butter, and sugar! This version is so healthy, nutritious, and ketogenic that you could enjoy them every day. See the recipe for Savory Brie, Mushroom, and Spinach Crêpes with Sugar-Free Glaze on page 364 for a tasty savory option.

5 eggs

⅔ cup (5⅓ fluid ounces/160 ml) almond milk

2 tablespoons coconut flour

3 or 4 drops liquid stevia

¼ teaspoon almond extract

¼ teaspoon vanilla extract

3 tablespoons coconut oil or unsalted butter, for the pan

FOR SERVING (OPTIONAL):

Butter

Ground Ceylon cinnamon or regular cinnamon

Freshly squeezed lemon juice

Powdered stevia

1. Using an electric mixer, beat together the eggs, milk, coconut flour, stevia, and extracts until well incorporated.

2. In a small skillet over high heat, melt the coconut oil.

3. Pour ¼ cup of the batter into the pan to make a crêpe, rotating the pan to spread the batter into a thin layer. When cooked on one side (about 1 minute), flip and cook on the other side. Remove from the pan and keep warm. Repeat with the remaining batter, making a total of 6 crêpes.

4. If desired, serve the crêpes with butter and cinnamon or with lemon juice and stevia.

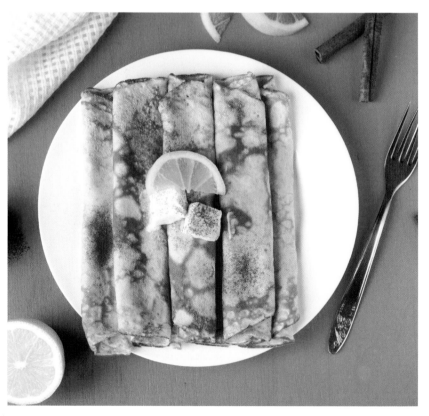

MACRONUTRIENTS
(per serving)

Fat	Protein	Carbs	Fiber	Energy
23.3g	11.3g	3.7g	2g	277 cal
78%	17%	5%		

Egg, Bacon, Sun-Dried Tomato, and Feta
Breakfast Muffins

Prep Time: **5 minutes** | Cook Time: **25 minutes**
Yield: **12 muffins (2 per serving)**

These muffins are the best grab-and-go breakfast for busy weekday mornings. Make them on Sunday and you'll have breakfast for the whole week! They are perfect for picnics or hikes, and they can even be frozen. Add some chopped fresh spinach or kale to increase the carb content.

Coconut oil, for the pan

20 slices thick-cut bacon, diced

10 eggs

1 cup (4 ounces/115 g) crumbled feta cheese

1 ounce (28 g) sun-dried tomatoes in oil, drained and sliced

¼ cup plus 2 tablespoons (3 ounces/85 g) coconut cream (see note, page 108) or heavy whipping cream

¼ teaspoon onion powder

¼ teaspoon garlic powder

¼ teaspoon fine sea salt

¼ teaspoon ground black pepper

1. Preheat the oven to 350°F (177°C). Grease a 12-cup muffin pan with coconut oil.

2. In a skillet over medium heat, fry the bacon for 5 to 7 minutes, until slightly crispy; do not overcook. Transfer to a bowl to cool, reserving the bacon fat in the pan.

3. In a medium bowl, whisk the eggs. Add the rest of the ingredients, including the bacon, to the bowl and stir gently to combine.

4. Divide the egg mixture among the greased muffin cups, using ¼ to ⅓ cup per muffin.

5. Bake until set, about 20 minutes.

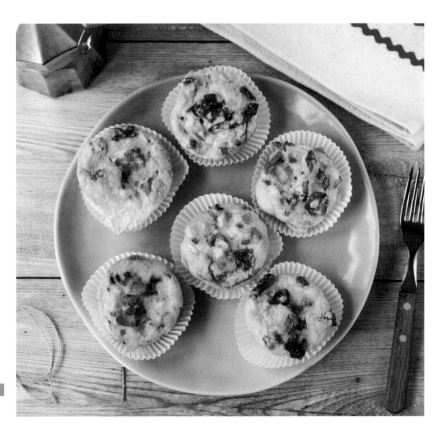

MACRONUTRIENTS
(per serving)

Fat	Protein	Carbs	Fiber	Energy
34.5g	25g	3.5g	1.5g	432 cal
73%	24%	3%		

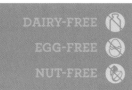

DAIRY-FREE

EGG-FREE

NUT-FREE

Savory Brie, Mushroom, and Spinach Crêpes with Sugar-Free Glaze

Prep Time: **10 minutes** | Cook Time: **30 minutes**
Yield: **2 servings (3 crêpes per serving)**

I love cheese and mushrooms together—especially in a savory crêpe! This recipe reminds me of a cheese and mushroom quesadilla as well. I use regular white or brown mushrooms, but you can use varieties like chanterelles or morels if you prefer. Eat these crêpes for break-fast or dinner!

CRÊPES:

5 eggs

⅔ cup (5½ fluid ounces/160 ml) almond milk

2 tablespoons coconut flour

1 or 2 drops liquid stevia (optional)

3 tablespoons coconut oil or unsalted butter, for the pan

FILLING:

1 tablespoon coconut oil

1 clove garlic, crushed

1 cup (2.6 ounces/75 g) sliced mushrooms

1 cup (1¼ ounces/35 g) fresh spinach, chopped

¼ teaspoon fine sea salt

¼ teaspoon ground black pepper

4 ounces (115 g) triple cream Brie, sliced into 12 sections

2 tablespoons Sugar-Free Glaze (page 364), for drizzling

1. Prepare the crêpes: In a mixing bowl or the bowl of a stand mixer, combine the eggs, milk, coconut flour, and stevia, if using. Beat together with a handheld electric mixer or stand mixer.

2. In a small skillet over high heat, melt 3 tablespoons of coconut oil. When hot, pour 2 tablespoons to ¼ cup of the batter into the pan, rotating the pan to spread the batter into a thin layer. When cooked on one side (about 1 minute), flip and cook on the other side. Remove from the pan and keep warm. Repeat with the remaining batter, making a total of 6 crêpes.

3. Make the filling: In a medium skillet over medium heat, melt 1 tablespoon of coconut oil. Add the garlic and cook for 1 to 2 minutes, until fragrant. Add the mushrooms and cook for 4 to 5 minutes, until nicely browned; be careful not to overcrowd the mushrooms as you cook them. Once browned, add the spinach and cook for 2 to 3 minutes, until cooked. Season with the salt and pepper.

4. Return the pan in which you cooked the crêpes to the stovetop over medium-low heat. Lay a crêpe flat in the pan. Add about one-sixth of the mushroom and spinach filling and layer with 2 slices of Brie. Fold the crêpe in half or into a triangle by folding in both sides. Flip over and cook until the cheese is melted. Repeat with the remaining crêpes and filling.

5. Plate the crêpes and drizzle 1 tablespoon of the glaze over each serving.

MACRONUTRIENTS
(per serving)

Fat	Protein	Carbs	Fiber	Energy
65.5g	28g	11g	3g	729 cal
79%	15%	6%		

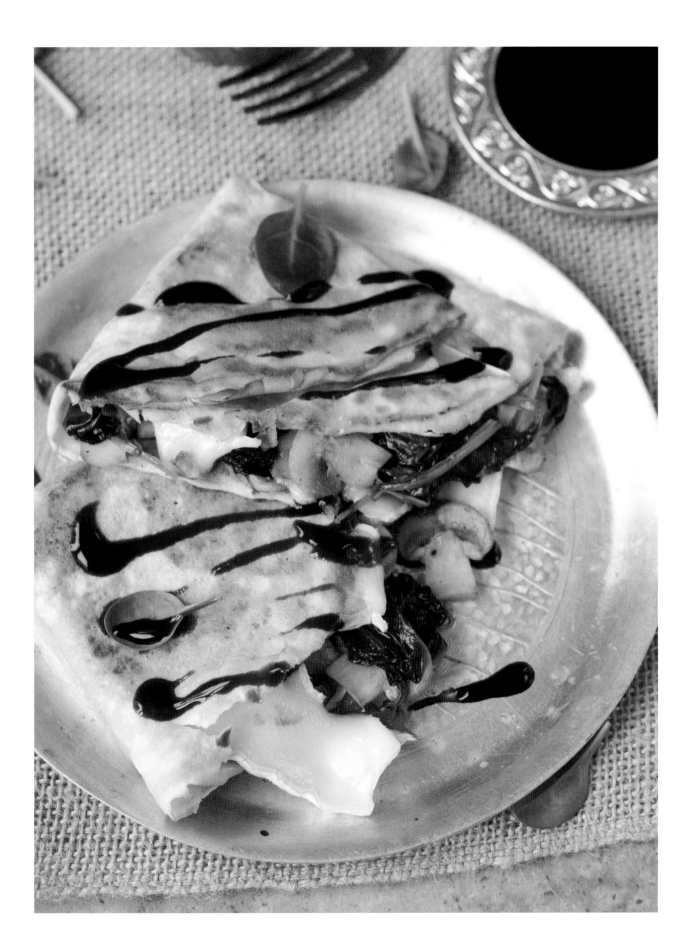

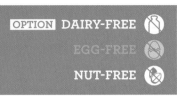

OPTION **DAIRY-FREE**

EGG-FREE

NUT-FREE

Eggs
with Sausage Stuffing

Prep Time: 5 minutes | **Cook Time: 10 minutes**
Yield: 1 serving

Stuffing is not just for the holidays! This is one of my favorite ways to start the day. You'll love this unexpected breakfast of savory stuffing and eggs.

2 eggs

2 tablespoons coconut oil or butter

1 serving Cauliflower Sausage Herb Stuffing (page 232), warm

Chopped fresh parsley, for garnish (optional)

1. Fry or scramble the eggs in the coconut oil over medium heat.

2. Serve the eggs on top of the reheated stuffing, garnished with parsley, if desired.

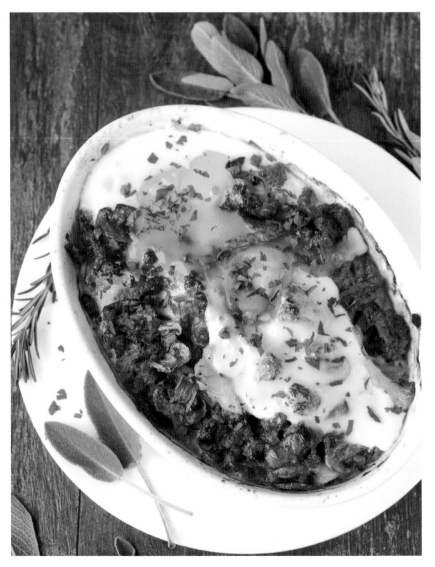

MACRONUTRIENTS
(per serving)

Fat	Protein	Carbs	Fiber	Energy
61g	25g	9g	3g	684 cal
80%	15%	5%		

Eggs, Bacon, and Roasted Rosemary Radishes

Prep Time: **10 minutes** | Cook Time: **20 minutes**
Yield: **2 servings**

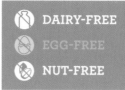

- DAIRY-FREE
- EGG-FREE
- NUT-FREE

I used to love rosemary potatoes for breakfast. It's so great to be able to enjoy similar textures and flavors using radishes in this dish. As with potatoes, duck fat adds a wonderful rich flavor to the radishes! If you don't have duck fat, try bacon fat or lard instead.

3 ounces (85 g) duck fat, melted

1 tablespoon chopped fresh rosemary, or 1 teaspoon dried rosemary

2 cups (7½ ounces/210 g) halved or quartered radishes, depending on size

½ teaspoon fine sea salt

¼ teaspoon ground black pepper

¼ teaspoon garlic powder

4 slices bacon

4 eggs

1. Preheat the oven to 450°F (232°C). Line a rimmed baking sheet with aluminum foil.

2. In a bowl, combine the melted duck fat and rosemary. Add the radishes and toss to coat. Add the salt, pepper, and garlic powder and mix together.

3. Distribute the radishes across the prepared pan. Bake for 20 minutes, until fork-tender.

4. Meanwhile, in a skillet over medium heat, fry the bacon for 5 to 7 minutes, until slightly crispy; do not overcook.

5. Poach or fry the eggs, according to your preference.

6. Divide the radishes between 2 plates. Add 2 slices of bacon and 2 eggs to each plate and serve.

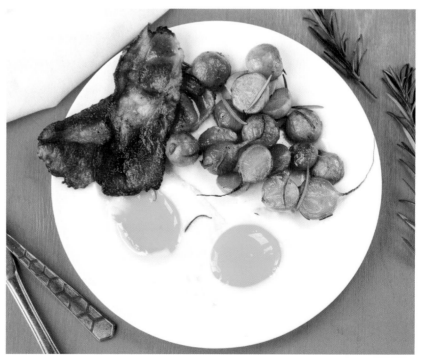

MACRONUTRIENTS
(per serving)

Fat	Protein	Carbs	Fiber	Energy
59g	18.5g	5.5g	2g	618 cal
85%	12%	3%		

DAIRY-FREE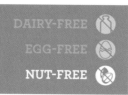

EGG-FREE

NUT-FREE

Eggs Benedict

Prep Time: **2 minutes** | Cook Time: **15 minutes**
Yield: **2 servings**

This is the classic brunch favorite: eggs Benedict with keto-friendly English muffins and Canadian bacon. If you like, serve with some mushrooms fried in butter.

4 eggs

4 Keto Chive and Onion "English Muffins" (page 158)

4 ounces (115 g) Canadian bacon or sliced ham

¼ cup plus 3 tablespoons Hollandaise (page 354)

Paprika, for garnish (optional)

Chopped fresh parsley, for garnish (optional)

1. Poach the eggs: Bring some water to a boil in a small saucepan. Meanwhile, crack an egg into a small bowl. When the water is boiling, remove the saucepan from the heat and use a spoon to swirl the water clockwise around the pan. Slide the egg into the "whirlpool" you created in the pan. Poach for 3 to 4 minutes, until the white is set. Spoon out the egg and keep warm in a warm water bath while you repeat with the remaining eggs.

2. Place 2 muffins on each of 2 plates; place 1 ounce of Canadian bacon and 1 poached egg on each muffin. Pour about 3½ tablespoons of hollandaise over each serving of eggs. If desired, garnish with paprika and/or chopped parsley.

tip

Have the muffins and hollandaise made before you poach the eggs.

MACRONUTRIENTS
(per serving)

Fat	Protein	Carbs	Fiber	Energy
55.5g	38g	4g	0g	670 cal
75%	23%	2%		

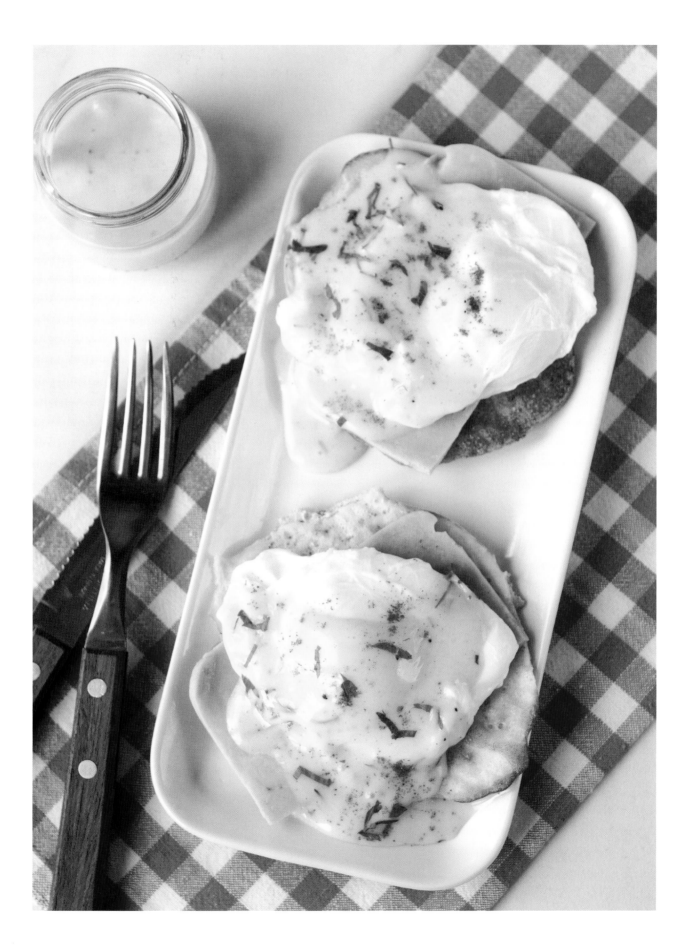

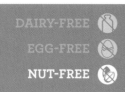

DAIRY-FREE

EGG-FREE

NUT-FREE

Eggs Benedict Royale

Prep Time: **2 minutes** | Cook Time: **15 minutes**
Yield: **2 servings**

This is probably my favorite breakfast of all time. At only 1 percent carbohydrate, this recipe is fantastically low-carb and just as delicious as the original, but much more nutritious. Enjoy this once-decadent breakfast as a healthy and nourishing regular meal. If you like, serve it with some cherry tomatoes and arugula on the side.

4 eggs

4 Keto Chive and Onion "English Muffins" (page 158)

4 ounces (115 g) sugar-free smoked salmon

½ batch Hollandaise (page 354)

Paprika, for garnish (optional)

Chopped fresh parsley, for garnish (optional)

1. Poach the eggs: Bring some water to a boil in a small saucepan. Meanwhile, crack an egg into a small bowl. When the water is boiling, remove the saucepan from the heat and use a spoon to swirl the water clockwise around the pan. Slide the egg into the "whirlpool" you created in the pan. Poach for 3 to 4 minutes, until the white is set. Spoon out the egg and keep warm in a warm water bath while you repeat with the remaining eggs.

2. Place 2 English muffins on each of 2 plates; place 1 ounce of smoked salmon and 1 poached egg on each muffin. Pour about 3⅓ tablespoons of hollandaise over each serving of eggs. If desired, garnish with paprika and/or chopped parsley.

tip

Have the muffins and hollandaise made before you poach the eggs.

MACRONUTRIENTS
(per serving)

Fat	Protein	Carbs	Fiber	Energy
56.5g	37.5g	2g	0g	676 cal
76%	23%	1%		

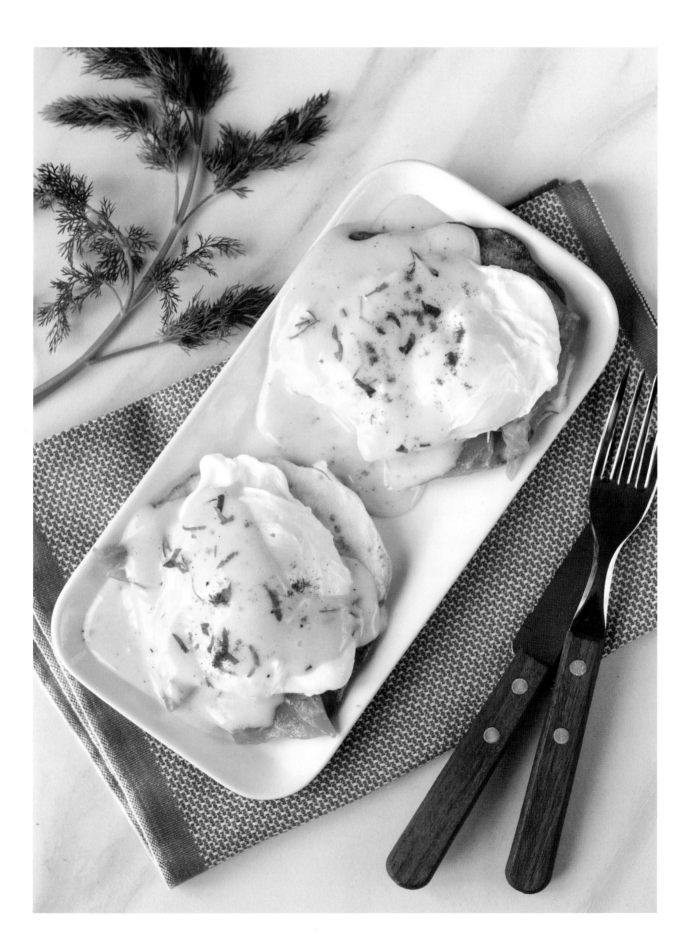

Chapter 8
Appetizers, Snacks & Breads

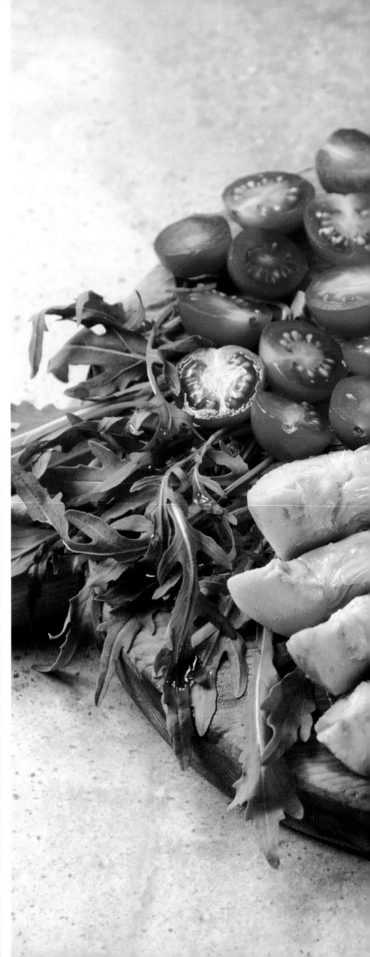

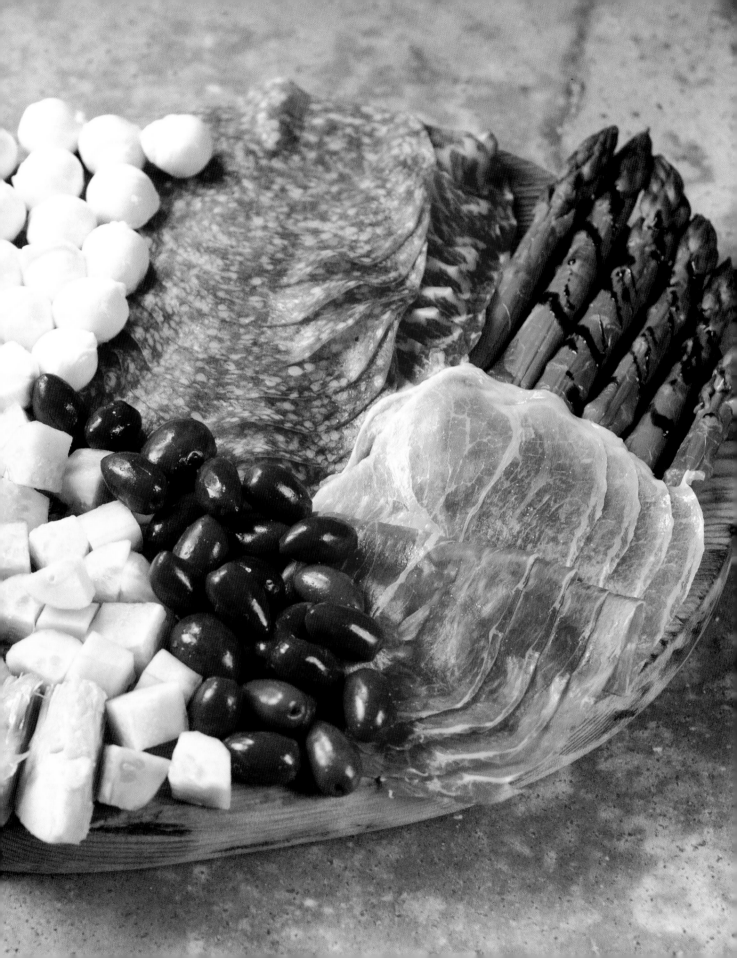

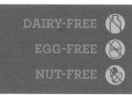

DAIRY-FREE

EGG-FREE

NUT-FREE

Deep-Fried Goat Cheese Balls
with Sugar-Free Glaze

Prep Time: 15 minutes | Cook Time: **10 minutes**
Yield: **9 balls (3 per serving)**

I am a goat cheese fanatic. I never would have dreamed of a recipe like this being healthy, yet when it's made with coconut oil and nut flours, it is! This is a very ketogenic recipe as well, with only 6 grams of carbohydrates (or 2 grams of net carbs) per serving.

7 ounces (200 g) medium-firm plain goat cheese

½ cup (2 ounces/55 g) almond flour

2 tablespoons coconut flour

½ teaspoon fine sea salt

¼ teaspoon ground black pepper

2 eggs

2 tablespoons club soda

Refined coconut oil, lard, or duck fat, for frying

1 batch Sugar-Free Glaze (page 364)

1. Cut the goat cheese into 9 slices. Roll each slice between your palms to shape into a ball.

2. In a mixing bowl or food processor, mix together the almond flour, coconut flour, salt, and pepper. Spread this mixture in a shallow bowl.

3. In a separate bowl, whisk together the eggs and club soda.

4. Dip the cheese balls one at a time into the egg mixture, then roll in the flour mixture until well covered. Set on a plate covered with wax paper or aluminum foil. Refrigerate for 15 to 20 minutes.

5. In a medium skillet that is at least 2 inches (5 cm) deep, over medium-high heat, heat enough coconut oil to go about 1 inch (2.5 cm) up the sides of the skillet.

6. When the oil is hot, lower each cheese ball into the oil and move it around gently to fry on all sides. Don't overcrowd the pan or the cheese balls will become soggy. Fry the balls until golden brown, then remove to a paper towel–lined plate to drain.

7. Serve warm with the glaze.

tip

For more even frying, use a deep-fryer rather than a skillet.

note

The nutritional information assumes that each serving of cheese balls retains 2 tablespoons of coconut oil from frying.

MACRONUTRIENTS
(per serving)

Fat	Protein	Carbs	Fiber	Energy
48.6g	29g	16.3g	3.6g	574 cal
71%	19%	10%		

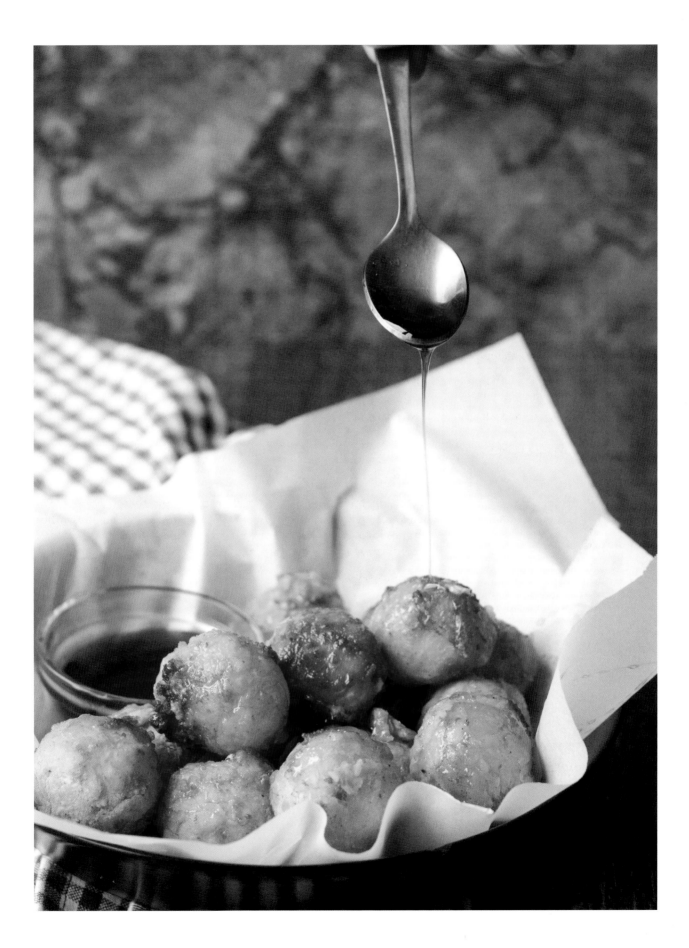

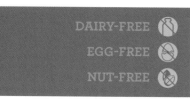

Fried Eggplant
Mozzarella Balls

Prep Time: 15 minutes | **Cook Time:** 40 minutes
Yield: 36 balls (6 per serving)

On a recent trip to Italy, I tasted a dish similar to this one, and it blew my mind! I knew I had to re-create it once I got back home—and I had to include it in this book. I like to deep-fry these savory little mozzarella balls, but you can also make them in an air-fryer.

4 cups (1 pound/455 g) cubed eggplant (about 1½ whole)

2 tablespoons plus 1 teaspoon fine sea salt, divided

2 egg yolks

¼ cup plus 2 tablespoons (1½ ounces/40 g) grated Parmesan cheese

⅓ cup plus ¼ cup (2¼ ounces/ 65 g) almond meal, divided

2 tablespoons chopped fresh parsley, plus more for garnish

½ teaspoon garlic powder

½ teaspoon ground black pepper, divided

36 mini bocconcini mozzarella balls (12.7 ounces/360 g)

2 whole eggs

Lard, duck fat, or refined coconut oil, for frying

1. Place the eggplant in a colander or on a bed of paper towels. Sprinkle on both sides with 2 tablespoons of the salt and let sit for 10 to 15 minutes. Wipe well with paper towels to remove the salt and to dry the eggplant.

2. Preheat the oven to 350°F (177°C). Spray a rimmed baking sheet with cooking spray.

3. Spread the cubed eggplant in a single layer on the prepared baking sheet. Bake for 30 to 35 minutes, until softened.

4. Transfer the cooked eggplant to a food processor and pulse for a few minutes to puree.

5. Scrape the pureed eggplant into a mixing bowl, then add the egg yolks, Parmesan, ¼ cup (1 ounce/28 g) of the almond meal, parsley, garlic powder, ½ teaspoon of the salt, and ¼ teaspoon of the pepper. Mix until well combined.

6. Using a small spoon, make 36 small balls of the eggplant mixture. With moistened hands, place one bocconcino inside each ball, rolling so the cheese is well covered. Set aside on a plate.

7. In a bowl, whisk the whole eggs with a fork. In a shallow dish, combine the remaining ⅓ cup (1¼ ounces/35 g) of almond meal, remaining ½ teaspoon of salt, and remaining ¼ teaspoon of pepper.

8. Dip each ball into the eggs, then roll in the almond meal mixture. Place the coated balls on a plate and refrigerate for 15 to 20 minutes.

9. In a deep-fryer or heavy skillet, heat about ¾ inch (2 cm) of lard to 338°F (170°C). Fry the cheese balls for 2 to 3 minutes, then remove from the oil.

10. Increase the oil temperature to 375°F (190°C) and fry the balls again for 1 to 2 minutes, until golden brown. Remove from the oil and set on paper towels to drain. Garnish with chopped parsley before serving.

MACRONUTRIENTS
(per serving)

Fat	Protein	Carbs	Fiber	Energy
23g	20.2g	5.8g	3g	314 cal
67%	26%	7%		

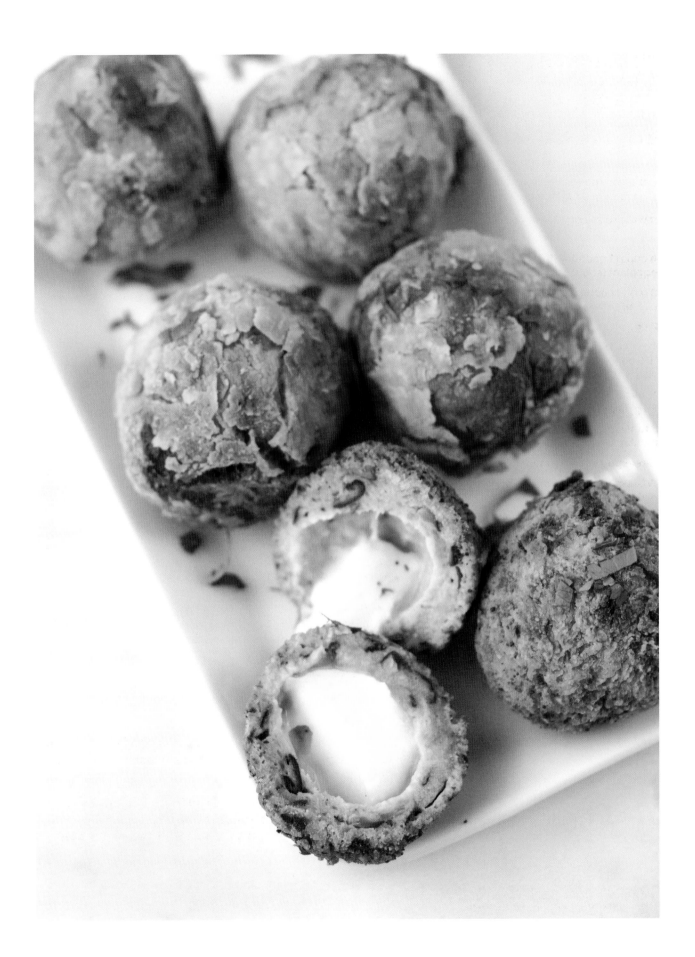

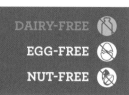

DAIRY-FREE

EGG-FREE

NUT-FREE

Prosciutto Baked Brie

Prep Time: 10 minutes | **Cook Time: 14 minutes**
Yield: 4 servings as an appetizer or 2 servings as a meal

How delicious is baked Brie? It's even more delicious—and keto—when it's wrapped in prosciutto! This amazing starter is great to serve at a party or as a filling keto meal. The glaze recipe makes more than you'll need for the Brie. Enjoy the leftover glaze on meat, fish, vegetables, or even salads.

1 (8-ounce/225-g) wheel Brie

2 ounces (55 g) sliced prosciutto

1 cup (1½ ounces/40 g) arugula

¼ batch Sugar-Free Glaze (page 364)

Chopped fresh parsley, cilantro, or basil, for garnish (optional)

1. Preheat the oven to 375°F (190°C).

2. Line a rimmed baking sheet with parchment paper. Alternatively, you can bake the Brie in an earthenware baking dish.

3. Wrap the Brie in the prosciutto and place on the prepared baking sheet. Bake for 12 to 14 minutes, until bubbly on top and golden brown. Remove from the oven and let cool for 3 to 4 minutes.

4. Plate the Brie on top of the arugula. Drizzle with the glaze and garnish with parsley, if desired.

MACRONUTRIENTS
(per serving)

Fat	Protein	Carbs	Fiber	Energy
41g	12.3g	0.3g	0g	431 cal
88%	12%	0%		

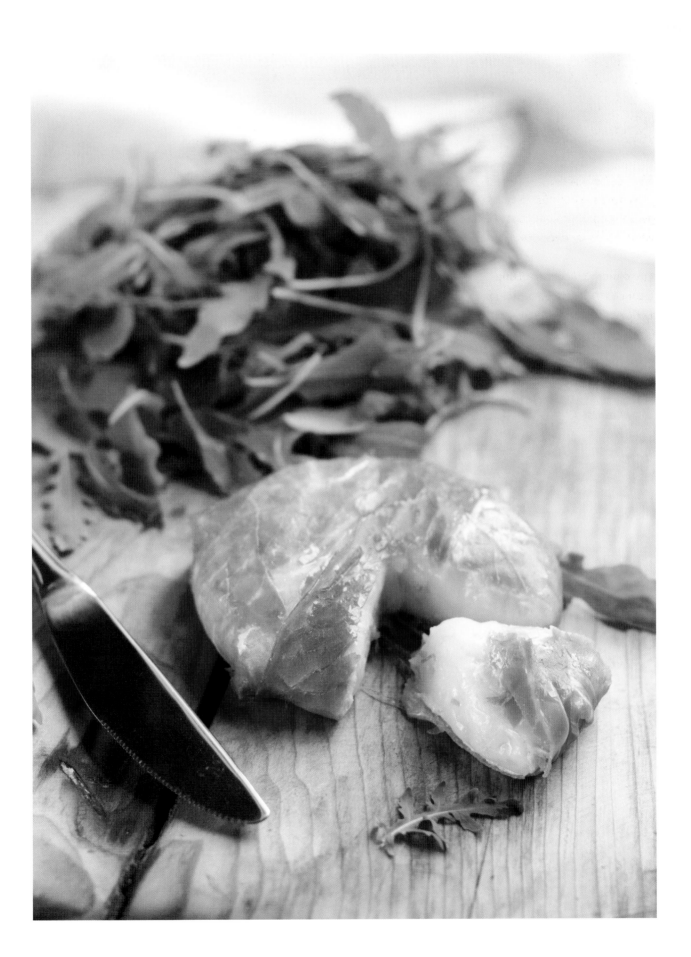

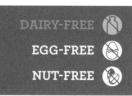

DAIRY-FREE
EGG-FREE
NUT-FREE

Keto Antipasto Plate

Prep Time: **10 minutes** | Cook Time: **10 minutes**
Yield: **4 servings**

This delicious dish was inspired by my recent trip to Puglia, which lies at the heart of Italian gastronomy. Antipasto is a great option for entertaining; it's perfect for a summer evening cookout or a picnic. For the salami and prosciutto, uncured and unsweetened are ideal for keto. Artichoke hearts marinated in oil or brine are great. If you prefer, use sun-dried tomatoes instead of cherry tomatoes. For a change, garnish with shaved Parmesan and pine nuts, or serve with Pesto (page 142).

10 asparagus spears, woody ends trimmed

4 tablespoons (2 fluid ounces/ 60 ml) olive oil, divided

1 cup (1½ ounces/40 g) arugula

½ cup (3 ounces/90 g) artichoke hearts, drained

4 ounces (115 g) mini buffalo mozzarella cheese balls

4 ounces (115 g) sliced prosciutto

4 ounces (115 g) sliced salami

20 mixed Kalamata olives

5 cherry tomatoes, halved

2 cups (7 ounces/200 g) peeled and cubed cucumbers

Fresh basil leaves, whole or torn, for garnish

1. To grill the asparagus, preheat a grill to high heat. Brush the asparagus with 2 tablespoons of the olive oil. Wrap the spears in aluminum foil and grill for 2 to 3 minutes, until cooked through and slightly blackened.

   Alternatively, broil the asparagus. Preheat the oven broiler to medium-high heat. Line a rimmed baking sheet with foil and spread out the asparagus in the pan. Drizzle the asparagus with 2 tablespoons of the olive oil. Broil for 9 to 11 minutes, until cooked but still crisp.

2. Artfully plate the grilled asparagus, arugula, artichoke hearts, cheese, meats, olives, tomatoes, and cucumbers on a large platter. Drizzle with the remaining 2 tablespoons of olive oil and garnish with basil. Serve with small plates and toothpicks or forks.

MACRONUTRIENTS
(per serving)

Fat	Protein	Carbs	Fiber	Energy
34.5g	20.8g	5.8g	1.5g	434 cal
75%	20%	5%		

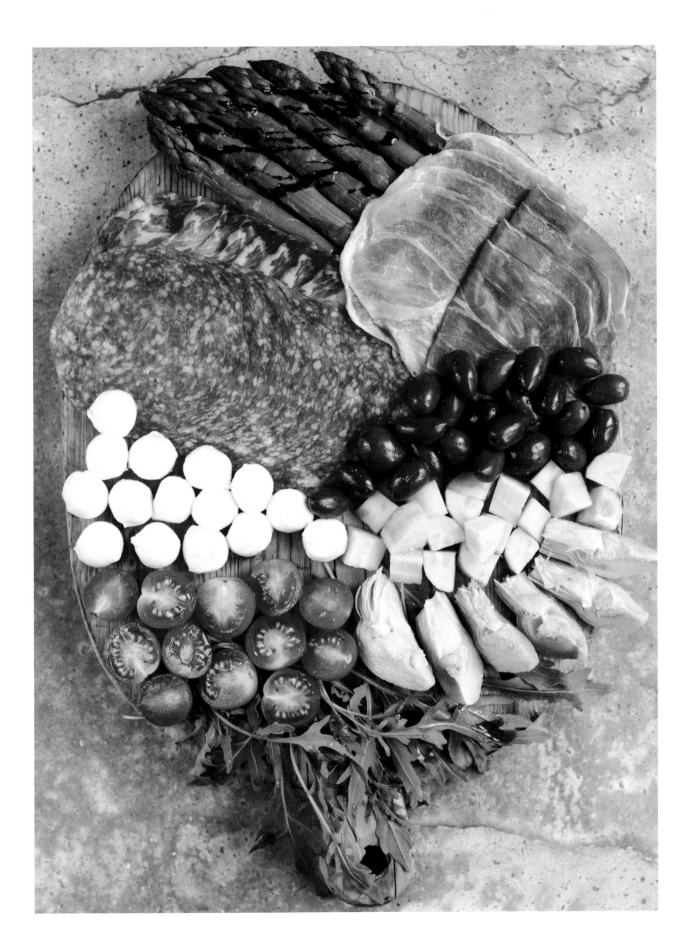

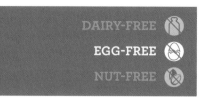

DAIRY-FREE

EGG-FREE

NUT-FREE

Prosciutto Mozzarella Sticks
with Pesto Dipping Sauce

Prep Time: 15 minutes
Yield: 16 sticks (4 per serving)

You will need 16 small to medium-length wooden skewers for this fun and easy summer dish. Try it when entertaining, or enjoy it as a lunch or dinner in the garden.

PESTO:

2 cups (2¾ ounces/80 g) arugula

1 cup (1 ounce/28 g) fresh basil leaves

½ cup (2.4 ounces/70 g) pine nuts

⅓ cup (2½ fluid ounces/80 ml) MCT oil or olive oil

1 clove garlic, or ¼ teaspoon garlic powder

½ teaspoon fine sea salt

Ground black pepper, to taste

16 cherry tomatoes

16 mini bocconcini mozzarella balls

16 fresh basil leaves, plus more for garnish

1½ to 2 cucumbers, peeled and cut into 16 (½-inch/1.25-cm) cubes

3 ounces (85 g) prosciutto, sliced into 16 pieces

16 pitted Kalamata olives

Pine nuts, for garnish (optional)

1. Place all the pesto ingredients in a food processor and process until smooth.

2. Onto a wooden skewer, slide on a cherry tomato, a bocconcino, a basil leaf, a cucumber cube, a piece of prosciutto, and an olive. Repeat to make a total of 16 skewers and arrange the skewers on a plate.

3. Dollop some of the pesto onto the skewers and decorate the plate with additional fresh basil and pine nuts, if desired. Serve with the remaining pesto.

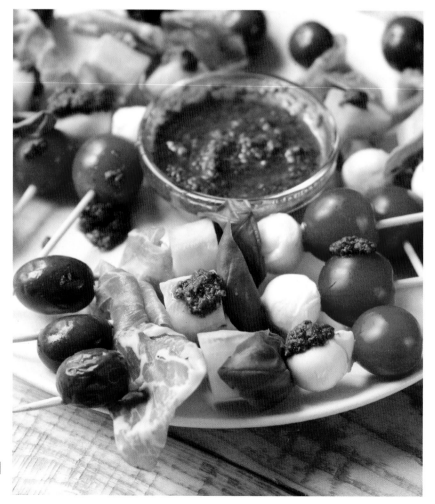

MACRONUTRIENTS (per serving)				
Fat	Protein	Carbs	Fiber	Energy
43g 80%	17.5g 14%	7.5g 6%	2g	484 cal

Guacamole
with Cabbage "Chips"

Prep Time: 15 minutes
Yield: 2 servings

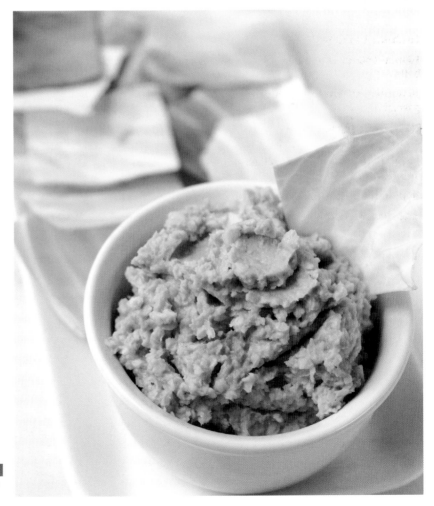

Guacamole is a tasty and healthy keto snack. I love it with cabbage chips or pork rinds, and of course as a side with Mexican food! Avocados contain a lot of carbs, but because they are so rich in fiber, they are one of the only foods from which I subtract the fiber. Virtually all the carbs in avocados are in the form of fiber.

2 medium-sized ripe avocados, halved and pitted

1 tablespoon MCT oil

1 tablespoon freshly squeezed lime juice

½ teaspoon fine sea salt

¼ teaspoon garlic powder

¼ teaspoon hot sauce, or a pinch of cayenne pepper or chili powder

¼ small head green cabbage, cut into "chips," for serving

1. Scoop the avocado flesh into a bowl, then add the MCT oil.

2. In another bowl, combine the lime juice, salt, garlic powder, and hot sauce. Add to the avocado mixture and use an immersion blender to mix thoroughly. Taste and add more salt, if needed.

3. Serve with the cabbage chips.

MACRONUTRIENTS (per serving)				
Fat	Protein	Carbs	Fiber	Energy
25g	1.5g	17.5g	10g	288 cal
83%	2%	15%		

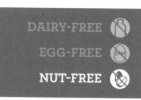

DAIRY-FREE

EGG-FREE

NUT-FREE

Spinach, Kale, and Artichoke Dip

Prep Time: **15 minutes** | Cook Time: **25 minutes**
Yield: **5 servings**

This hot dip is fantastic for entertaining or bringing to a party, and it's always a hit. At 82 percent fat, 12 percent protein, and 6 percent carbohydrate, it is nice and keto, and one of the few full-fat dairy recipes that I include in this book. Serve it with pork rinds or cucumber slices.

½ (10-ounce/285-g) box frozen chopped spinach, thawed

½ (10-ounce/285-g) box frozen chopped kale, thawed

12 large artichoke hearts, drained

4 ounces (115 g) cream cheese, softened

1 cup (4 ounces/115 g) shredded mozzarella cheese

1 cup (4 ounces/115 g) grated Parmesan cheese, divided

1 cup (8 ounces/225 g) mayonnaise

2 cloves garlic, minced

½ teaspoon fine sea salt

¼ teaspoon ground black pepper

Cucumber slices or pork rinds, for serving (optional)

1. Preheat the oven to 325°F (163°C).

2. Drain as much water as possible from the frozen spinach and kale, using a colander and/or paper towels to remove the excess moisture.

3. Cut one of the artichoke hearts lengthwise into quarters and set aside. Coarsely chop the remaining artichoke hearts, then place in a food processor.

4. To the food processor with the artichoke hearts, add the cream cheese, mozzarella, three-quarters of the Parmesan, mayonnaise, garlic, salt, pepper, spinach, and kale. Process for several minutes to thoroughly combine the ingredients.

5. Pour the dip into a 1-quart (1-L) ovenproof baking dish. Arrange the reserved artichoke heart quarters on top of the dip, then sprinkle with the remaining one-quarter of the Parmesan.

6. Bake for 20 minutes, then turn the oven to broil and broil for 3 to 5 more minutes to brown the top and make it nice and crispy.

7. Serve with cucumber slices or pork rinds for dipping, if desired.

MACRONUTRIENTS
(per serving)

Fat	Protein	Carbs	Fiber	Energy
52.6g	16.8g	9g	2.6g	560 cal
82%	12%	6%		

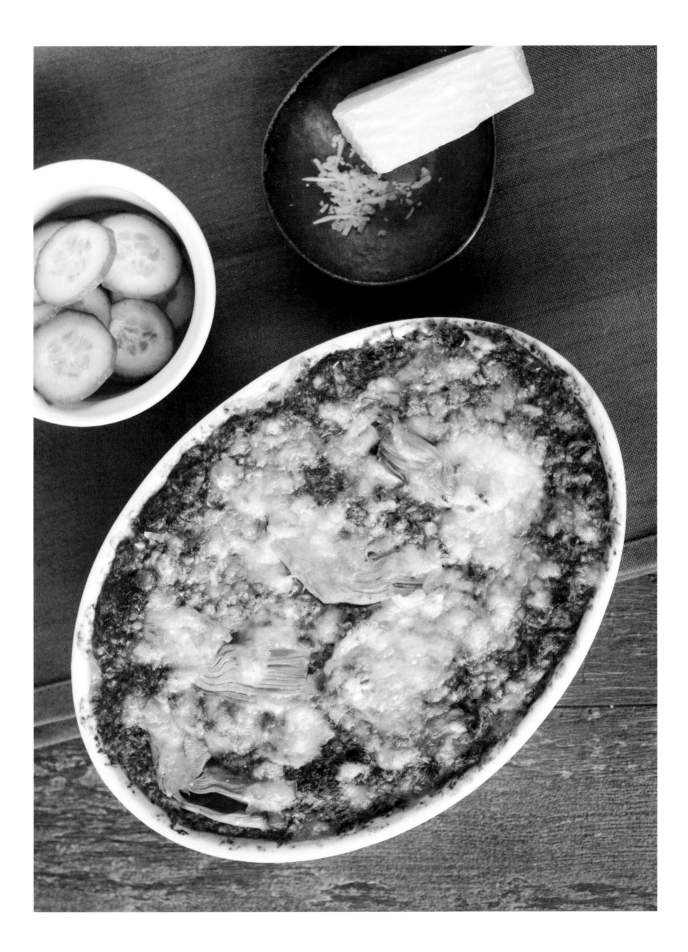

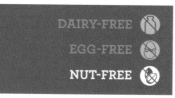

DAIRY-FREE

EGG-FREE

NUT-FREE

Sun-Dried Tomato Dip

Prep Time: 10 minutes
Yield: 3 servings

This dip is so quick and easy to whip up from a handful of ingredients, and it's one the most delicious dips you'll ever eat! Enjoy it as a meal or a party appetizer. I love it with celery, pork rinds, or cucumber slices.

½ cup (2½ ounces/70 g) drained sun-dried tomatoes in oil

1 (8-ounce/225-g) package cream cheese, softened

½ cup (4 ounces/115 g) mayonnaise

½ cup (2 ounces/55 g) crumbled feta cheese

½ teaspoon fine sea salt

1 tablespoon thinly sliced green onions (optional)

Celery sticks or cucumber slices, for serving (optional)

1. Combine the sun-dried tomatoes, cream cheese, mayonnaise, feta, and salt in a food processor; pulse until well combined and creamy. Transfer to a serving bowl and top with the green onions, if using.

2. Serve with celery sticks or cucumber slices, if desired. The dip will keep in the refrigerator for up to a week.

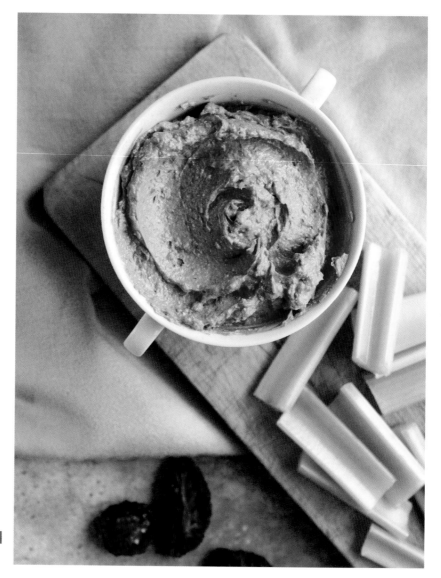

MACRONUTRIENTS
(per serving, dip only)

Fat	Protein	Carbs	Fiber	Energy
56.6g	9.3g	4.3g	.6g	585 cal
90%	7%	3%		

Ketogenic Girl
Hummus

Prep Time: 10 minutes | **Cook Time: 15 minutes**
Yield: 3 servings

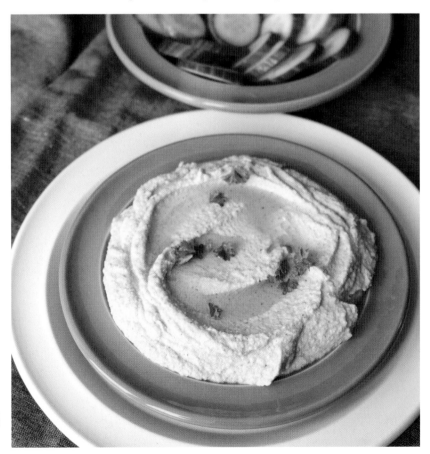

DAIRY-FREE

EGG-FREE

NUT-FREE

The recipe makes three servings, but it is very low in calories and moderate in carbs, so it could be divided into two servings instead of three. Pork rinds or cucumber crackers make a delicious pairing. If you prefer a sweeter, less-intense garlic flavor, roast a couple of garlic cloves whole in their skins in a covered baking dish in a 400°F (205°C) oven for 45 minutes before making the hummus.

2½ cups (10 ounces/285 g) chopped cauliflower florets (about ½ medium head)

1 cup (5 ounces/140 g) sliced zucchini (about 1 medium)

¼ cup (1¼ ounces/35 g) tahini

3 tablespoons freshly squeezed lemon juice

3 tablespoons olive oil, divided

1 clove garlic (or more to taste)

½ teaspoon fine sea salt

¼ teaspoon ground black pepper

¼ teaspoon paprika, for garnish

Chopped fresh parsley, for garnish (optional)

Cucumber slices, for serving (optional)

1. Boil the cauliflower in a medium to large saucepan full of water until soft, about 10 minutes. Add the zucchini and cook for another 5 minutes. Remove and drain.

2. Transfer the cauliflower and zucchini to a food processor. Add the tahini, lemon juice, 1 tablespoon of the olive oil, garlic, salt, and pepper and blend until smooth. Taste and adjust for seasoning.

3. Place the hummus on a serving plate. Garnish with the paprika and parsley, if using, and drizzle with the remaining 2 tablespoons of olive oil. Serve with cucumber slices for dipping, if desired. The hummus will keep in the refrigerator for up to a week.

MACRONUTRIENTS
(per serving)

Fat	Protein	Carbs	Fiber	Energy
19g	3.3g	8.3g	3g	211 cal
79%	6%	15%		

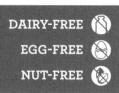

DAIRY-FREE

EGG-FREE

NUT-FREE

Keto Baba Ghanoush

Prep Time: **15 minutes** | Cook Time: **12 minutes**
Yield: **2 servings**

Mediterranean food emphasizes low-carb and high-fat—concepts that are keto-friendly and provide a ton of recipe inspiration for me! This baba ghanoush is great with cucumber slices or pork rinds. The standard eggplant for baba ghanoush is a globe eggplant, which is generally 7 to 8 inches long (18 to 20 cm) and weighs about 1 pound (2.5 kg).

½ globe eggplant (8 ounces/225 g), top removed, sliced into 6 long sections

1 teaspoon fine sea salt, divided

1 cup (4¼ ounces/120 g) quartered and sliced zucchini

2 cloves garlic

5 tablespoons (2½ fluid ounces/ 75 ml) olive oil, divided

2 tablespoons tahini

1 tablespoon freshly squeezed lemon juice

¼ teaspoon ground cumin

¼ teaspoon ground black pepper

¼ teaspoon paprika, for garnish

1 tablespoon chopped fresh parsley, for garnish

1. Preheat the broiler to medium.

2. Place the eggplant in a colander or on a bed of paper towels. Sprinkle on both sides with ½ teaspoon of the salt and let sit for 10 to 15 minutes. Wipe well with paper towels to dry the eggplant and remove the salt.

3. Arrange the salted eggplant, zucchini, and garlic on a rimmed baking sheet. Drizzle with 1 tablespoon of the olive oil.

4. Broil the vegetables for 10 to 12 minutes, until softened. Using a spoon, scrape the flesh of the eggplant out of the skin and into a food processor.

5. To the food processor, add the roasted zucchini and garlic cloves, along with the remaining ½ teaspoon of salt, 3 tablespoons of the olive oil, tahini, lemon juice, cumin, and pepper. Blend until smooth. Taste and adjust for seasoning.

6. Transfer the baba ghanoush to a serving bowl. Drizzle with the remaining 1 tablespoon of olive oil, sprinkle with the paprika, and garnish with parsley. The baba ghanoush will keep in the refrigerator for up to 3 days.

MACRONUTRIENTS
(per serving)

Fat	Protein	Carbs	Fiber	Energy
42.5g	4.5g	11.5g	6g	430 cal
86%	4%	10%		

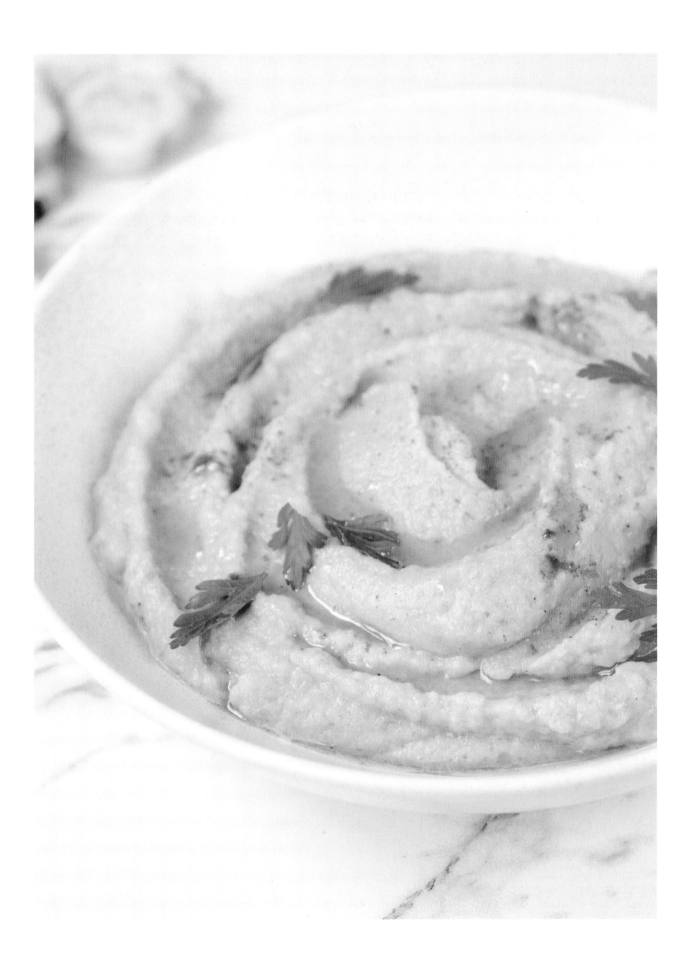

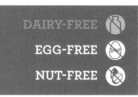

DAIRY-FREE

EGG-FREE

NUT-FREE

Tzatziki Dip

Prep Time: 15 minutes
Yield: 4 servings

Full-fat Greek yogurt is a creamy treat that can be enjoyed in moderation on a ketogenic diet, as it provides tons of fat and probiotics. This is a fantastic dip or dinner side; it's great in my Pork Gyro Lettuce Wraps with Quick Pickled Red Onions (page 302), as a dip with endive leaves or crudités, or simply served alongside grilled meat or a tossed salad.

½ large cucumber, peeled

½ teaspoon fine sea salt

1 cup (8 ounces/225 g) plain Greek yogurt

1 cup (8 ounces/225 g) sour cream

2 tablespoons finely chopped fresh dill, plus more for garnish

1 tablespoon finely chopped fresh mint, plus more for garnish

1 tablespoon freshly squeezed lemon juice

1 clove garlic, minced

¼ teaspoon ground black pepper

¼ cup (2 fluid ounces/60 ml) olive oil

¼ cup (1¼ ounces/35 g) slivered Kalamata olives (optional)

1. Peel the cucumber and scrape out the seeds. Grate the seeded cucumber, then place it in a colander and set over a bowl to drain. Stir in the salt and allow to sit, stirring occasionally, until the moisture drains out, 10 to 15 minutes. Wrap in a clean dish towel or paper towels and squeeze out the excess water.

2. In another bowl, stir together the salted cucumber, yogurt, sour cream, dill, mint, lemon juice, garlic, and pepper. Taste and season with additional salt, if needed.

3. Transfer the dip to a wide serving bowl. Drizzle with the olive oil and sprinkle with the olives, if using. Garnish with additional dill and mint.

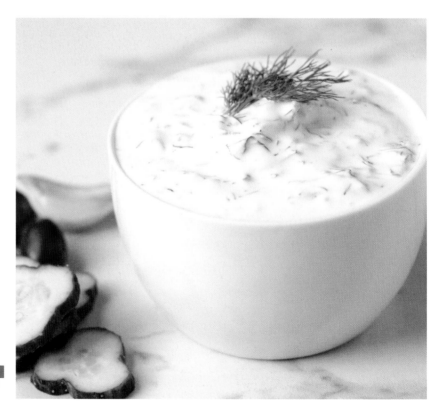

MACRONUTRIENTS
(per serving)

Fat	Protein	Carbs	Fiber	Energy
19g	5.3g	7.3g	0.8g	217 cal
77%	10%	14%		

Avocado Tzatziki Dip

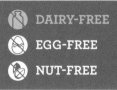

- DAIRY-FREE
- EGG-FREE
- NUT-FREE

Prep Time: 15 minutes
Yield: 4 servings

Mediterranean diets incorporate wonderful fats, including lots of olive oil. I created a version of tzatziki with avocado and avocado oil for a fun twist on this Greek favorite. It makes for a great alternative to guacamole!

½ large cucumber, peeled

½ teaspoon fine sea salt

1 medium-sized ripe avocado, halved and pitted

½ cup (4 ounces/115 g) Greek yogurt

½ cup (4 ounces/115 g) sour cream

2 tablespoons finely chopped fresh dill

1 tablespoon freshly squeezed lemon juice

1 clove garlic, minced

¼ teaspoon ground black pepper

¼ cup (2 fluid ounces/60 ml) avocado oil

¼ cup (1¼ ounces/35 g) slivered Kalamata olives (optional)

Fresh mint leaves, for garnish (optional)

1. Peel the cucumber and scrape out the seeds. Grate the seeded cucumber, then place it in a colander and set over a bowl to drain. Stir in the salt and allow to sit, stirring occasionally, until the moisture drains out, 10 to 15 minutes. Wrap in a clean dish towel or paper towels and squeeze out the excess water.

2. Scoop the avocado flesh into another bowl and mash until very smooth. Stir in the salted cucumber, yogurt, sour cream, dill, lemon juice, garlic, and pepper. Taste and season with additional salt, if needed.

3. Transfer the dip to a wide serving bowl. Drizzle with the avocado oil and sprinkle with the olives, if using. Garnish with mint leaves, if desired.

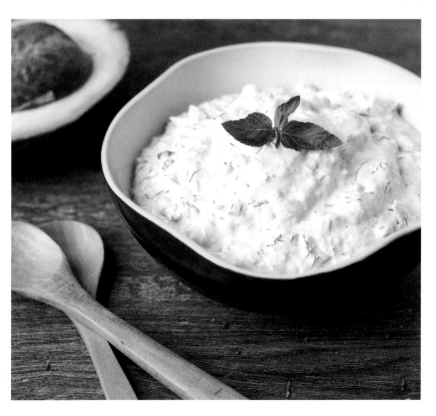

MACRONUTRIENTS (per serving)				
Fat	Protein	Carbs	Fiber	Energy
31.3g	4.8g	10.8g	4.3g	332 cal
82%	6%	12%		

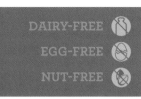

DAIRY-FREE

EGG-FREE

NUT-FREE

Stuffed Mushrooms

Prep Time: 15 minutes | **Cook Time: 18 minutes**
Yield: 4 servings

Who doesn't love stuffed mushrooms? This is a super-cute and fun appetizer for a party, and it's easy to double or triple the recipe if you need a big batch. Or just make these for yourself for a yummy keto snack!

16 large cremini or porcini mushrooms

1 tablespoon MCT oil

4 slices bacon, chopped

1 (just-under-2-ounce/55-g) bag pork rinds

½ cup (4 ounces/115 g) mayonnaise

2 ounces (55 g) cream cheese

1 ounce (28 g) raw cashews

2 tablespoons sliced green onions, plus more for garnish

2 tablespoons chopped fresh basil, plus more for garnish (optional)

1 tablespoon chopped fresh mint, plus more for garnish (optional)

1 clove garlic

½ teaspoon fine sea salt

¼ cup (1 ounce/28 g) grated Parmesan cheese

1. Preheat the oven to 400°F (205°C).

2. Remove the stems from the mushrooms and brush the caps with the MCT oil.

3. Fry the bacon in a skillet over medium heat until crispy, 5 to 6 minutes; remove the bacon from the pan.

4. In a food processor, grind the pork rinds for 5 to 6 minutes, until extremely fine. Add the bacon, mayonnaise, cream cheese, cashews, green onions, basil, mint, garlic, and salt. Pulse for about 1 minute, until well combined.

5. Stuff the mushroom caps with the pork rind mixture and place on a rimmed baking sheet. Sprinkle with the Parmesan.

6. Bake for 10 to 12 minutes, until nicely browned on top. Serve garnished with extra green onions, basil, and/or mint, if desired.

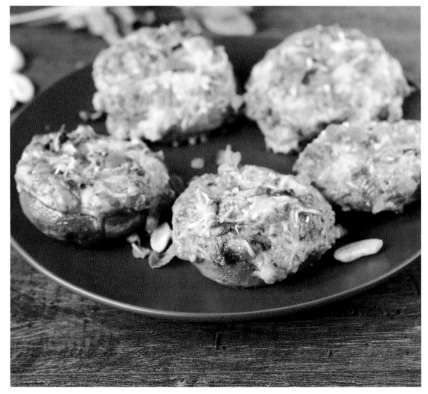

MACRONUTRIENTS
(per serving)

Fat	Protein	Carbs	Fiber	Energy
42.3g	17.3g	6.3g	1.3g	465 cal
80%	15%	5%		

Stuffed Tomatoes

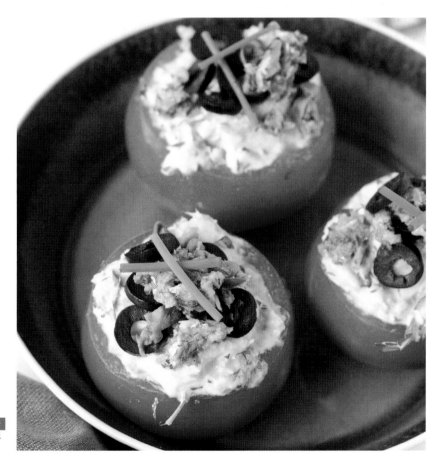

DAIRY-FREE

EGG-FREE

NUT-FREE

Prep Time: 15 minutes
Yield: 4 servings

Ripe, firm tomatoes straight off the vine are the essence of summer meals. This dish, French in origin, is a fun way to serve up a ketogenic summer tomato dish with a low-carb twist.

4 medium tomatoes

1 teaspoon fine sea salt, divided

2 eggs, hard-boiled

1 cup (8 ounces/225 g) mayonnaise

1 (4-ounce/115-g) can tuna, drained and flaked

¼ cup (¼ ounce/7 g) chopped fresh parsley

1 tablespoon chopped fresh chives, plus more for garnish

¼ teaspoon garlic powder

¼ teaspoon onion powder

¼ teaspoon ground black pepper

10 black olives, pitted and sliced

6 anchovies, drained and finely chopped

1 tablespoon capers

1. Slice the tops off the tomatoes and remove the pulp with a spoon. To remove the excess moisture, sprinkle ½ teaspoon of the salt over the tomatoes, then flip them upside down on a bed of paper towels to absorb the moisture as it drains.

2. Make the filling: Roughly chop the hard-boiled eggs. In a mixing bowl, mash together the eggs and mayonnaise. Add the tuna, parsley, chives, garlic powder, onion powder, remaining ½ teaspoon of salt, and pepper.

3. Use dry paper towels to wipe the salt off the tomatoes. Divide the filling between the tomatoes. Top with the olives, anchovies, capers, and snipped fresh chives.

MACRONUTRIENTS
(per serving)

Fat	Protein	Carbs	Fiber	Energy
47.5g	11.3g	3.3g	0.6g	485 cal
88%	9%	3%		

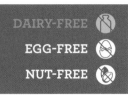

Eggplant Cherry Tomato

Pizzas

Prep Time: **10 minutes** | Cook Time: **30 minutes**
Yield: **4 servings**

My favorite pizza is topped with buffalo mozzarella, cherry tomatoes, and arugula. You can make it with this eggplant crust or use another ketogenic pizza crust for a divine-tasting Italian-inspired dish!

1 large eggplant (approximately 1 pound/455 g), cut lengthwise into ¼-inch (6-mm)-thick slices

1 teaspoon fine sea salt, divided

¼ cup (2 fluid ounces/60 ml) olive oil

½ teaspoon garlic powder

8 ounces (225 g) buffalo mozzarella cheese, shredded

1 cup (5½ ounces/155 g) cherry or grape tomatoes, quartered

½ cup (¾ ounce/20 g) arugula, plus more for garnish

1 tablespoon dried oregano leaves

Handful of fresh basil leaves, for garnish

1. Preheat the oven to 400°F (205°C).

2. To remove the excess moisture from the eggplant, spread the eggplant slices in a single layer on a bed of paper towels. Sprinkle on both sides with ½ teaspoon of the salt and let sit for 10 to 15 minutes. Wipe well with paper towel to dry the eggplant and remove the salt.

3. Spray a rimmed baking sheet with cooking spray and spread the eggplant slices in a single layer on the pan.

4. In a bowl, combine the olive oil, garlic powder, and remaining ½ teaspoon of salt. Coat each slice of eggplant with the olive oil mixture. Top the slices evenly with the mozzarella, tomatoes, arugula, and oregano.

5. Bake for 25 to 30 minutes, until the eggplant is cooked through. Sprinkle with additional arugula and basil before serving.

MACRONUTRIENTS
(per serving)

Fat	Protein	Carbs	Fiber	Energy
40g	11.8g	10g	4.5g	447 cal
81%	10%	9%		

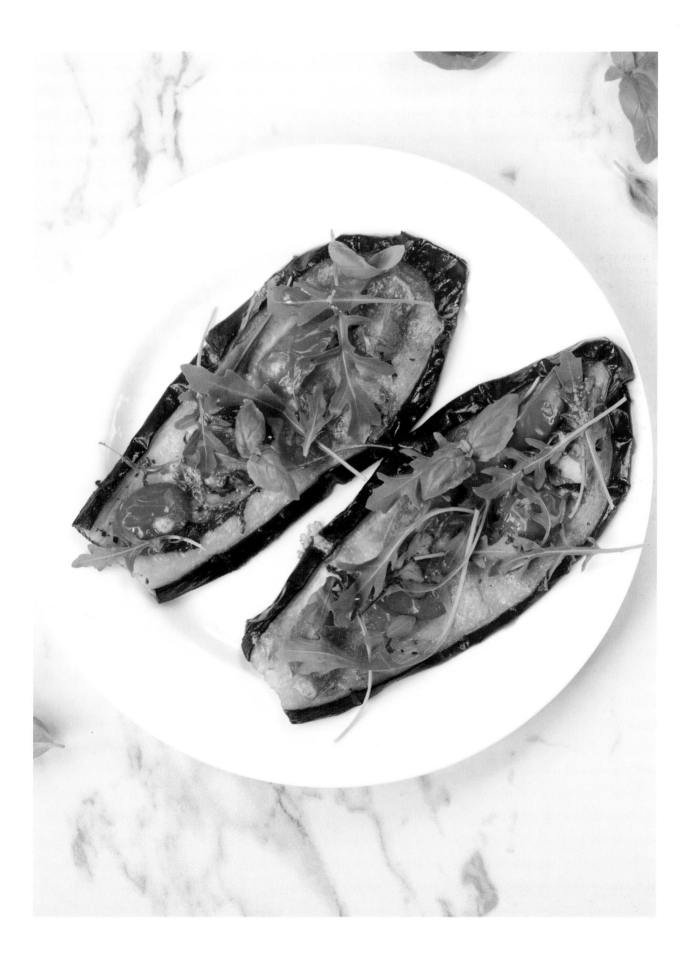

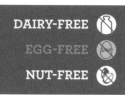

DAIRY-FREE

EGG-FREE

NUT-FREE

Keto Bread Loaf

Prep Time: 10 minutes, plus time to rest and dry overnight | **Cook Time:** 45 minutes
Yield: one 9 by 5-inch (23 by 13-cm) loaf (15 servings)

Eating keto doesn't mean you can't enjoy flavorful homemade bread every day of the week! This loaf relies on omega-3–rich flax meal, which absorbs liquid effectively, as well as eggs to bind, to produce a hearty and nutty-tasting loaf. Unlike glutinous bread, this is incredibly easy to make; a quick mix and bake in the oven, and you have a bread for every occasion.

½ cup (4 ounces/115 g) flax meal

1 cup (8 fluid ounces/240 ml) filtered water

½ cup (2 ounces/55 g) coconut flour

1 teaspoon baking soda

½ teaspoon fine sea salt

¼ teaspoon onion powder

½ cup (4 ounces/115 g) coconut oil, melted, plus more for the pan

3 eggs

1 tablespoon apple cider vinegar

2 to 4 drops liquid stevia

1. Preheat the oven to 350°F (177°C). Grease a 9 by 5-inch (23 by 13-cm) loaf pan with coconut oil.

2. In a small bowl, combine the flax meal and water; set aside.

3. In another bowl, use a whisk to combine the coconut flour, baking soda, salt, and onion powder. Add the melted coconut oil and blend with the whisk. Add the eggs and flax mixture and blend well. Mix in the vinegar and stevia until a thick batter forms.

4. Spoon the batter into the greased loaf pan. Bake for 40 to 45 minutes, until nicely browned.

5. Let cool in the pan for at least an hour or overnight. Once cool, remove the loaf gently from the pan and let it dry out overnight.

6. To serve, cut into 15 slices. Store the slices in a resealable plastic bag in the refrigerator for up to 3 days. For longer life, freeze the slices, then remove from the freezer the night before using.

tip

When ready to eat this bread, I recommend placing the slices on a baking sheet and toasting them under the broiler for 2 to 3 minutes, turning them halfway through. Watch them carefully, as the slices can burn quickly!

MACRONUTRIENTS
(per serving)

Fat	Protein	Carbs	Fiber	Energy
10g	2.6g	3.2g	2.4g	116 cal
80%	9%	11%		

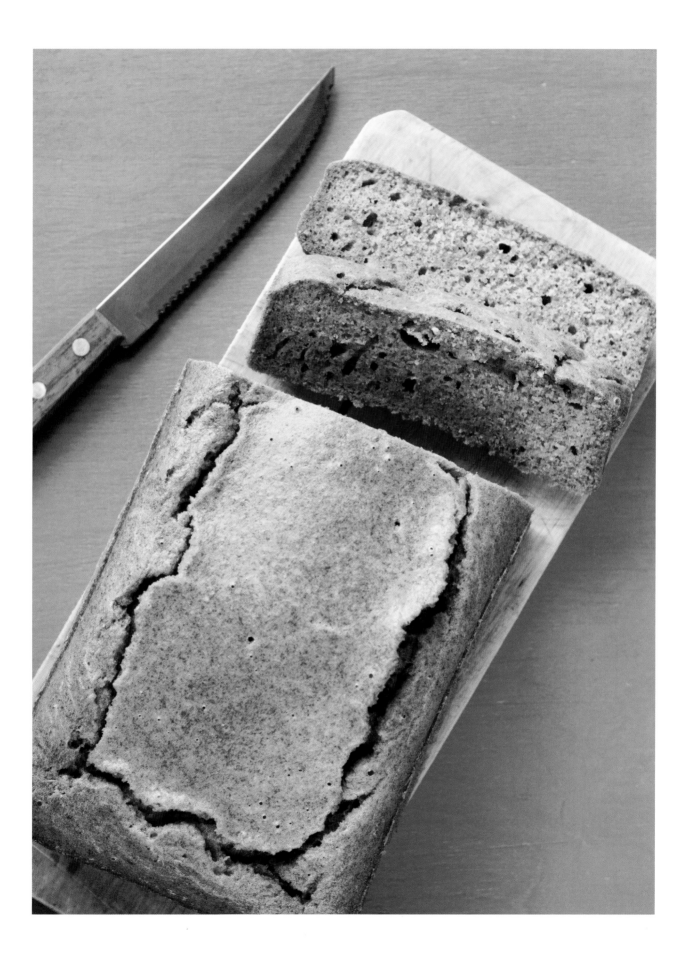

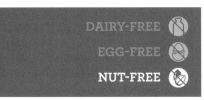

DAIRY-FREE

EGG-FREE

NUT-FREE

Keto Chive and Onion
"English Muffins"

Prep Time: 10 minutes | **Cook Time: 25 minutes**
Yield: 4 muffins (2 per serving)

This fantastic keto bread is free of gluten, wheat, nuts, and sugar and has only 1 percent carbohydrate or less. These muffins are great for Eggs Benedict (page 128) or as sandwich or burger buns. For versatile unflavored muffins, simply omit the chives and onion powder.

4 eggs

½ teaspoon baking powder

2 ounces (55 g) cream cheese, softened

2 tablespoons finely chopped fresh chives

¼ teaspoon onion powder

Pinch of sea salt

1. Preheat the oven to 350°F (177°C). Line a baking sheet with parchment paper cut to the size of the pan. (A small dot of egg white under each corner of the parchment will help it adhere to the pan.)

2. Separate the eggs, placing the yolks in a mixing bowl and the whites in the bowl of a stand mixer or another mixing bowl.

3. Add the baking powder to the egg whites and, using an electric mixer, whip until stiff peaks form, 5 to 6 minutes.

4. Add the cream cheese to the bowl with the egg yolks and use a whisk to combine them. Add the chives, onion powder, and salt and stir until very smooth.

5. With a rubber spatula, gently fold the whipped egg yolk mixture into the egg whites, being careful not to deflate the whites.

6. Carefully spoon 4 large buns onto the prepared baking sheet, gently shaping each bun into a round like an English muffin. Bake for 20 to 25 minutes, until golden brown.

7. Remove from the oven and let cool on the pan. Once cool, use a spatula to gently lift the buns from the pan. Store in a resealable plastic bag or airtight container for up to 3 days.

tip

If you forgot to soften the cream cheese ahead of time, you can gently soften it by warming it in a low oven for several minutes or by microwaving it for 30 seconds.

MACRONUTRIENTS
(per serving)

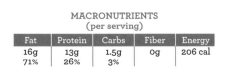

Fat	Protein	Carbs	Fiber	Energy
16g	13g	1.5g	0g	206 cal
71%	26%	3%		

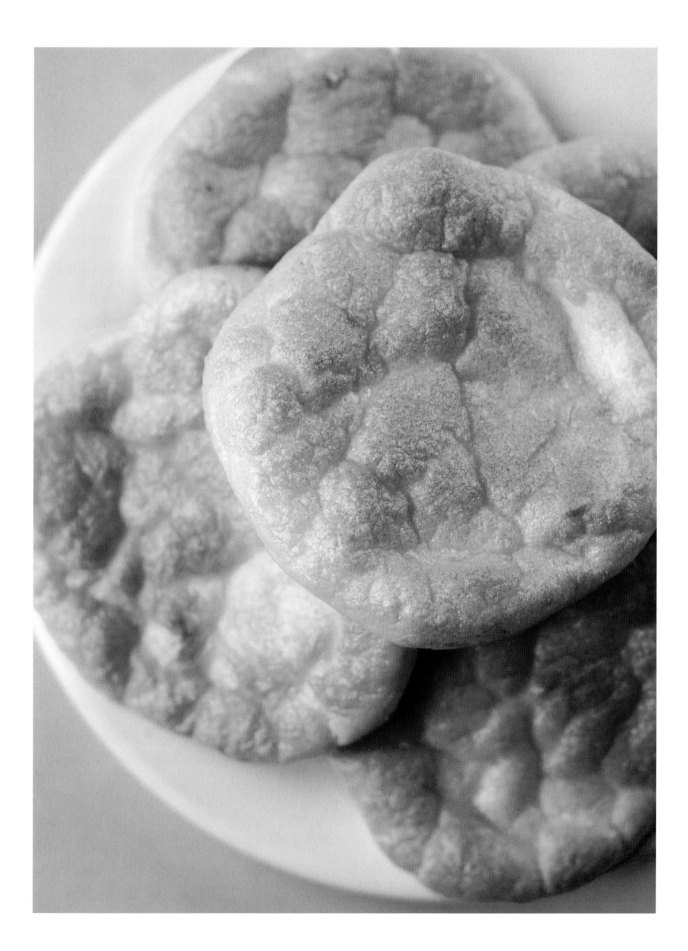

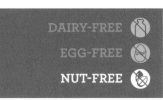

DAIRY-FREE

EGG-FREE

NUT-FREE

Cinnamon Muffins

Prep Time: 4 minutes | **Cook Time: 25 minutes**
Yield: 4 servings

I love cinnamon and its magical ability to lower blood sugar, and flax is possibly the best source of omega-3 fatty acids out there. Combined, they make these muffins superfood muffins!

½ cup (4 ounces/110 g) flax meal

¼ cup plus 2 tablespoons (1½ ounces/42 g) coconut flour

1 teaspoon baking powder

1 teaspoon ground Ceylon cinnamon or regular cinnamon

½ teaspoon fine sea salt

4 eggs

¼ cup (2 ounces/55 g) unsalted butter, melted but not hot

1 cup (8 fluid ounces/240 ml) filtered water

½ to 1 teaspoon liquid stevia, to taste

1 tablespoon plus 1 teaspoon erythritol or powdered stevia (optional)

¼ cup (2 ounces/55 g) butter, softened, for serving

1. Preheat the oven to 350°F (177°C). Spray 4 wells of a standard-size muffin pan with coconut oil spray.

2. In a small bowl, use a fork to combine the flax meal, coconut flour, baking powder, cinnamon, and salt.

3. In a separate bowl, combine the eggs, melted butter, water, liquid stevia, and erythritol, if using.

4. Add the dry ingredients to the wet ingredients and stir with a wooden spoon to combine. Spoon the batter into the prepared muffin cups and bake for 20 to 25 minutes, until a toothpick inserted in the middle of a muffin comes out clean.

5. Serve each muffin with a tablespoon of room-temperature butter.

MACRONUTRIENTS (using stevia only)				
Fat	Protein	Carbs	Fiber	Energy
34.3g	11g	9.3g	5.8g	386 cal
80%	11%	9%		

MACRONUTRIENTS (using stevia and erythritol)				
Fat	Protein	Carbs	Fiber	Energy
34.3g	11g	13.3g	9.8g	406 cal
76%	11%	13%		

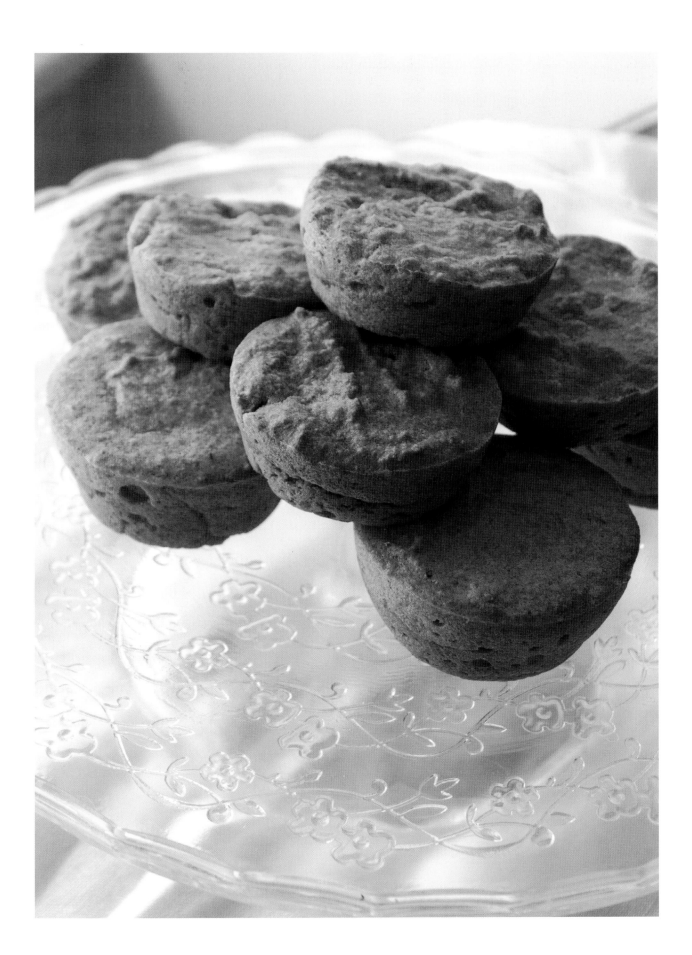

Chapter 9
Salads & Soups

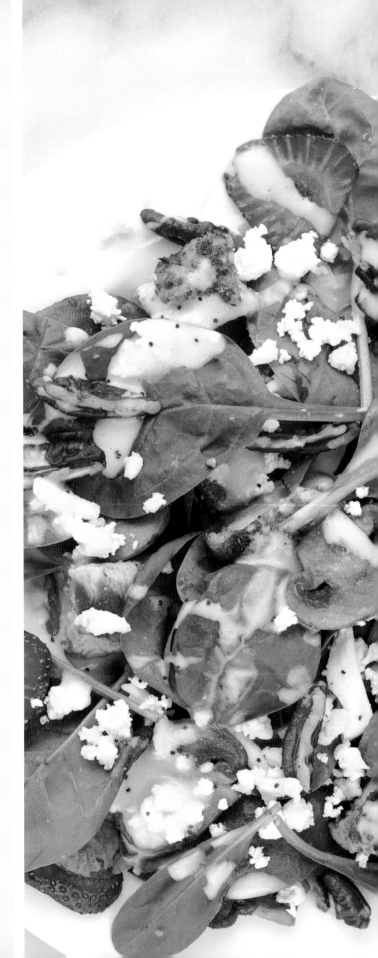

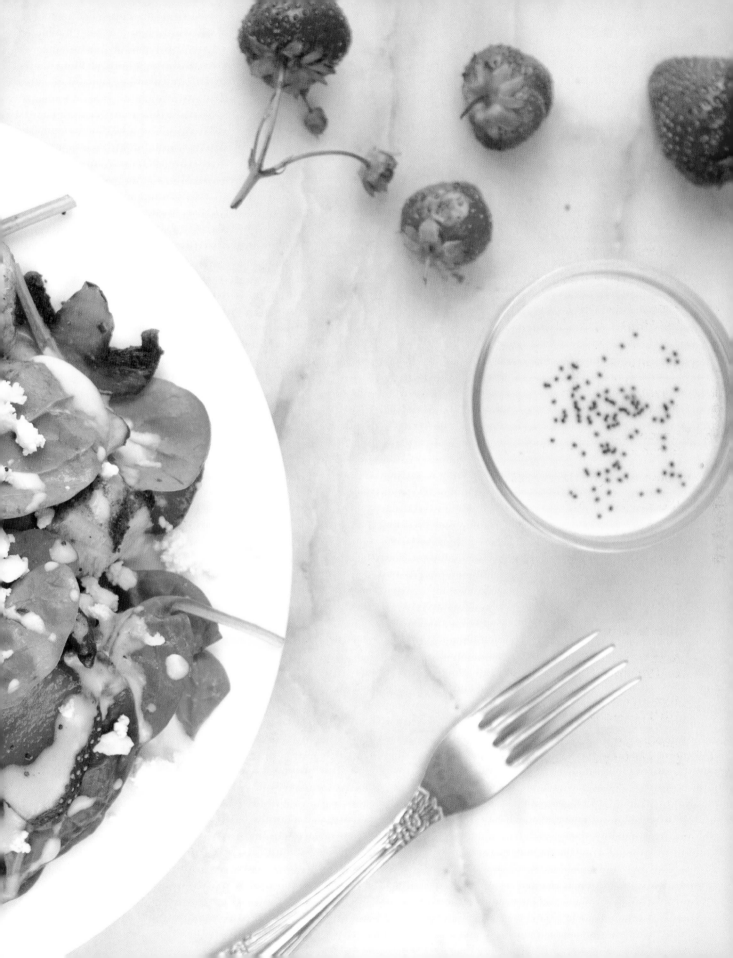

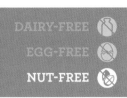

DAIRY-FREE

EGG-FREE

NUT-FREE

Bacon Wedge Salad

Prep Time: 10 minutes (not including time to cook bacon) | Yield: **4 servings**

This delicious salad has been regaining in popularity, and for good reason. It is a classic steakhouse salad offering, and it's very ketogenic.

2 small heads iceberg lettuce, cored, 1 or 2 outer layers removed

1 cup (8 fluid ounces/240 ml) Blue Cheese Dressing (page 357)

1 pound (455 g) bacon, cooked and chopped into small pieces

1 medium tomato, diced

2 tablespoons thinly sliced green onions

1½ cups (6 ounces/170 g) crumbled blue cheese

1. Chop the lettuce into 8 wedges. Place 2 wedges on each of 4 plates.

2. Top the lettuce wedges on each plate with one-quarter of the dressing, bacon, tomato, green onions, and blue cheese.

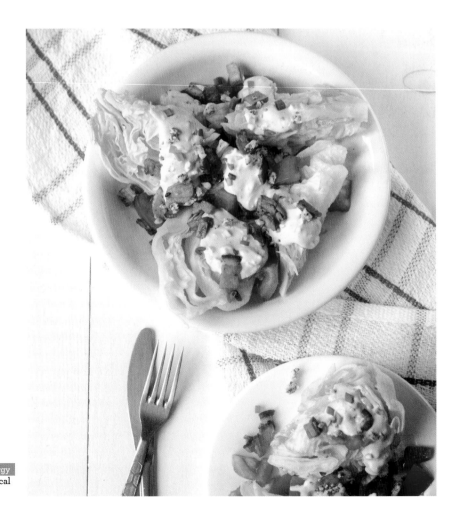

MACRONUTRIENTS
(per serving)

Fat	Protein	Carbs	Fiber	Energy
59g	21.5g	5g	3.3g	639 cal
83%	14%	4%		

Cobb Salad

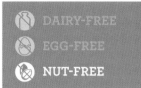

Prep Time: **10 minutes** | Cook Time: **20 minutes**
Yield: **2 servings**

I always thought of cobb salad as an indulgent dish. On a keto diet, it's a fantastic source of healthy fats! For a bit of a kick, top this classic salad with your favorite keto hot sauce.

6 slices bacon

1 (6-ounce/170-g) boneless chicken breast, preferably skin-on

½ teaspoon ground cumin

½ teaspoon paprika

½ teaspoon fine sea salt

¼ teaspoon ground black pepper

2 cups (2¾ ounces/80 g) chopped romaine lettuce

½ medium-sized ripe avocado, peeled and cut into ½-inch (1.25-cm) cubes

4 eggs, hard-boiled, peeled and sliced

1 medium tomato, cut into ½-inch (1.25-cm) cubes

½ cup (2 ounces/55 g) crumbled blue cheese

½ cup (4 fluid ounces/120 ml) Ranch Dressing (page 359)

1 tablespoon sliced green onions, for garnish (optional)

1. Fry the bacon in a pan over medium heat until cooked and slightly crispy, 6 to 7 minutes. Remove from the pan and chop, leaving the bacon fat in the pan.

2. Season the chicken with the cumin, paprika, salt, and pepper. Fry the chicken in the bacon fat for 6 to 7 minutes on each side, until nicely browned. Remove from the pan and cut into cubes.

3. Divide the lettuce between 2 plates. Arrange rows of avocado, eggs, chicken, tomato, blue cheese, and bacon on each plate. Top each plate with half of the dressing (or serve the dressing on the side, as shown) and garnish with the green onions, if desired.

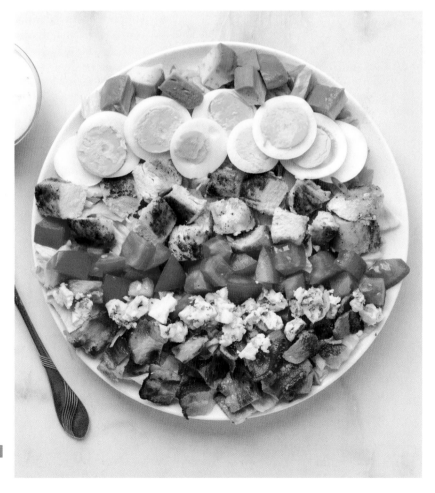

	MACRONUTRIENTS (per serving)			
Fat	Protein	Carbs	Fiber	Energy
67g	46.5g	8.5g	3g	831 cal
73%	23%	4%		

DAIRY-FREE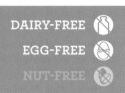
EGG-FREE
NUT-FREE

Spinach Gomae Salad

Prep Time: 5 minutes, plus time to cool spinach | **Cook Time:** 5 minutes
Yield: 2 servings

This dish is one of my favorites when we go out for sushi; my homemade version is keto-compliant and healthier, with no sugar or peanut butter—and it tastes just as good! I love making this salad with kale as well as spinach—or a combination of the two.

6 ounces (170 g) fresh baby spinach (about 6 cups)

GOMAE SAUCE:

3 tablespoons light sesame oil

2 tablespoons unsweetened almond butter

2 tablespoons filtered water

2 tablespoons tamari

1 tablespoon tahini

2 to 4 drops liquid stevia, to taste

1 tablespoon sesame seeds

1. Cook the spinach in boiling-hot water or steam it.

   If boiling, bring a pot of salted water to a boil. Add the spinach and turn off the heat. Leave the spinach in the hot water for 2 to 3 minutes, until cooked. Drain and place in a bowl lined with paper towels to absorb the excess water.

   If steaming, place a steamer basket or metal steamer insert over a pot of boiling water. Put the spinach in the basket or insert and steam for 3 to 4 minutes, until wilted. Remove from the steamer and drain.

2. Refrigerate the spinach for 30 minutes or place in the freezer for 10 minutes to cool.

3. Meanwhile, make the gomae sauce: In a small bowl, thoroughly combine the sesame oil, almond butter, water, tamari, tahini, and stevia.

4. In a dry pan over very low heat, toast the sesame seeds for 30 seconds to 1 minute, stirring constantly, until fragrant and lightly toasted.

5. Serve the cooled spinach with the gomae sauce on top, sprinkled with the toasted sesame seeds.

MACRONUTRIENTS
(per serving)

Fat	Protein	Carbs	Fiber	Energy
33g	11.5g	7.5g	5g	347 cal
80%	12%	8%		

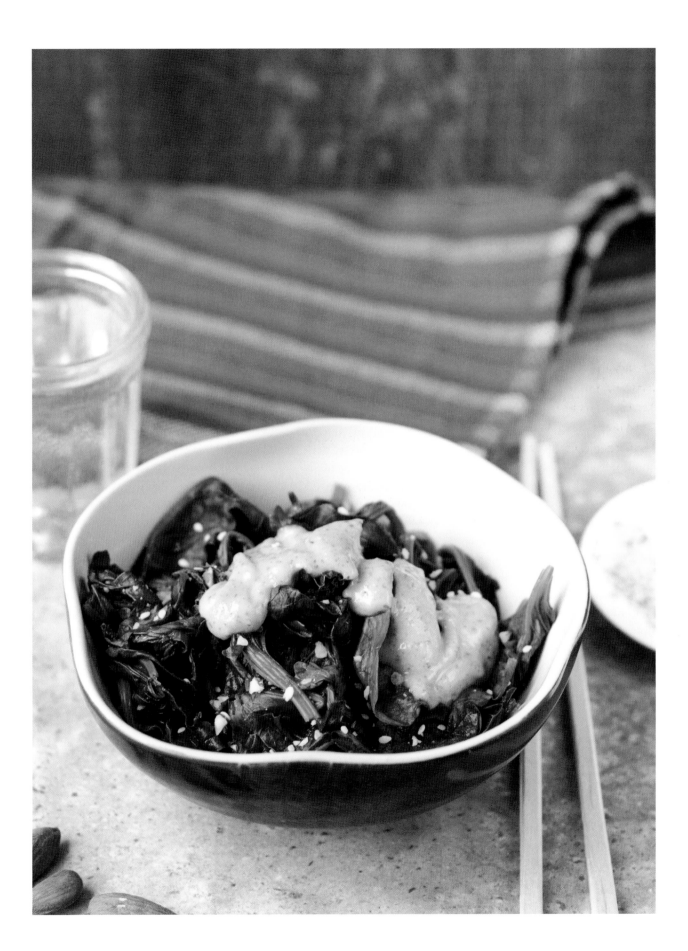

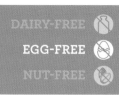

DAIRY-FREE

EGG-FREE

NUT-FREE

Fennel, Asparagus, and Goat Cheese Salad

Prep Time: 15 minutes | **Cook Time:** 20 minutes
Yield: 2 servings

The cheese that I use in this recipe is one of my favorites—a Brie goat cheese round. This unusual cheese has a bloomy Brie rind and a creamy but firm goat cheese center. I find it at Costco and at health-food stores and local cheese markets. You can make this salad using any kind of firm or soft goat cheese. Baking the cheese is optional, too. With an abundance of omega-3 fatty acids, walnut oil provides one of the most important fats; however, you can also use avocado oil or MCT oil in this recipe. If you cannot locate lamb's lettuce, substitute another green lettuce. I find that a mandoline is very handy for thinly slicing the fennel.

2 (4-ounce/115 g) wheels firm goat Brie cheese

2 asparagus spears, woody ends trimmed

2 cups (2¾ ounces/80 g) arugula

1 cup (1½ ounces/40 g) lamb's lettuce

1 cup (3 ounces/85 g) thinly sliced fennel

2 tablespoons chopped raw hazelnuts or pecans, for garnish

WALNUT VINAIGRETTE:

3 tablespoons walnut oil

2 tablespoons apple cider vinegar

1 teaspoon Dijon mustard

1 teaspoon freshly squeezed lemon juice

1 teaspoon onion powder

¼ teaspoon garlic powder

¼ teaspoon liquid stevia

½ teaspoon fine sea salt

1. Preheat the oven to 350°F (177°C).

2. Place the cheese rounds in a small baking pan and bake for 15 to 20 minutes, until warmed and slightly browned. If desired, broil on medium-high for 2 to 3 minutes to brown the tops.

3. In a bowl, whisk together the ingredients for the vinaigrette.

4. Using a vegetable peeler, carefully shave the asparagus into ribbons.

5. Place the arugula, lettuce, fennel, and asparagus ribbons in a bowl. Toss in the vinaigrette to coat well. Divide between 2 plates. Place a warm goat cheese round in the middle of each salad and garnish each plate with 1 tablespoon of the nuts.

tip

To really take this salad over the top, roast the nuts in butter for 1 to 3 minutes before garnishing.

MACRONUTRIENTS
(per serving)

Fat	Protein	Carbs	Fiber	Energy
39g	15g	9g	3g	444 cal
79%	13%	8%		

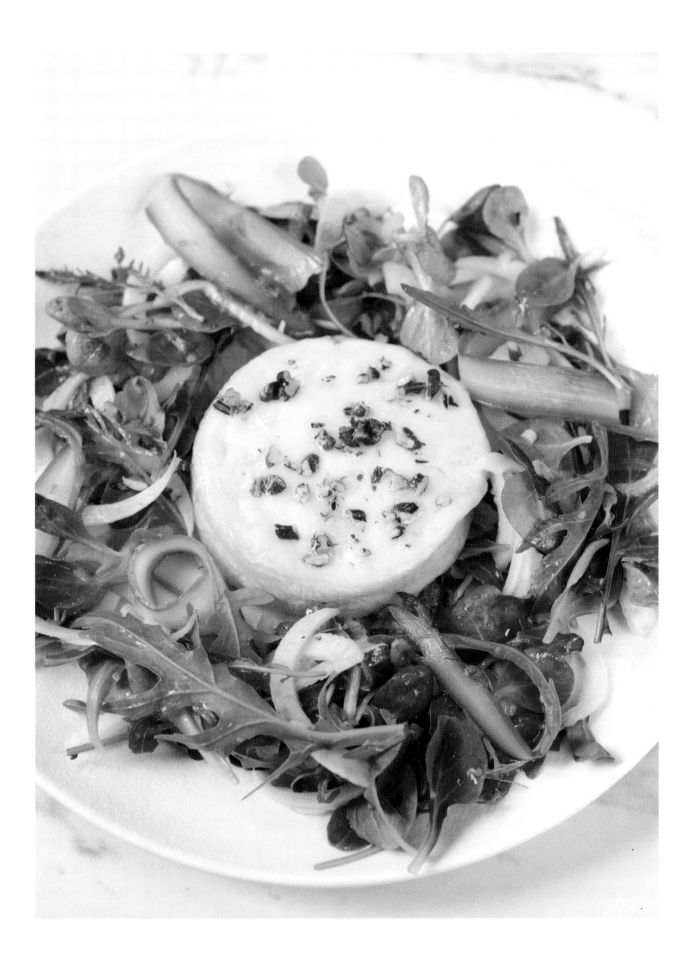

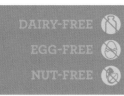

DAIRY-FREE

EGG-FREE

NUT-FREE

Spinach, Goat Cheese, Pecan, and Strawberry Salad

Prep Time: 10 minutes | Cook Time: **8 minutes**
Yield: **4 servings**

This is a wonderful ketogenic meal full of rich fatty acids, vitamins, and fiber. When I first tried a spinach salad at a summer job at the university in Vancouver, it was love at first bite. Using my 50 percent staff discount, I ordered the spinach and mushroom salad every day on my lunch break. The poppy seed dressing is perfect with this salad—and my version doesn't contain the sugar normally found in this dressing. For a refreshing summer salad, enjoy the mushrooms raw rather than cooked.

2 tablespoons butter

1 cup (4 ounces/115 g) sliced white mushrooms

¼ cup (1 ounce/28 g) raw pecans, halved

2 eggs, hard-boiled

6 ounces (170 g) fresh baby spinach (about 6 cups)

10 ounces (285 g) cubed skin-on rotisserie chicken

½ cup (2 ounces/55 g) crumbled fresh (soft) goat cheese

¼ cup (1¼ ounces/35 g) thinly sliced strawberries

POPPY SEED DRESSING:

⅔ cup (5¼ fluid ounces/150 ml) MCT oil

¼ cup (2 fluid ounces/60 ml) apple cider vinegar

1 tablespoon Dijon mustard

1 teaspoon freshly squeezed lemon juice

1 teaspoon onion powder

½ teaspoon fine sea salt

¼ teaspoon garlic powder

¼ teaspoon liquid stevia (or to taste) or other keto sweetener of choice

2 tablespoons poppy seeds

1. In a medium skillet over medium heat, melt the butter. Add the mushrooms and cook for 5 to 6 minutes, turning occasionally, until nicely browned on both sides. Remove the mushrooms from the pan.

2. Reduce the heat to low and add the pecans; cook for 1 to 2 minutes, until the nuts are lightly toasted and the oils release a bit. Set aside.

3. Peel the eggs and place in a large bowl; use a fork to crumble them.

4. Prepare the dressing: In a food processor, combine all the dressing ingredients except for the poppy seeds. Process until well combined. Stir in the poppy seeds.

5. Add the spinach, chicken, mushrooms, pecans, goat cheese, and strawberries to the bowl with the eggs and toss gently to combine. Divide the salad between 4 bowls. Top with the dressing or serve the dressing on the side.

MACRONUTRIENTS
(per serving)

Fat	Protein	Carbs	Fiber	Energy
57.3g	25.8g	6.3g	2.8g	648 cal
80%	16%	4%		

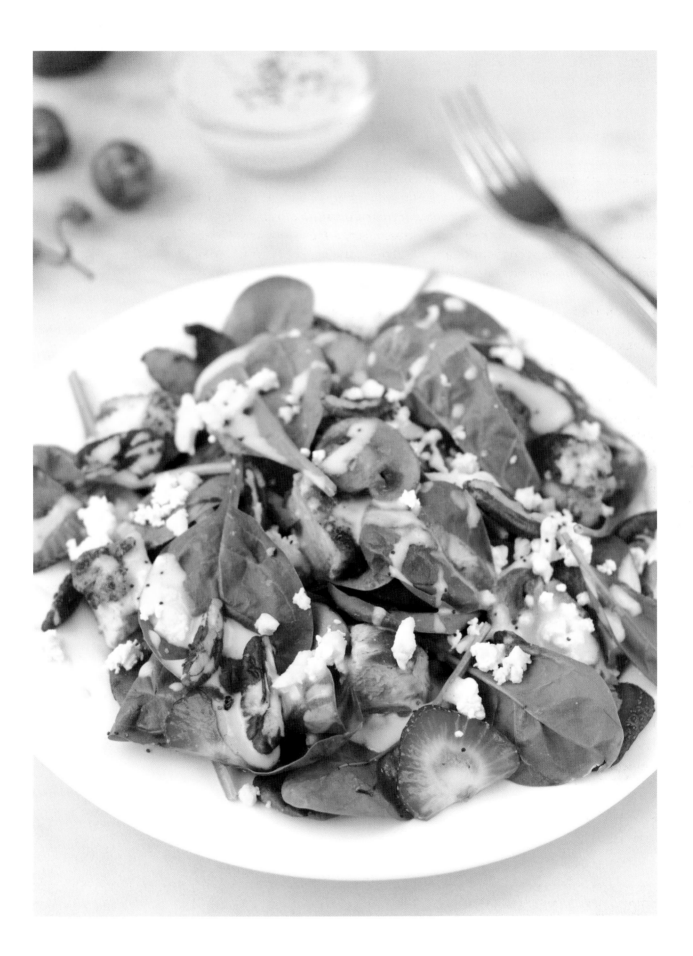

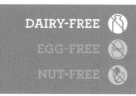

DAIRY-FREE

EGG-FREE

NUT-FREE

Oriental Salad
with Japanese Ginger Dressing

Prep Time: **15 minutes**
Yield: **2 servings**

My main reason for going out for sushi was always the creamy ginger dressing! There's something about this sweet, zesty dressing that I just adore. I love it on a green salad, and I even like to dip sushi rolls into it. Re-creating it at home was one of my all-time cooking-related joys. My version has zero sugar or guilt, but all the flavor!

8 ounces (225 g) sushi-grade salmon

2 cups (4 ounces/115 g) shredded iceberg lettuce

1 cup (4 ounces/115 g) radishes, grated

1 cup (5½ ounces/155 g) cucumber ribbons

½ medium tomato, diced

½ medium avocado, diced

1 teaspoon sesame seeds

1 batch Restaurant-Style Keto Japanese Ginger Dressing (page 361), chilled

1. Cut the salmon into ¼-inch (6-mm) slices.

2. Arrange the lettuce, radishes, cucumber ribbons, and tomato on a plate or in a salad bowl. Top with the salmon and avocado and sprinkle with the sesame seeds.

3. Drizzle the chilled dressing over the salad. If you prefer, toss to combine.

	MACRONUTRIENTS (per serving)			
Fat	Protein	Carbs	Fiber	Energy
53.5g	28.5g	8.5g	4g	646 cal
80%	15%	5%		

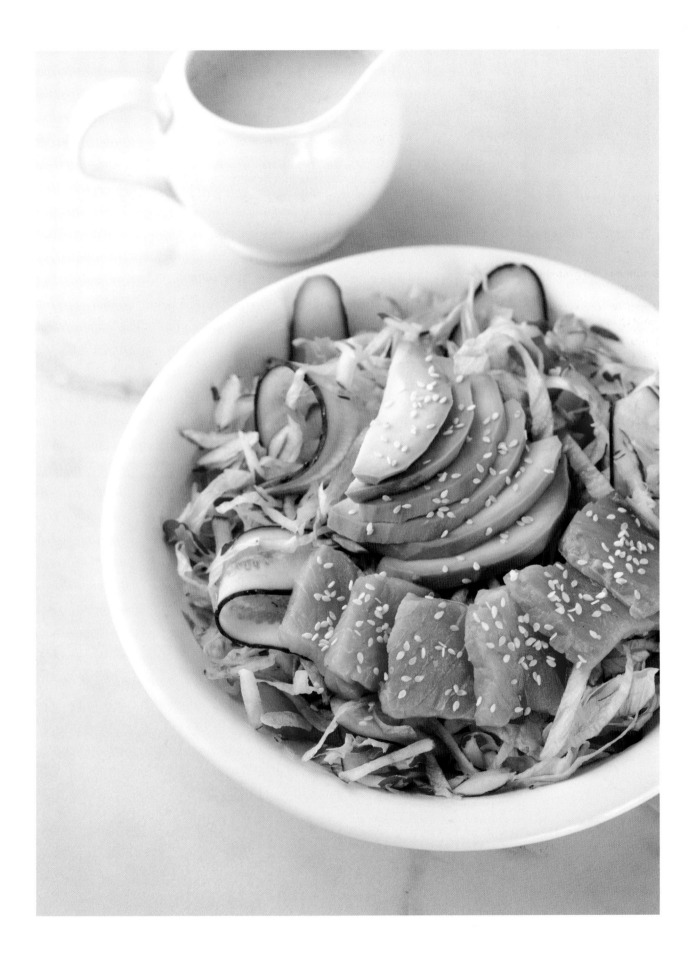

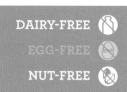

DAIRY-FREE

EGG-FREE

NUT-FREE

Deconstructed
Bacon Burger Salad

Prep Time: 10 minutes (not including time to grill burger patty)
Yield: 1 serving

My Special Burger Sauce is hands-down the most popular recipe I have ever published! Who would have imagined a burger salad could be such a healthy meal? When prepared ketogen-ically, it is a whole-food meal with nourishing greens and avocado, and it provides essential fatty acids, essential amino acids, and plenty of key nutrients, like vitamin E and potassium.

2 cups (4 ounces/115 g) shredded butter lettuce, iceberg lettuce, or romaine lettuce

¼ medium tomato, cut into ½-inch (1.25-cm) cubes

½ medium-sized ripe avocado, peeled and chopped

3 slices bacon, cooked and chopped

1 (4-ounce/115-g) beef burger patty (meat only; no breadcrumbs or other additives), grilled and cooled to room temperature

2 tablespoons Special Burger Sauce (page 363)

1. Arrange the lettuce, tomato, and avocado in a salad bowl.

2. Top with the bacon and burger patty.

3. Dress the salad with the burger sauce and enjoy!

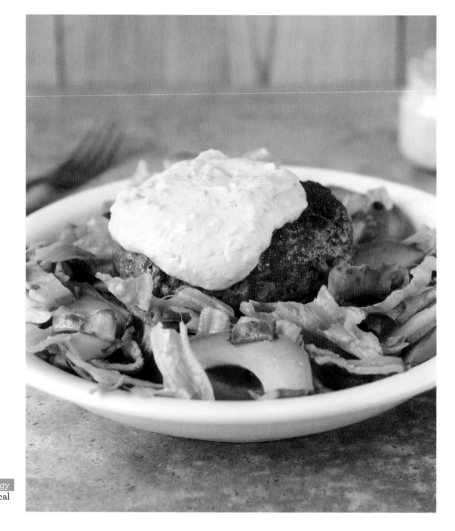

MACRONUTRIENTS (per serving)				
Fat	Protein	Carbs	Fiber	Energy
66g	37g	8g	3g	724 cal
77%	18%	5%		

Keto Gado-Gado Bowl

DAIRY-FREE

EGG-FREE

NUT-FREE

Prep Time: **15 minutes**
Yield: **2 servings**

This is my keto twist on a traditional Indonesian comfort food; it's a great way to incorporate the flavors of Southeast Asia into a ketogenic dish!

ALMOND BUTTER DRESSING:

¼ cup (2 fluid ounces/60 ml) MCT oil

2 tablespoons unsweetened almond butter

2 tablespoons tamari

1 tablespoon freshly squeezed lime juice

½ teaspoon ginger juice, or 1 teaspoon grated fresh ginger

½ teaspoon liquid stevia, erythritol, or xylitol

½ teaspoon fine sea salt

¼ teaspoon garlic powder

¼ teaspoon hot sauce, or a pinch of cayenne pepper or chili powder

2 cups (2½ ounces/70 g) mixed spring lettuces

½ cup (1¾ ounces/50 g) Braised Red Cabbage (page 216), or 1 cup (4 ounces/115 g) shredded raw red cabbage

4 eggs, hard-boiled, peeled and halved

½ English cucumber, sliced

1 tablespoon crushed almonds, for garnish

1 tablespoon chopped fresh cilantro, for garnish

1. Place the dressing ingredients in a small food processor and process until well blended. Alternatively, place the ingredients in a bowl and whisk by hand.

2. Divide the lettuces, cabbage, eggs, and cucumber slices between 2 bowls.

3. Pour half of the dressing over each salad. Garnish each bowl with half of the almonds and cilantro.

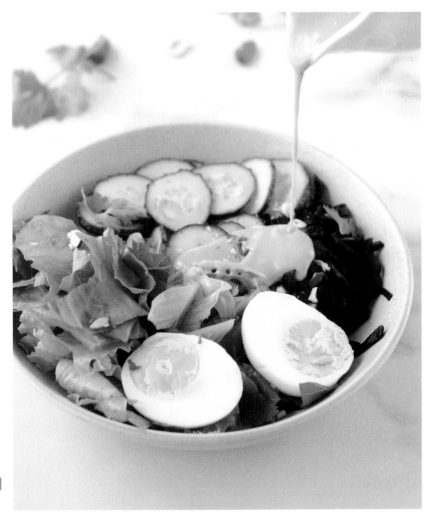

MACRONUTRIENTS (per serving)				
Fat	Protein	Carbs	Fiber	Energy
51g	20.5g	11.5g	5g	589 cal
78%	14%	8%		

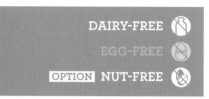

DAIRY-FREE

EGG-FREE

OPTION NUT-FREE

Niçoise Salad

Prep Time: **15 minutes** | Cook Time: **4 minutes**
Yield: **2 servings**

Tuna is a great source of omega-3 fatty acids, which are important for balancing out the omega-6 fats in our diets. This recipe combines olive oil with walnut or flax oil—two top sources of omega-3s. With the oil, eggs, tuna, and olives, this salad contains so many healthy fats! Look for organic tuna with low levels of mercury.

2.6 ounces (75 g) French green beans, whole or chopped

2 cups (2¾ ounces/80 g) chopped romaine lettuce or butter lettuce, mixed spring lettuces, or arugula

1 (5-ounce/142-g) can tuna, drained and flaked

½ cup (2¼ ounces/65 g) pitted black olives, drained

½ cup (2½ ounces/70 g) grape or cherry tomatoes, quartered

4 medium radishes, quartered

2 eggs, hard-boiled and peeled

1 tablespoon sliced green onions

VINAIGRETTE:

½ cup (½ ounce/15 g) fresh parsley leaves, chopped

¼ cup (2 fluid ounces/60 ml) olive oil

¼ cup (2 fluid ounces/60 ml) walnut or flax oil

3 tablespoons apple cider vinegar

1 tablespoon Dijon mustard

1 tablespoon chopped fresh tarragon

1 clove garlic, minced or crushed in a garlic press

½ teaspoon onion powder

4 anchovies

1. Bring a saucepan of water to a boil over high heat. Add the green beans and turn off the heat, leaving the pan on the burner. Let the beans sit in the hot water for 2 to 4 minutes, until crisp-tender and bright green in color. Drain the beans and plunge into a bowl of ice water to stop the cooking and keep the beans crisp. When chilled, drain again and set aside.

2. Place the vinaigrette ingredients in a food processor and process until well blended.

3. Divide the lettuce, tuna, olives, tomatoes, radishes, eggs, green onions, and green beans between 2 plates. Pour half of the vinaigrette over each salad and serve.

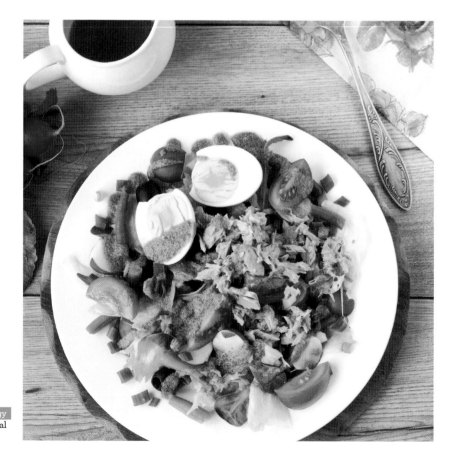

MACRONUTRIENTS
(per serving)

Fat	Protein	Carbs	Fiber	Energy
68.5g	30.5g	9g	3g	777 cal
80%	16%	4%		

Seaweed Salad

DAIRY-FREE

EGG-FREE

NUT-FREE

Prep Time: **15 minutes**
Yield: **2 servings**

Seaweed is one of the world's most densely nutritious foods. It is a great source of iodine, which helps relieve fatigue. As an integral part of the Japanese diet, seaweed is thought to play a huge role in the health and longevity of the Japanese people.

½ cup (4 fluid ounces/120 ml) filtered water

½ cup (½ ounce/15 g) dried wakame seaweed, broken into pieces

3 tablespoons apple cider vinegar

3 tablespoons tamari

1 tablespoon light sesame oil

½ teaspoon ginger juice, or 1 teaspoon grated fresh ginger

¼ teaspoon liquid stevia

1 to 3 drops hot sauce, to taste

½ teaspoon garlic powder

½ teaspoon onion powder

2 green onions, thinly sliced

2 tablespoons chopped fresh cilantro

1 tablespoon sesame seeds

1. Place the water and dried wakame in a bowl and let sit for 5 to 6 minutes to rehydrate.

2. Meanwhile, make the dressing: In a small bowl, mix together the vinegar, tamari, sesame oil, ginger juice, stevia, hot sauce, garlic powder, and onion powder.

3. Drain the wakame well. Add the dressing to the wakame and mix thoroughly. Top with the green onions, cilantro, and sesame seeds. Serve chilled or at room temperature.

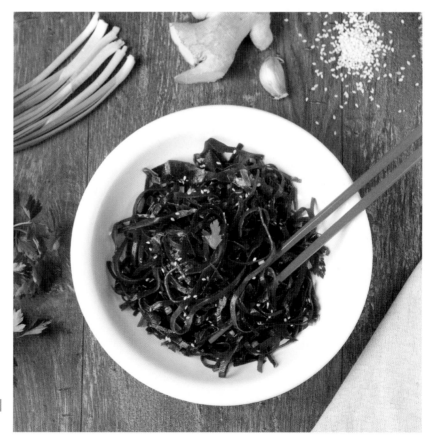

MACRONUTRIENTS (per serving)				
Fat	Protein	Carbs	Fiber	Energy
15.5g	7g	5g	3.5g	182 cal
74%	15%	11%		

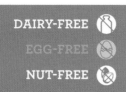

DAIRY-FREE

EGG-FREE

NUT-FREE

Superfood
Buddha Bowl

Prep Time: 15 minutes | **Cook Time: 4 minutes**
Yield: 1 serving

Filled with prebiotics and cruciferous veggies, this bowl is a powerful meal for gut health! The recipe makes more tahini sauce than you will need for the bowl—you will use only about one-fifth of the sauce as prepared. Refrigerate the extra sauce and enjoy it on salads, as a dip for vegetables, or over seafood. It will keep for up to a week.

TAHINI SAUCE:

½ cup (4 ounces/115 g) mayonnaise

½ cup (2½ ounces/70 g) tahini

¼ cup (2 fluid ounces/60 ml) freshly squeezed lemon juice

¼ cup (2 fluid ounces/60 ml) olive oil

3 tablespoons filtered water

1 to 3 cloves garlic, to taste

½ teaspoon fine sea salt

½ teaspoon paprika

¼ teaspoon turmeric powder

¼ teaspoon ground black pepper

½ cup (1 ounce/30 g) chopped broccoli florets

3 tablespoons filtered water

1 ounce (28 g) dried wakame seaweed, broken into pieces

1 cup (2 ounces/55 g) shredded iceberg lettuce

¼ cup (1 ounce/28 g) shredded red cabbage

2 tablespoons sugar–free sauerkraut

¼ avocado, peeled and sliced

2 medium radishes, thinly sliced

1 tablespoon chopped fresh cilantro

¼ teaspoon sesame seeds

1. Make the sauce: Place the mayonnaise, tahini, lemon juice, olive oil, 3 tablespoons of water, and garlic in a blender and blend until smooth. Add the salt and spices and blend to combine. Set aside.

2. Bring a saucepan of water to a boil over high heat. Add the broccoli, then turn off the heat. Leave the broccoli in the hot water for 3 to 4 minutes, until the broccoli is bright green. Drain, then plunge into a bowl of ice water to stop the cooking. When chilled, drain again and set aside.

3. Meanwhile, place 3 tablespoons of water in a bowl with the dried wakame and let it sit for 5 to 6 minutes to rehydrate. Drain the wakame well.

4. In a bowl, arrange the shredded lettuce as a bed; top with the cabbage, sauerkraut, avocado, radishes, and wakame. Sprinkle with the cilantro and sesame seeds. Drizzle with one-fifth of the tahini sauce.

note

This salad will keep in the refrigerator for up to 4 days.

MACRONUTRIENTS
(per serving)

Fat	Protein	Carbs	Fiber	Energy
36.8g	7.8g	13.6g	10g	418 cal
79%	8%	13%		

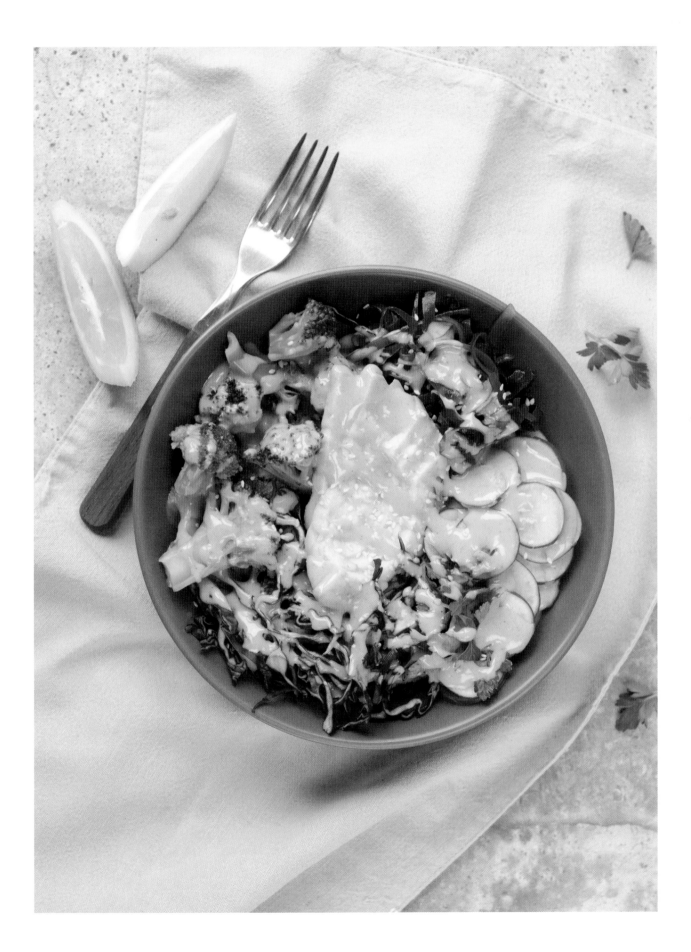

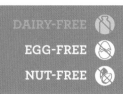

French Onion Soup
with Keto Croutons

Prep Time: **10 minutes** | Cook Time: **35 minutes**
Yield: **4 servings**

There's nothing warmer and more comforting in winter than a bowl of hot French onion soup with caramelized onions. Enjoy this version with keto "croutons"!

¾ cup (6 ounces/170 g) salted butter

½ cup (3 ounces/80 g) sliced yellow onions

¼ cup (1½ ounces/40 g) sliced green onions

1 teaspoon erythritol, or 2 to 4 drops liquid stevia

2 cloves garlic, minced

⅛ teaspoon guar gum or xanthan gum

4 cups (32 fluid ounces/1 L) beef bone broth

1 tablespoon apple cider vinegar

1 to 2 sprigs fresh thyme

1 bay leaf

½ teaspoon fine sea salt

¼ teaspoon ground black pepper

2 (1¾-ounce/50–g) packages pork rinds

½ cup (4 ounces/115 g) shredded Gruyère cheese

½ cup (2 ounces/55 g) grated Parmesan cheese

1. In a medium saucepan over medium-low heat, melt the butter. Add the yellow and green onions and cook for 8 to 10 minutes, until translucent. Add the erythritol and continue to cook, stirring frequently with a wooden spoon, until the onions brown, about 5 minutes.

2. Add the garlic and guar gum and blend well, then add the broth, vinegar, thyme, bay leaf, salt, and pepper. Cover and simmer on low heat for about 20 minutes.

3. Meanwhile, preheat the broiler. Cut each pork rind into 3 or 4 "croutons."

4. Divide the broth between 4 ovenproof bowls. Cover each bowl with one-quarter of the pork rinds and 2 tablespoons of each of the cheeses. Broil until the cheese is melted.

MACRONUTRIENTS
(per serving)

Fat	Protein	Carbs	Fiber	Energy
48.8g	33.5g	5.8g	0.5g	589 cal
74%	22%	4%		

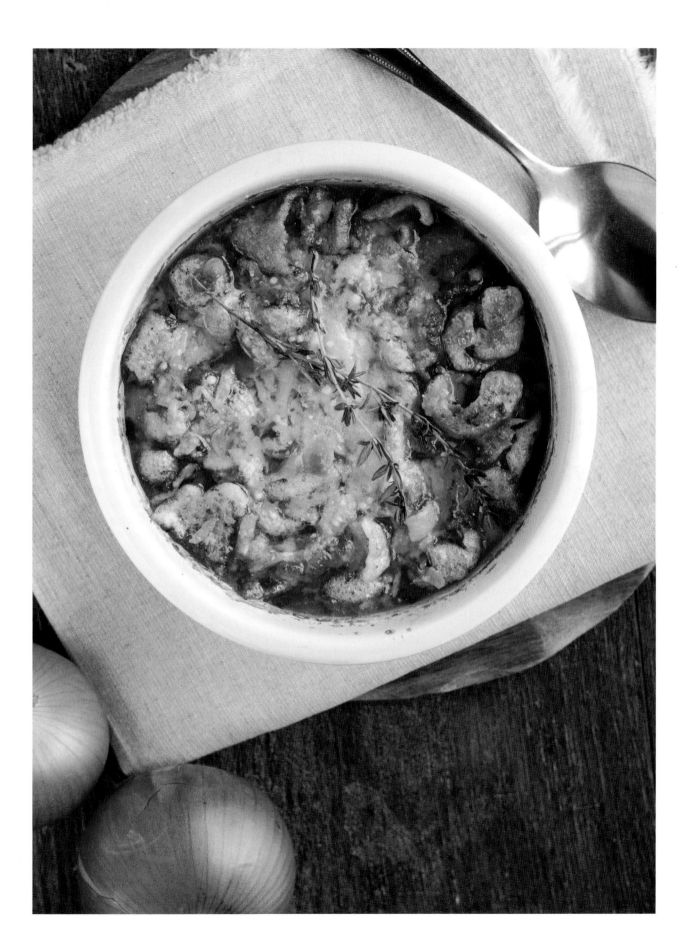

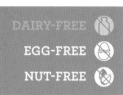

DAIRY-FREE

EGG-FREE

NUT-FREE

Lobster Bisque

Prep Time: **10 minutes** | Cook Time: **1 hour**
Yield: **4 servings**

One of the first recipes I was excited to re-create when I first started working with ketogenic ingredients was lobster bisque. It was a dish that I'd always loved to order at restaurants; it seemed so indulgent and rich. Lobster bisque is wonderful for entertaining; it will delight and impress your guests.

8 ounces (225 g) precooked lobster meat (fresh lump or frozen, or canned lobster tails, precooked and frozen or fresh and uncooked)

½ cup (4 ounces/115 g) unsalted butter

1 medium tomato, coarsely chopped

½ cup (4 ounces/115 g) chopped celery

½ cup (1.3 ounces/40 g) chopped white or brown mushrooms

¼ cup (1.3 ounces/40 g) chopped yellow onions

¼ cup (1 ounce/30 g) sliced green onions

1 clove garlic, minced

2 cups (16 fluid ounces/480 ml) seafood or chicken bone broth

1 tablespoon chopped fresh tarragon

1 sprig thyme

1 bay leaf

½ teaspoon fine sea salt

¼ teaspoon ground black pepper

¼ teaspoon cayenne pepper

1 cup (8 fluid ounces/240 ml) heavy whipping cream

1 tablespoon apple cider vinegar

2 to 4 drops liquid stevia (optional)

¼ cup (2 fluid ounces/60 ml) olive oil

1. If you are using frozen precooked lobster tails, defrost the tails by placing them in a colander and running cold water over them. When the tails are defrosted, drain and remove the meat from the shells.

2. Melt the butter in a medium saucepan over medium-low heat. Add the tomato, celery, mushrooms, yellow and green onions, and garlic. Cook, stirring occasionally, until softened, 8 to 10 minutes.

3. Add the broth and bring to a boil over high heat. Add the tarragon, thyme, bay leaf, salt, black pepper, and cayenne. Lower the heat and simmer for 10 to 12 minutes to allow the flavors to meld.

4. If you are using fresh uncooked lobster tails, fill a stockpot about half full with water and bring to a boil over high heat. Add the tails and simmer for 10 to 12 minutes, until they are bright red. Drain and remove the meat from the shells.

5. Pour the soup into a blender, add half of the lobster meat, and blend until smooth. Chop the remaining lobster meat, if desired, and set aside.

6. Strain the blended soup, then pour it back into the saucepan. Add the cream, vinegar, stevia (if using), and remaining lobster meat. Cook on low for 20 to 25 minutes to allow the flavors to meld.

7. To serve, divide the soup between 4 bowls and drizzle each bowl with 1 tablespoon of olive oil.

MACRONUTRIENTS
(per serving)

Fat	Protein	Carbs	Fiber	Energy
51.5g	17.5g	7.5g	1.5g	575 cal
82%	13%	5%		

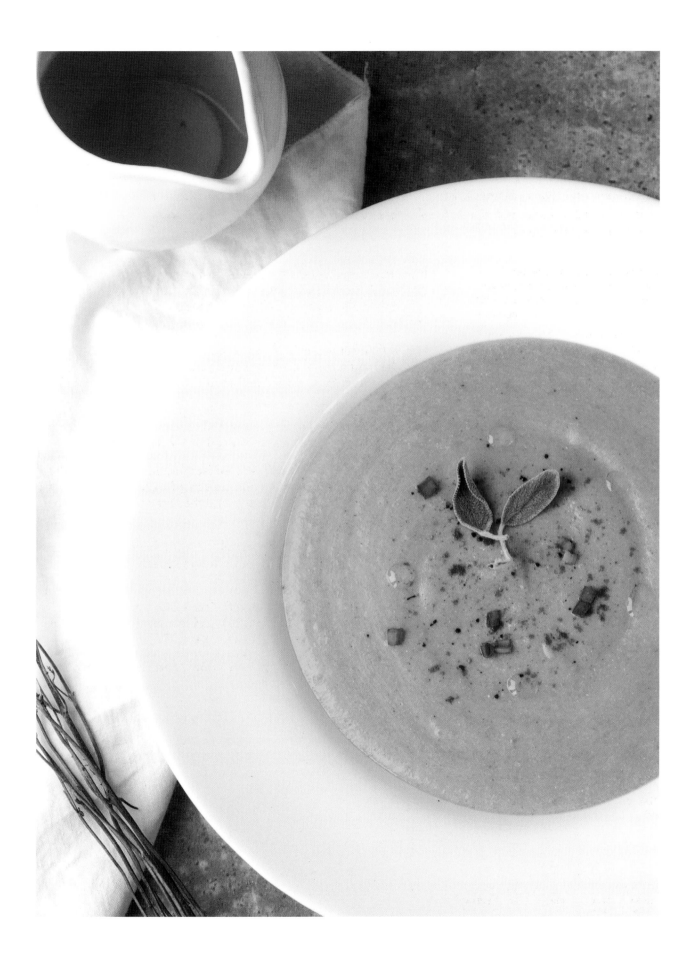

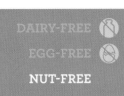

DAIRY-FREE

EGG-FREE

NUT-FREE

Keto "Kulajda" Dill and
Poached Egg Soup

Prep Time: **10 minutes** | Cook Time: **1 hour 20 minutes**
Yield: **4 servings**

My husband introduced me to this fantastic creamy Czech soup made with soft-poached eggs. I love the combination of dill and lemon, so I was enthusiastic to try it. The soup is made with foraged wild mushrooms—and mushroom foraging is practically a Czech national sport! This comforting soup traditionally has a potato base, but I have replaced the potatoes with low-carb cauliflower, and the result is just as creamy as the original. I am so excited to share this beautiful Czech dish with you.

¼ cup plus 2 tablespoons (3 ounces/85 g) salted butter

1 small head (about 10½ ounces/ 300 g) cauliflower, diced

¼ cup (1.3 ounces/40 g) finely chopped yellow onions or thinly sliced green onions

2 quarts (64 fluid ounces/2 L) filtered water

7 ounces (200 g) fresh wild porcini mushrooms, or 1 ounce (25 g) dried wild porcini mushrooms, cleaned and sliced

4 sprigs fresh dill, plus more for garnish

2 bay leaves

1 teaspoon ground cumin

1 teaspoon fine sea salt

1 tablespoon coconut flour, or ½ teaspoon guar gum or xanthan gum

1 cup (8 ounces/225 g) sour cream

1 tablespoon freshly squeezed lemon juice

4 eggs

1 tablespoon apple cider vinegar or white wine vinegar

¼ teaspoon ground black pepper

1. In a large saucepan over low heat, melt the butter. Add the cauliflower and onions and cook for 5 to 6 minutes, until the onions are translucent.

2. Add the water, mushrooms, dill, bay leaves, cumin, and salt. Bring to a boil over high heat, then reduce the heat to low and simmer for about 1 hour to thicken the soup.

3. In a mixing bowl, whisk the coconut flour into the sour cream. Stir in the lemon juice. Add this mixture to the soup and whisk until well combined, then turn off the heat.

4. Poach the eggs: Bring some water to a boil in a small saucepan. Meanwhile, crack an egg into a small bowl. When the water is boiling, remove the saucepan from the heat and use a spoon to swirl the water clockwise around the pan. Slide the egg into the "whirlpool" you created in the pan. Poach for 3 to 4 minutes, until the white is set. Spoon out the egg and keep warm in a warm water bath while you repeat with the remaining eggs.

5. Using an immersion blender, blend the soup to a creamy consistency. Add the vinegar and pepper and combine well.

6. Divide the soup between 4 serving bowls. Serve hot with one poached egg per bowl, garnished with fresh dill.

note

If you can't find porcini mushrooms, feel free to substitute another type. The soup will still be delicious!

MACRONUTRIENTS
(per serving)

Fat	Protein	Carbs	Fiber	Energy
31g	10.8g	9g	5g	116 cal
78%	12%	10%		

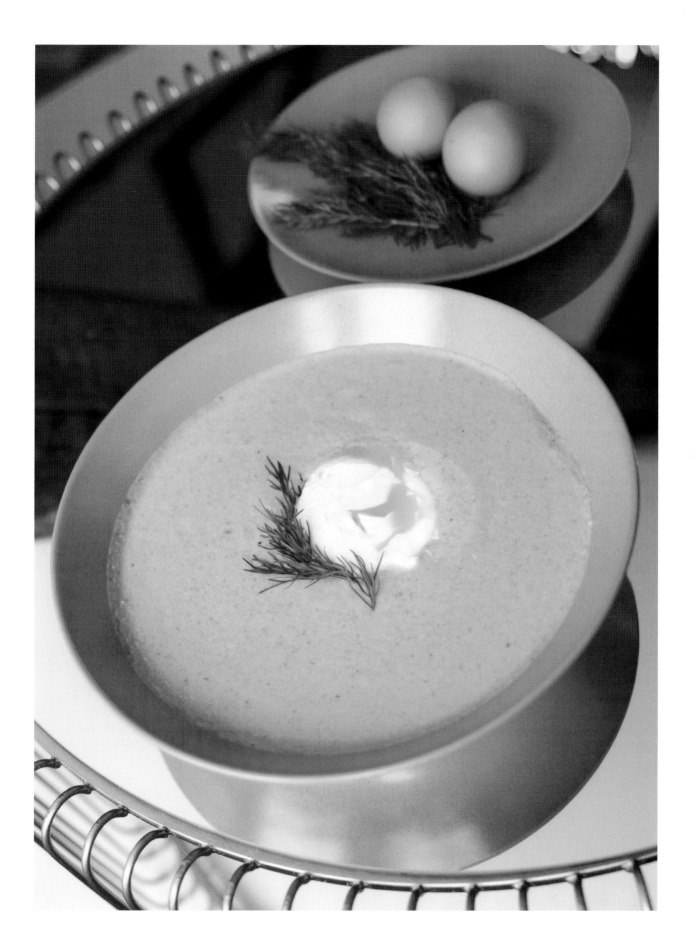

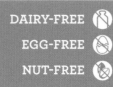

DAIRY-FREE

EGG-FREE

NUT-FREE

Tom Yum Koong
(Thai Shrimp Soup)

Prep Time: **10 minutes** | Cook Time: **1 hour 5 minutes**
Yield: **4 servings**

This soup is so delicious, I could eat it every night! It is creamy, satisfying, and filling. This version of the Thai classic features shrimp instead of chicken. To make it a full meal, add some shirataki noodles.

5 cups (40 fluid ounces/1.2 L) chicken bone broth

2 (1- to 2-inch/2.5- to 5-cm) pieces galangal, sliced

2 shallots, sliced

2 stalks lemon grass, sliced

6 kaffir lime leaves

6 white mushrooms, sliced

24 medium-sized raw shrimp, thawed if frozen, peeled and deveined

3 cups (24 ounces/680 g) coconut cream (see note, page 108)

1 red chili pepper, sliced in half lengthwise (optional)

1 tablespoon freshly squeezed lime or lemon juice

1 tablespoon fish sauce

2 to 4 drops liquid stevia, to taste

¼ cup (1 ounce/30 g) fresh cilantro leaves

1. Bring the broth and galangal to a boil in a medium saucepan over high heat. Reduce the heat to a simmer and cook until the broth absorbs the flavor of the galangal, 25 to 30 minutes.

2. Add the shallots, lemon grass, and lime leaves. Reduce the heat to medium-low and add the mushrooms; simmer for 20 to 30 minutes, until the mushrooms are tender.

3. Add the shrimp, coconut cream, chili pepper (if using), lime juice, fish sauce, and stevia. Simmer for 4 to 5 minutes more, until the shrimp is cooked and the flavors are well combined. Remove from the heat and top with the cilantro.

tip

Galangal is a root similar to ginger; you can find it at most markets and at Asian food stores.

MACRONUTRIENTS
(per serving)

Fat	Protein	Carbs	Fiber	Energy
32g	17.5g	6.3g	0g	382 cal
75%	18%	7%		

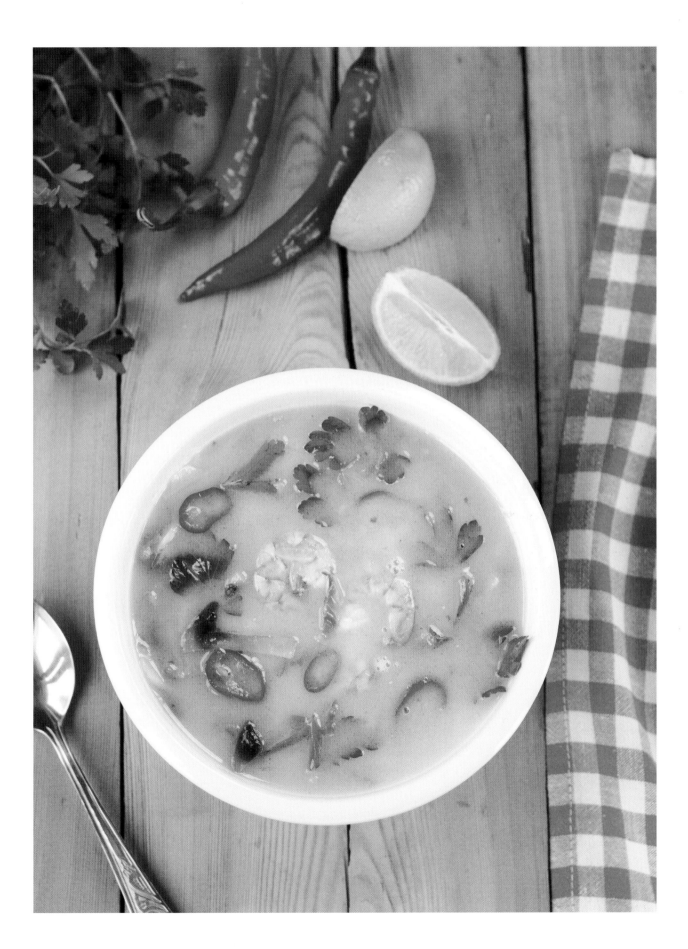

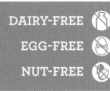

DAIRY-FREE

EGG-FREE

NUT-FREE

Tom Kha Gai
(Thai Chicken Coconut Soup)

Prep Time: **10 minutes** | Cook Time: **55 minutes**
Yield: **4 servings**

This creamy soup is the quintessential Thai soup. Thai cuisine makes the most of fragrant spices and incorporates saturated fat-filled coconut milk in wonderful ways, and this soup is no exception. It features the full spectrum of what makes Thai food so tasty—sweet, sour, salty, and spicy flavors. The first time I tried Tom Kha Gai was in Bangkok, and it quickly became a dish that I had to master at home so that I could enjoy it regularly.

5 cups (40 fluid ounces/1.2 L) chicken bone broth

2 (1- to 2-inch/2.5- to 5-cm) pieces galangal, sliced

2 shallots, sliced

2 stalks lemon grass

8 kaffir lime leaves

6 ounces (170 g) boneless, skinless chicken breast, thinly sliced

8 ounces (225 g) white mushrooms, sliced

4 cups (32 ounces/1 L) coconut cream (see note, page 108)

10 cherry tomatoes, halved

1 red chili pepper, sliced in half lengthwise (optional)

1 tablespoon freshly squeezed lime juice

1 tablespoon fish sauce

2 to 4 drops liquid stevia, to taste

¼ cup (1 ounce/30 g) fresh cilantro leaves

1. Bring the broth and galangal to a boil in a medium saucepan over high heat. Reduce the heat to a simmer and cook until the broth absorbs the flavor of the galangal, 25 to 30 minutes.

2. Add the shallots, lemon grass, and lime leaves. Reduce the heat to medium-low and add the chicken and mushrooms; simmer for 15 to 20 minutes, until the chicken is cooked.

3. Add the coconut cream, tomatoes, chili pepper (if using), lime juice, fish sauce, and stevia. Cook for 4 to 5 minutes more, until the flavors are well combined. Remove from the heat and top with the cilantro.

tip

You can make this soup with shrimp instead of chicken (see Tom Yum Koong, page 186), which is equally delicious. To make it a full meal, add some shirataki noodles.

MACRONUTRIENTS
(per serving)

Fat	Protein	Carbs	Fiber	Energy
42g	20g	10g	2g	486 cal
76%	16%	8%		

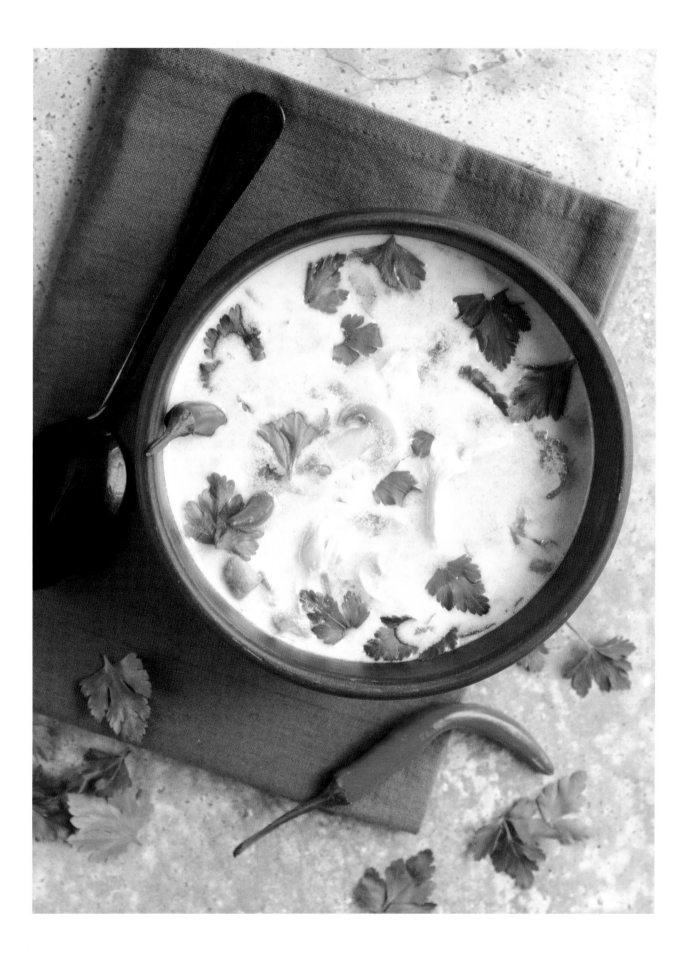

Chapter 10
Noodles & Rice

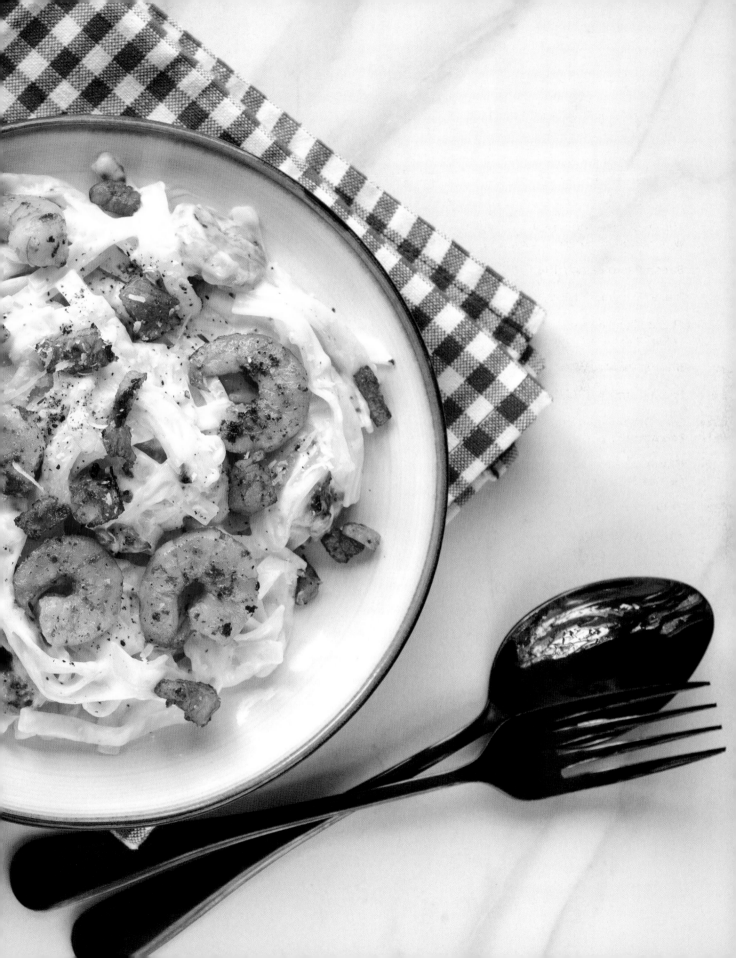

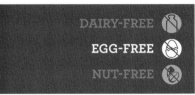

DAIRY-FREE

EGG-FREE

NUT-FREE

Three-Cheese Macaroni
with Bacon au Gratin

Prep Time: 15 minutes | **Cook Time:** 15 minutes
Yield: 4 servings

This recipe uses a French sauce called béchamel as a base, but substitutes keto-friendly al-mond flour for the traditional all-purpose flour. Just like the quick and easy boxed version, this dish is made entirely on the stovetop, although there is a short broiling step to get the top brown and delicious. If you can't find macaroni-style shirataki noodles, use the fettuc-cine style and cut them into 1-inch (2.5-cm) pieces.

4 (7-ounce/200-g) packages macaroni-style zero-carb shirataki noodles

6 slices bacon

¾ cup (6 ounces/170 g) unsalted butter

¼ cup plus 2 tablespoons (1½ ounces/40 g) almond flour

1 cup (8 fluid ounces/240 ml) almond milk, warmed

1 cup (8 ounces/230 g) shredded Gruyère cheese

½ cup (4 ounces/115 g) shredded cheddar cheese

1 teaspoon onion powder

½ teaspoon coarse sea salt

¼ teaspoon ground nutmeg

¼ cup (1 ounce/28 g) grated Parmesan cheese

1. Rinse and drain the noodles. In a saucepan over high heat, boil the noodles in water for 1 to 2 minutes. Drain and set on paper towels to absorb the excess water.

2. In a medium skillet over medium heat, fry the bacon for 4 to 5 minutes, until medium crisp; remove to a cutting board to cool. Slice or crumble the bacon into rough bits and set aside.

3. In a medium saucepan over medium-low heat, melt the butter. Add the almond flour and stir to combine. Continue to cook, stirring frequently, for 1 to 2 minutes, until well combined and smooth and starting to bubble lightly.

4. Slowly pour in the almond milk, combining well with a whisk.

5. Add the Gruyère and cheddar and stir until just melted, then remove from the heat. Stir in the onion powder, salt, and nutmeg.

6. In a bowl, combine the noodles and sauce. Divide the sauced noodles between 4 individual oven-safe ramekins or 1 large baking dish. Top evenly with the Parmesan.

7. Set the oven to broil and broil the macaroni for 3 to 4 minutes, until a browned crust forms. Top with the crumbled bacon before serving.

tip

You can find zero-carb shirataki noodles at health-food stores or on-line.

MACRONUTRIENTS
(per serving)

Fat	Protein	Carbs	Fiber	Energy
58.5g	21g	4.8g	3g	622 cal
84%	13%	3%		

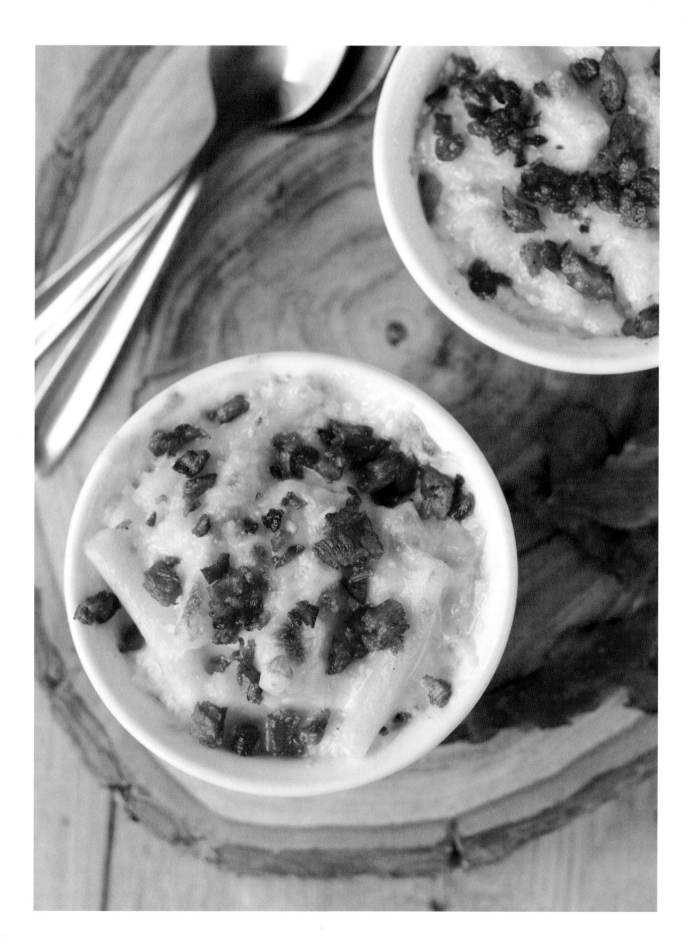

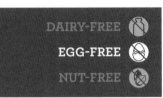

DAIRY-FREE

EGG-FREE

NUT-FREE

Bacon Pesto Pasta

Prep Time: 10 minutes | **Cook Time: 8 minutes**
Yield: 1 serving

This is one of the easiest recipes I have written, requiring only a handful of ingredients and only 20 minutes from start to finish. You will need only half of the pesto; save the rest for use as a dip, a topper for eggs, a condiment for burgers, or anything that needs a little pizzazz. Pesto is traditionally made with basil, pine nuts, Parmesan cheese, and olive oil, but I've updated the recipe with power-packed MCT oil and kale for antioxidants and vitamin C. If you like a creamier, even cheesier pesto, use cashews along with or instead of the pine nuts.

This is a super-keto recipe, with the MCT oil generating fat-burning ketones and the macro-nutrient percentages being on target. It is delicious and extremely satiating for all-day fuel. Warning: You may not be able to finish it all!

1 (7-ounce/200-g) package angel hair–style or other long zero-carb shirataki noodles

6 slices bacon

PESTO:

1 cup (1 ounce/30 g) fresh basil leaves

½ cup (1 ounce/35 g) stemmed and chopped fresh kale

½ cup (2½ ounces/70 g) pine nuts or raw cashews

½ cup (4 fluid ounces/120 ml) MCT oil

1½ tablespoons grated Parmesan cheese

1 clove garlic, or ¼ teaspoon garlic powder (see note)

½ teaspoon fine sea salt

Ground black pepper, to taste

FOR GARNISH:

1½ teaspoons grated or shaved Parmesan cheese

Toasted pine nuts

1. Rinse and drain the noodles. In a saucepan over high heat, boil the noodles in water for 1 to 2 minutes. Drain and set on paper towels to absorb the excess water.

2. In a medium skillet over medium heat, fry the bacon for 3 to 4 minutes, until cooked but not crispy. Chop into ½-inch (1.25-cm) pieces.

3. Place the pesto ingredients in a food processor and process until fully combined and smooth.

4. Add the noodles to the skillet with the bacon and cook over medium heat for 1 to 2 minutes to remove any remaining moisture. Add half of the pesto to the pan and mix well; reserve the remainder for another use. Plate the sauced noodles and garnish with Parmesan and toasted pine nuts.

note

If you like a strong garlic flavor, add raw garlic to the pesto. If you prefer a milder flavor, use garlic powder. You can also add sautéed kale to this dish.

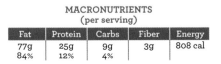

MACRONUTRIENTS
(per serving)

Fat	Protein	Carbs	Fiber	Energy
77g	25g	9g	3g	808 cal
84%	12%	4%		

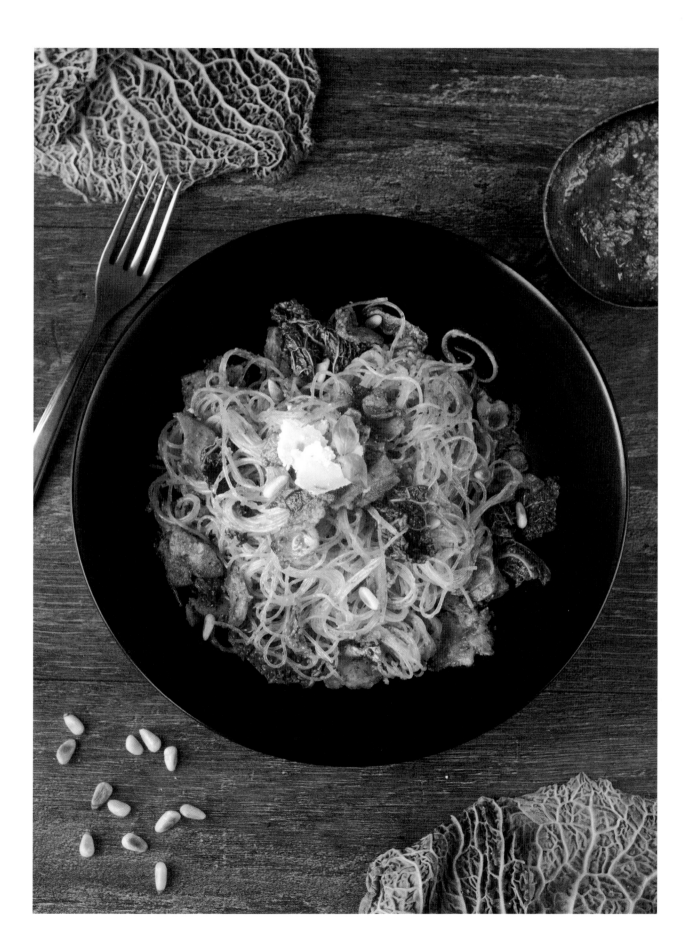

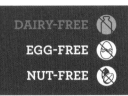

DAIRY-FREE

EGG-FREE

NUT-FREE

Pasta Bolognese

Prep Time: 10 minutes | **Cook Time:** 20 minutes
Yield: 4 servings

I like to serve this Bolognese on shirataki noodles. You can also serve it over shredded green cabbage or zucchini noodles.

5 slices bacon

4 (7-ounce/200-g) packages spaghetti-style zero-carb shirataki noodles

5 ounces (140 g) ground beef

5 ounces (140 g) ground pork

½ cup (4 ounces/115 g) butter

¼ cup chopped onions

1 clove garlic, minced

1 medium tomato, chopped

1 tablespoon chopped fresh parsley, plus more for garnish

1 tablespoon dried marjoram leaves

1 tablespoon dried oregano leaves

½ teaspoon fine sea salt

¼ teaspoon ground black pepper

2 tablespoons grated Parmesan cheese, for garnish

1. In a medium skillet over medium heat, fry the bacon for 3 to 4 minutes, until cooked but not crispy. Remove from the pan and set aside, leaving the bacon fat in the pan.

2. Rinse and drain the noodles. In a saucepan over high heat, boil the noodles in water for 1 to 2 minutes. Drain and set on paper towels to absorb the excess water.

3. In the skillet you used to cook the bacon, brown the ground beef and pork, breaking apart the meat with a wooden spoon as it cooks, 7 to 8 minutes.

4. In a saucepan over medium heat, melt the butter. Add the onions and garlic and sauté until lightly cooked, 3 to 4 minutes. Add the tomato and stir to combine.

5. Add the ground meat and bacon to the onion mixture and mix together. Add the parsley, marjoram, oregano, salt, and pepper and stir again. Simmer for 5 minutes to warm through.

6. Serve the sauce over the noodles, sprinkled with the Parmesan and chopped parsley.

MACRONUTRIENTS
(per serving)

Fat	Protein	Carbs	Fiber	Energy
47.8g	28g	5.3g	2.3g	563 cal
76%	20%	4%		

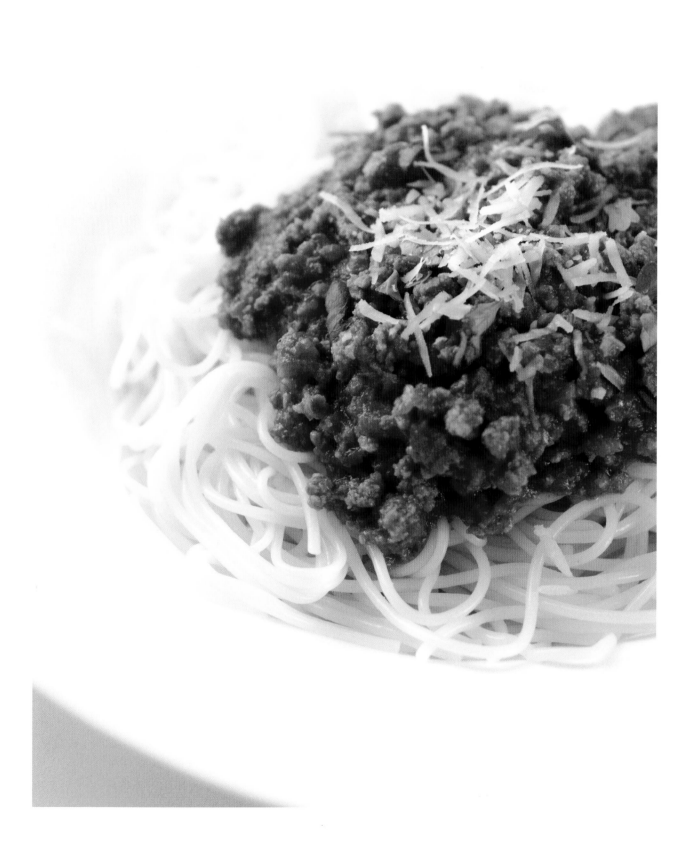

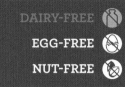

DAIRY-FREE

EGG-FREE

NUT-FREE

Fettuccine Alfredo
with Grilled Shrimp

Prep Time: 20 minutes | **Cook Time:** 15 minutes
Yield: 4 servings

My favorite Italian dish has always been fettuccine Alfredo. Between the rich cream and the decadent noodles, I always thought of it as an excessively indulgent dish, to be ordered once a year on a special occasion—if that. With zero-carb shirataki noodles, however, you can enjoy this rich and creamy dish without guilt.

4 (7-ounce/200-g) packages fettuccine-style zero-carb shirataki noodles

2 ounces (55 g) pancetta, diced

½ cup (4 ounces/115 g) butter

1 (8-ounce/225-g) package cream cheese

1 cup (8 fluid ounces/240 ml) heavy whipping cream

½ cup plus 2 tablespoons (2½ ounces/70 g) grated Parmesan cheese, divided

2 cloves garlic, minced

½ teaspoon fine sea salt

¼ teaspoon ground black pepper

20 large uncooked frozen or fresh shrimp, thawed, peeled, and deveined

1. Rinse and drain the noodles. In a saucepan over high heat, boil the noodles in water for 1 to 2 minutes. Drain and set on paper towels to absorb the excess water.

2. Place the noodles a cutting board and chop into 1-inch (2.5-cm) segments.

3. In a skillet over medium heat, fry the pancetta for 3 to 4 minutes, until cooked but not crisp. Slide the pan off the heat.

4. In a saucepan over low heat, melt the butter. Add the cream cheese, heavy cream, ½ cup of the Parmesan, garlic, salt, and pepper. Cook, stirring frequently, until the sauce starts to bubble; remove from the heat and cover to keep warm.

5. Return the pan with the pancetta to the stovetop over medium-low heat. Add the shrimp to the pan and cook for 2 to 3 minutes, until the shrimp is bright pink, being careful not to overcook. Remove from the heat.

6. Add the noodles to the Alfredo sauce and mix until the noodles are well coated. Divide between 4 plates. Top each plate with one-quarter of the pancetta and shrimp, then sprinkle each plate with 1½ teaspoons of the remaining Parmesan.

MACRONUTRIENTS
(per serving)

Fat	Protein	Carbs	Fiber	Energy
54.5g	22.8g	4.5g	4g	574 cal
82%	15%	3%		

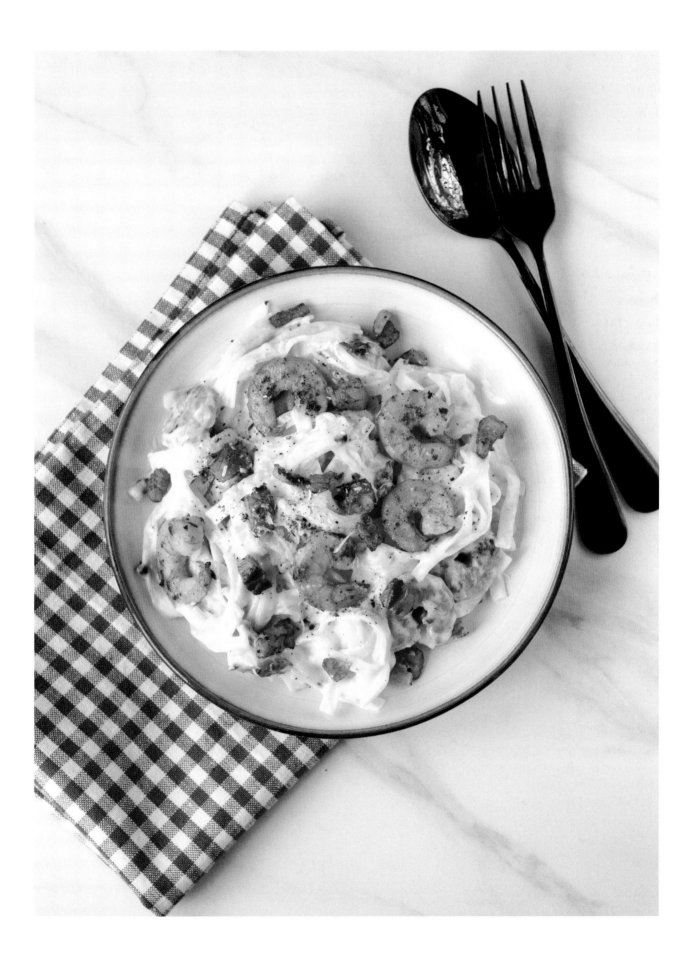

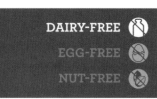

DAIRY-FREE

EGG-FREE

NUT-FREE

Shrimp Pad Thai

Prep Time: 20 minutes | Cook Time: 12 minutes
Yield: 2 servings

If I had to eat just one thing for the rest of my life, it would probably be Pad Thai. I've always loved this dish—especially when it comes from an open-air market in Bangkok, fresh and hot out of a wok and served in banana leaves and wrapped in newspaper. This recipe re-creates all those creamy, nutty, tangy, tart, sour, sweet, and spicy flavors without the palm sugar and tamarind in the original dish.

1 tablespoon coconut oil

2 eggs, whisked

½ cup (3½ ounces/100 g) mung beans, rinsed and drained

12 uncooked medium to large shrimp, thawed if frozen, peeled and deveined

2 (7-ounce/200-g) packages fettuccine-style zero-carb shirataki noodles

1 tablespoon crushed almonds

1 tablespoon chopped fresh cilantro

1 tablespoon sliced green onions

PAD THAI SAUCE:

2 tablespoons unsweetened almond butter

2 tablespoons coconut oil

2 tablespoons mayonnaise

2 tablespoons tahini

2 tablespoons tamari

1 tablespoon freshly squeezed lime juice

2 teaspoons fish sauce

½ teaspoon ginger juice, or 1 teaspoon grated fresh ginger

½ teaspoon liquid stevia (optional)

¼ teaspoon hot sauce, or a pinch of cayenne pepper

1 teaspoon granulated stevia or erythritol

½ teaspoon fine sea salt

¼ teaspoon garlic powder

1. In a small skillet over medium heat, melt 1 tablespoon of coconut oil. Add the eggs and cook through to make a thin omelet. Remove from the pan and set aside to cool. When cool, slice into thin ribbons.

2. In the same skillet over medium heat, fry the mung beans for 2 to 3 minutes. Add the shrimp and cook for 2 to 3 minutes, until bright pink and cooked through, being careful not to overcook.

3. Rinse and drain the noodles. In a saucepan over high heat, boil the noodles in water for 1 to 2 minutes. Drain the noodles and set on paper towels to absorb the excess water.

4. Put all the ingredients for the sauce in a food processor and process until well combined. Combine the noodles with the sauce.

5. Divide the sauced noodles between 2 plates. Top each plate with half of the egg ribbons, beans, shrimp, almonds, cilantro, and onions.

MACRONUTRIENTS
(per serving)

Fat	Protein	Carbs	Fiber	Energy
69.5g	27g	12.5g	5.5g	780 cal
80%	14%	6%		

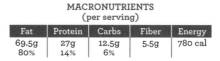

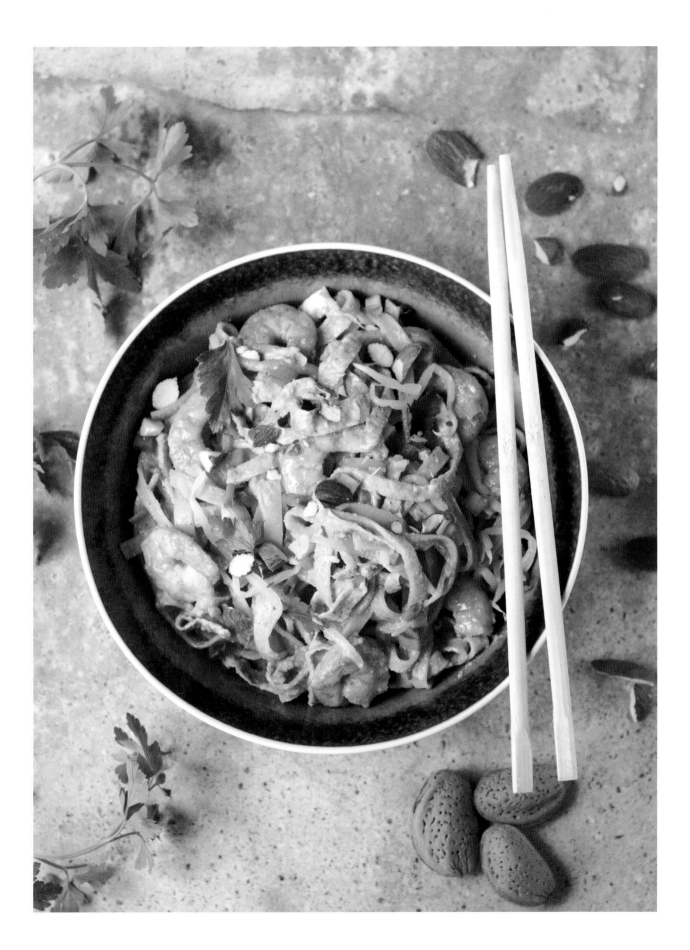

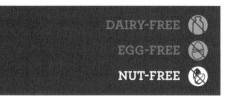

DAIRY-FREE

EGG-FREE

NUT-FREE

Pasta Carbonara

Prep Time: 5 minutes | Cook Time: 12 minutes
Yield: 4 servings

With zero-carb noodles, you can enjoy the rich and creamy flavor of this dish anytime.
Because the eggs don't fully cook in the hot sauce, it's important to use pasteurized eggs in
this recipe.

4 (7-ounce/200-g) packages
fettuccine-style zero-carb
shirataki noodles

6 egg yolks from pasteurized eggs

4 tablespoons (1 ounce/28 g)
grated Parmesan cheese, divided

½ teaspoon coarse sea salt

¼ teaspoon ground black pepper

¼ cup plus 2 tablespoons (3
ounces/85 g) butter or MCT oil,
divided

8 ounces (225 g) pancetta, diced

2 cloves garlic, peeled and
smashed (see note)

1 to 2 tablespoons filtered water

1. Rinse and drain the noodles. In a saucepan over high heat, boil the
   noodles in water for 1 to 2 minutes. Drain and set on paper towels
   to absorb the excess water.

2. In a bowl, whisk together the egg yolks, 3 tablespoons of the
   Parmesan, salt, and pepper. Set aside.

3. In a skillet over medium heat, heat 1 tablespoon of the butter. Add
   the pancetta and fry for 1 to 2 minutes. Add the garlic and sauté for
   about 1 minute, until fragrant. Add the remaining 5 tablespoons
   (2½ ounces/70 g) of butter and cook for 4 to 5 minutes, until the
   flavors are well absorbed. Remove the garlic cloves from the pan.

4. Add the noodles to the skillet and toss to coat. Remove from the
   heat and add 1 tablespoon of water, then pour in the egg yolk
   mixture. Gently but rapidly toss together the noodles and sauce,
   allowing the residual heat from the pan to gently cook the sauce
   without scrambling the eggs. If desired, add another 1 tablespoon
   of water to thin the sauce and make it smoother.

5. Divide the pasta between 4 bowls and top with the remaining 1
   tablespoon of Parmesan. Garnish with more pepper, if desired.

note

To smash garlic, lay the peeled cloves on a flat surface, such as your
kitchen counter. Lay the flat side of a chef's knife or other large knife
across the garlic. Use the edge of your fist to smack the top of the knife,
smashing the garlic.

| | MACRONUTRIENTS | | | |
| | (per serving) | | | |
Fat	Protein	Carbs	Fiber	Energy
41.3g	19.8g	4.8g	2g	469 cal
79%	17%	4%		

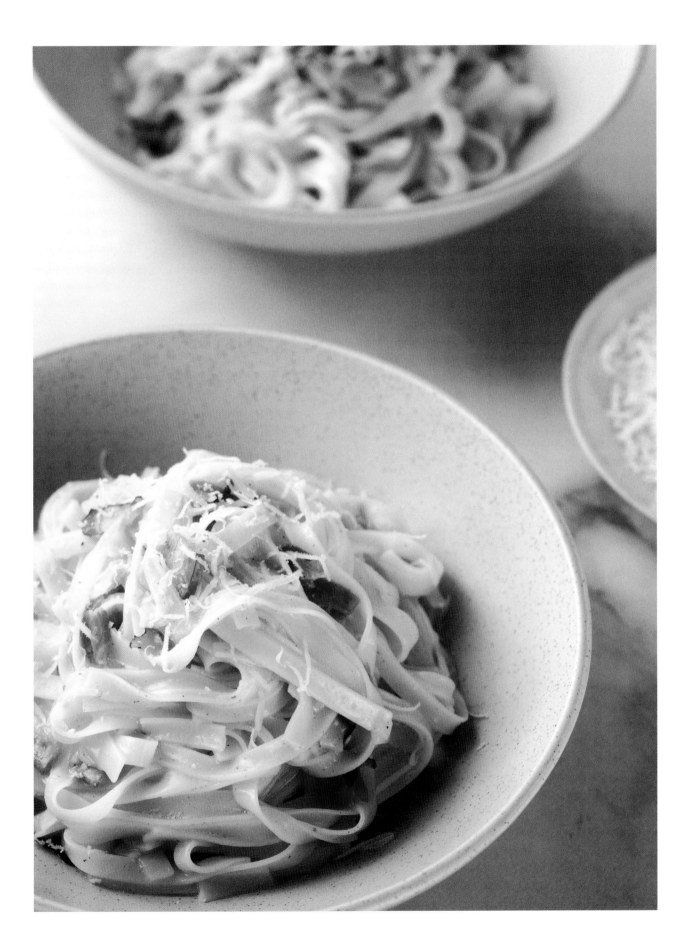

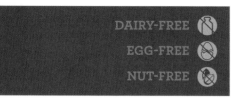

DAIRY-FREE

EGG-FREE

NUT-FREE

Sun-Dried Tomato
Fettuccine

Prep Time: **10 minutes** | Cook Time: **10 minutes**
Yield: **4 servings**

This is one of the most delicious pastas—and very filling! Use fettuccine-style shirataki noodles or omit the pasta altogether and serve the sauce over cooked green cabbage ribbons or zucchini noodles.

4 (7-ounce/200-g) packages fettuccine-style zero-carb shirataki noodles

⅓ cup (2⅔ fluid ounces/80 ml) almond milk

1 (8-ounce/225-g) package cream cheese

½ cup (4 ounces/115 g) mayonnaise

1 cup (5¼ ounces/150 g) crumbled feta cheese

2 ounces (56 g) sun-dried tomatoes in oil, drained

½ teaspoon fine sea salt

¼ teaspoon garlic powder

Cracked black pepper, for garnish (optional)

Red pepper flakes, for garnish (optional)

1. Rinse and drain the noodles. In a saucepan over high heat, boil the noodles in water for 1 to 2 minutes. Drain and set on paper towels to absorb the excess water.

2. If desired, transfer the noodles to a cutting board and chop into 2-inch (5-cm) segments. Set aside.

3. Place the milk, cream cheese, mayonnaise, feta, sun-dried tomatoes, salt, and garlic powder in a food processor and pulse until well combined and creamy.

4. Pour the sauce into a medium saucepan and cook over low heat until warmed through. Add the noodles and mix well.

5. Divide the sauced noodles between 2 plates. Serve topped with cracked black pepper and red pepper flakes, if desired.

MACRONUTRIENTS
(per serving)

Fat	Protein	Carbs	Fiber	Energy
48.8g	10.8g	9.3g	3g	520 cal
85%	8%	7%		

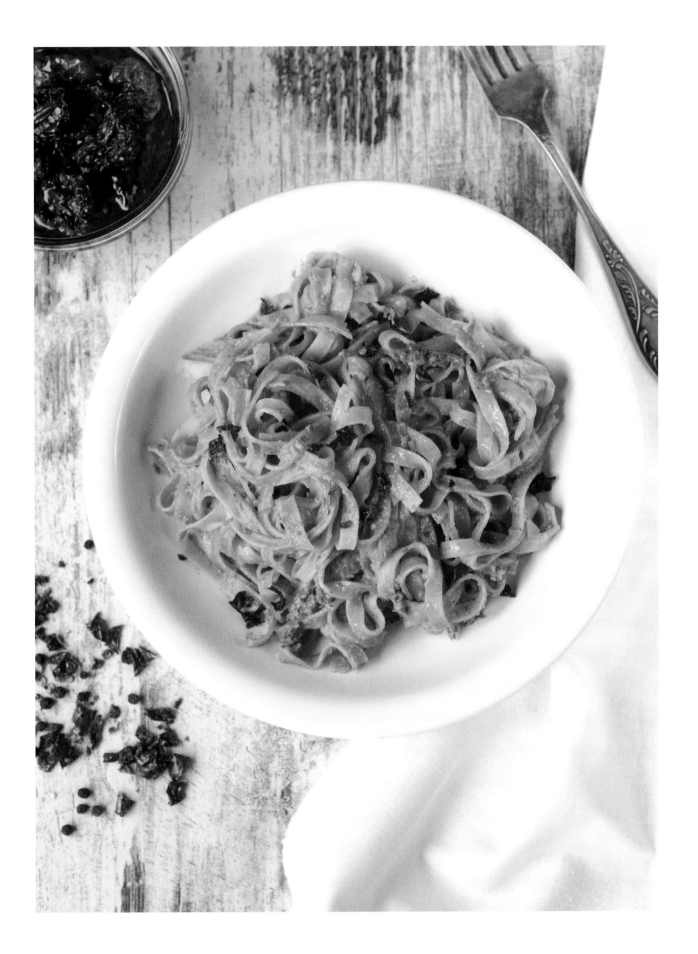

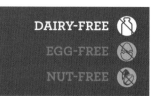

DAIRY-FREE

EGG-FREE

NUT-FREE

White Truffle
Fettuccine Alfredo

Prep Time: 5 minutes | Cook Time: 8 minutes
Yield: 2 servings

Nutritional yeast is one of the healthiest sources of B vitamins and other essential nutri-ents. Truffle is a quintessential Italian flavor. Most health-food stores and Italian food shops stock white truffle oil; I also have found it in small spray bottles on Amazon. A little goes a long way in this dairy-free and very keto take on a classic Italian dish.

DAIRY-FREE CHEESE BLEND:

2 tablespoons raw cashews

2 tablespoons nutritional yeast

½ teaspoon coarse sea salt

¼ teaspoon ground black pepper

¼ teaspoon garlic powder

¼ teaspoon onion powder

2 (7-ounce/200-g) packages fettuccine-style zero-carb shirataki noodles

2 tablespoons butter-flavored coconut oil

¼ cup plus 2 tablespoons (3 ounces/85 g) mayonnaise

2 teaspoons white truffle oil

¼ teaspoon red pepper flakes, for garnish (optional)

1. Make the cheese blend: In a food processor, pulse the cashews and nutritional yeast. Add the salt, pepper, garlic powder, and onion powder and blend well.

2. Rinse and drain the noodles. In a saucepan over high heat, boil the noodles in water for 1 to 2 minutes. Drain and set on paper towels to absorb the excess water.

3. Melt the coconut oil in a saucepan over low heat. Add the mayonnaise and blend well. Add the noodles and stir to combine.

4. Sprinkle the cheese blend over the noodles and stir to combine. Drizzle with the truffle oil.

5. Divide the noodles between 2 plates and sprinkle with the red pepper flakes, if desired.

tip

Although this dish is fabulous on its own, you can add sliced grilled chicken or shrimp to make it a full meal.

	MACRONUTRIENTS (per serving)			
Fat	Protein	Carbs	Fiber	Energy
57g	7g	9g	6g	577 cal
88%	6%	6%		

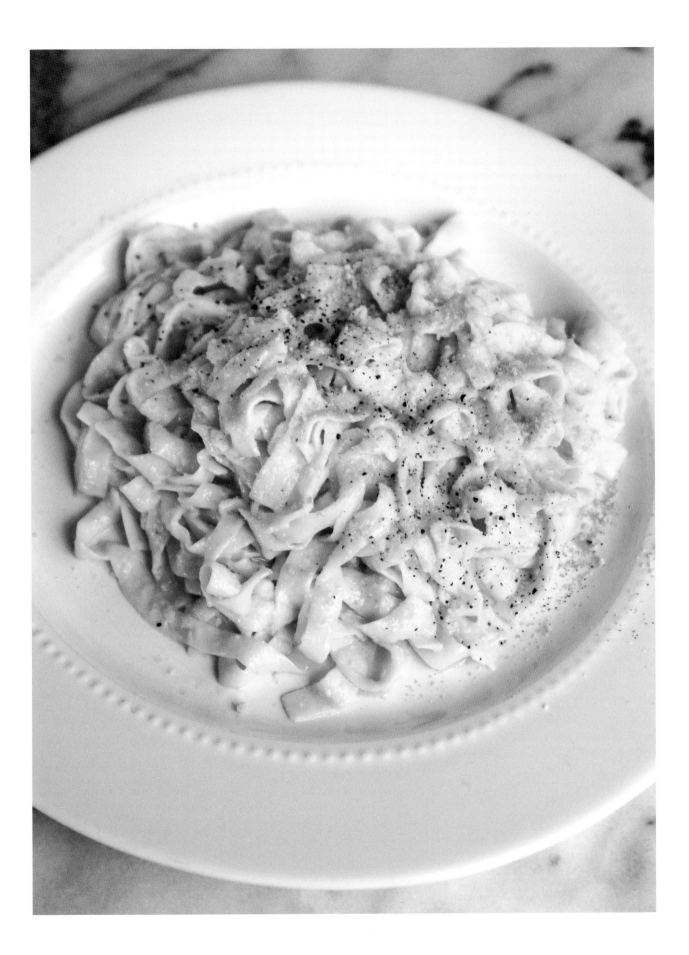

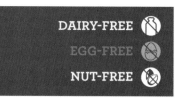

DAIRY-FREE

EGG-FREE

NUT-FREE

Shrimp Fried Rice

Prep Time: 10 minutes | **Cook Time:** 20 minutes
Yield: 4 servings

This easy and tasty low-carb version of restaurant-style fried rice uses cauliflower instead of white rice for a fun and healthy twist. The dish is great on its own or can be paired with Ginger Beef (page 294), Lemon Chicken (page 240), or one of the curry recipes in this book.

2 tablespoons coconut oil, divided

4 egg yolks, whisked

¼ cup (2 fluid ounces/60 ml) light sesame oil

½ cup (2¾ ounces/80 g) chopped French green beans

½ cup (2 ounces/55 g) sliced mushrooms

4 green onions, thinly sliced, plus 1 teaspoon for garnish

1 clove garlic, minced

4 cups (15 ounces/425 g) cauliflower florets, riced (see note)

½ cup (4 fluid ounces/120 ml) chicken bone broth

20 medium shrimp (7 ounces/200 g), thawed if frozen, peeled and deveined

2 ounces (55 g) canned water chestnuts, drained and diced

2 tablespoons apple cider vinegar

2 tablespoons tamari

1 teaspoon ginger juice, or 1 (1–inch/2.5–cm) piece fresh ginger, peeled and grated

3 or 4 drops liquid stevia, or 1 tablespoon erythritol

½ teaspoon fine sea salt

½ teaspoon sesame seeds, for garnish

1. In a small skillet over medium heat, melt 1 tablespoon of the coconut oil. Add the egg yolks and cook through to make a thin omelet. Remove to a cutting board and let cool. When cool, slice into thin ribbons.

2. Heat the sesame oil in a large saucepan or wok over medium heat. Add the green beans, mushrooms, green onions, and garlic and cook for 3 to 4 minutes, until lightly browned.

3. Add the riced cauliflower and stir-fry for a few minutes. Add the broth, shrimp, and water chestnuts and reduce the heat to low. Cover and let steam for 6 to 8 minutes, until the cauliflower has absorbed the liquid.

4. In a bowl, combine the vinegar, tamari, ginger juice, stevia, and salt. Add the tamari mixture to the cauliflower mixture and stir well.

5. Serve the fried rice topped with the green onions, sesame seeds, and cooked egg ribbons.

note

Use a food processor to chop the cauliflower to a ricelike consistency, pulsing the florets until the pieces are rice-sized. Do not use the puree button, or the pieces of cauliflower will become too tiny for this recipe.

MACRONUTRIENTS
(per serving)

Fat	Protein	Carbs	Fiber	Energy
25.8g	15g	8.3g	3.8g	318 cal
72%	18%	10%		

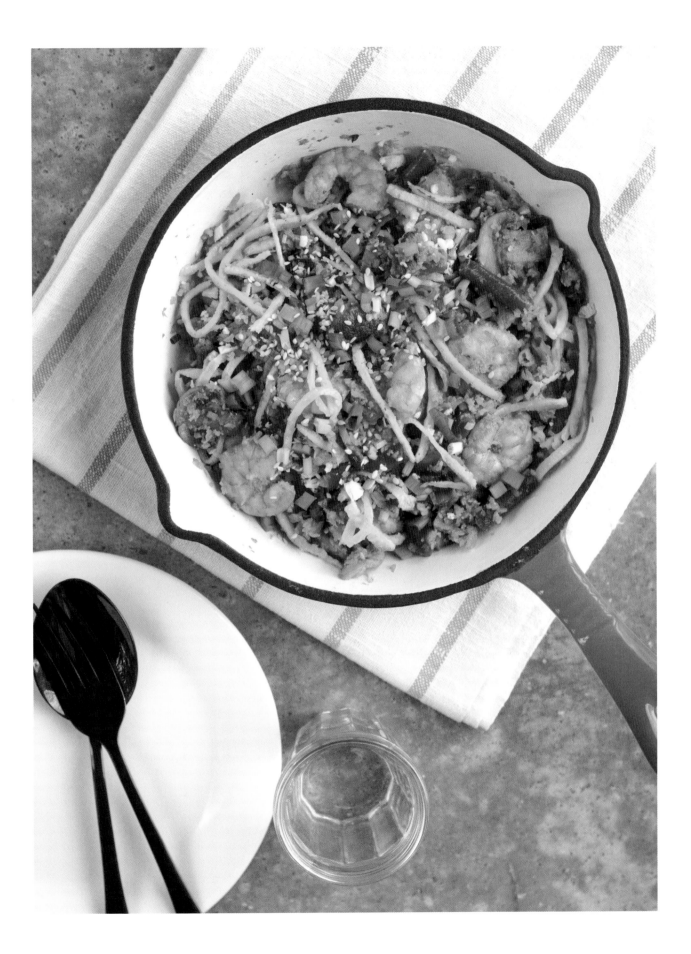

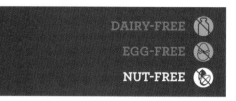

DAIRY-FREE

EGG-FREE

NUT-FREE

Truffle, Leek, and Mushroom
Risotto

Prep Time: **15 minutes** | Cook Time: **1 hour**
Yield: **5 servings**

Risotto is one of those beautiful, versatile, and heavenly-tasting dishes that can be amplified with various flavors. This is a more traditional approach, but it uses nontraditional "rice"—cauliflower and optional zero-carb rice or noodles. One large head of cauliflower makes about 5 cups of cauli-rice. This dish is fantastic with morel, chanterelle, or porcini mushrooms, but you can replace them with whatever is in season.

⅓ ounce (10 g) dried morel, chanterelle, or porcini mushrooms, or 3 ounces (85 g) fresh mushrooms, chopped

½ cup (4 ounces/120 ml) filtered water, boiling hot (if using dried mushrooms)

½ cup (4 ounces/115 g) salted butter

1 ounce (30 g) thinly sliced green onions

1 clove garlic, minced

5 cups (18 ounces/500 g) riced cauliflower (from 1 large head) (see note, page 292)

¼ cup plus 1 tablespoon (2½ fluid ounces/75 ml) white wine vinegar

2 cups (16 fluid ounces/480 ml) chicken or beef bone broth, heated

2 (7-ounce/200-g) packages zero-carb shirataki rice or shirataki noodles (optional)

1 cup (8 fluid ounces/240 ml) heavy whipping cream

⅓ cup (1¾ ounces/50 g) thinly sliced leeks

5 eggs

3½ ounces (100 g) grated Parmesan

1 teaspoon truffle oil, plus extra for drizzling, or ¼ teaspoon black truffle paste

1 teaspoon fine sea salt

Sea salt flakes, for garnish

Ground black pepper, for garnish

1. If using dried mushrooms, combine the dried mushrooms and hot water in a small bowl; let sit for 15 to 30 minutes for the mushrooms to reconstitute. Drain and chop the mushrooms.

2. In a medium saucepan over medium-low heat, melt the butter. Add the onions and garlic and sauté for 3 to 4 minutes, until lightly browned. Add the riced cauliflower and mix well with a wooden spoon until it is all coated and has absorbed the butter.

3. Add the vinegar to the cauliflower and stir. Pour in 1 cup of the broth and stir well. Lower the heat to a simmer. Simmer until the liquid is absorbed, stirring occasionally—15 to 20 minutes. Watch the risotto carefully so that the liquid evaporates but does not dry; otherwise, the bottom of the risotto will burn.

4. If using shirataki rice or noodles, rinse and drain the rice or noodles. In a saucepan over high heat, boil in water for 1 to 2 minutes. Drain and set on paper towels to absorb the excess water. If using noodles, place on a cutting board and cut into very small sections to create "rice." Add to the risotto.

5. Meanwhile, combine the cream and leeks in another saucepan. Bring to a boil over medium-high heat. Once boiling, remove from the heat and set aside.

6. When the rice has absorbed the first cup of broth, add the remaining cup of broth; simmer for 15 to 20 minutes, until the broth has been absorbed, stirring occasionally and keeping a close watch so that the risotto doesn't burn.

7. While the risotto is cooking, poach the eggs: Bring some water to a boil in a small saucepan. Meanwhile, crack an egg into a small bowl. When the water is boiling, remove the saucepan from the heat and use a spoon to swirl the water clockwise around the pan. Slide the egg into the "whirlpool" you created in the pan. Poach for 3 to 4 minutes, until the white is set. Spoon out the egg and keep warm in a warm water bath while you repeat with the remaining eggs.

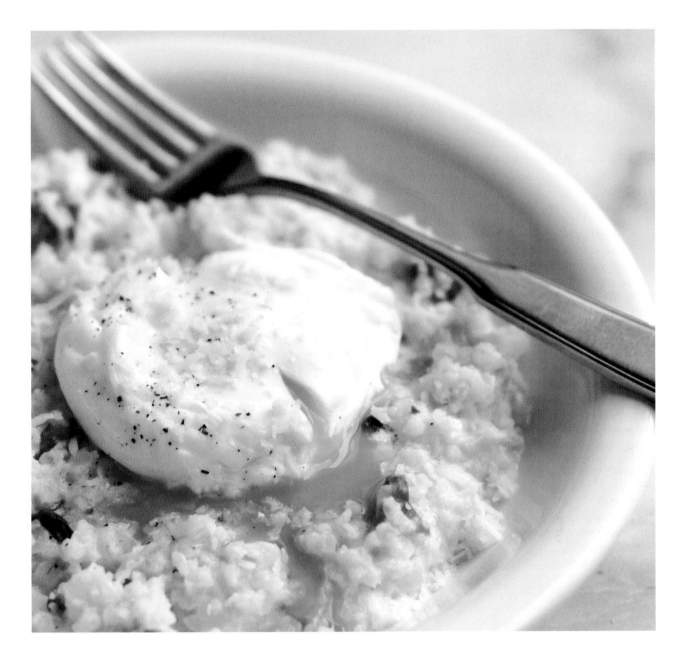

tip

Instead of poaching the eggs in Step 7, try my optional hack: Bake the eggs in a standard-size muffin pan. Preheat the oven to 350°F (177°C). Put 1 tablespoon of water in each of five cups of a muffin tin. Crack an egg into each cup and bake for 9 to 12 minutes, until the whites are set and the yolks are still soft and barely cooked.

8. Once most of the liquid in the risotto has evaporated (there should be just a little bit of moisture left in the pan), remove from the heat and add the mushrooms. Fold in the leek and cream mixture. Add three-quarters of the Parmesan and stir. Add the 1 teaspoon of truffle oil and season with 1 teaspoon of salt.

9. Divide the risotto among 5 plates and top each serving with a poached egg. Garnish with the remaining Parmesan, sea salt flakes, pepper, and 3 or 4 drops of truffle oil, if desired.

MACRONUTRIENTS
(per serving)

Fat	Protein	Carbs	Fiber	Energy
37g	18.2g	9.6g	6.3g	444 cal
75%	16%	9%		

Chapter 11
Sides

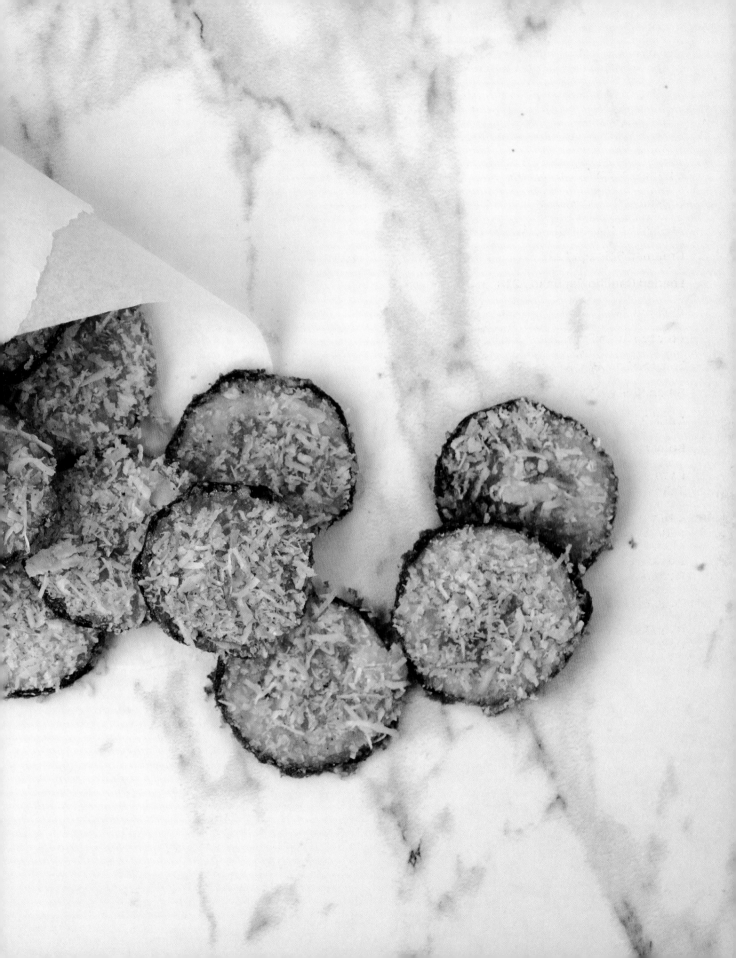

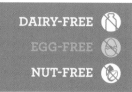

DAIRY-FREE

EGG-FREE

NUT-FREE

"Honey"-Mustard Slaw

Prep Time: **10 minutes**
Yield: **2 servings**

I love to serve this savory slaw as a side with sliced steak. If you have a higher carb threshold and are looking for some extra crunch, try topping this slaw with sunflower seeds.

1½ cups (6 ounces/170 g) shredded green cabbage

½ cup (2 ounces/55 g) shredded red cabbage

1 cup (3 ounces/85 g) broccoli slaw (thinly sliced broccoli stems)

1 cup (2¼ ounces/70 g) stemmed and chopped fresh kale

"HONEY"-MUSTARD DRESSING:

4½ tablespoons (2¼ ounces/65 g) mayonnaise

1 tablespoon prepared yellow mustard

¼ teaspoon fine sea salt

¼ teaspoon garlic powder

¼ teaspoon onion powder

2 to 4 drops liquid stevia, to taste

1. In a medium bowl, mix together the green and red cabbage, broccoli slaw, and kale.

2. In a small bowl, combine the ingredients for the dressing and blend well. Add to the slaw, mixing thoroughly.

3. Serve chilled or at room temperature.

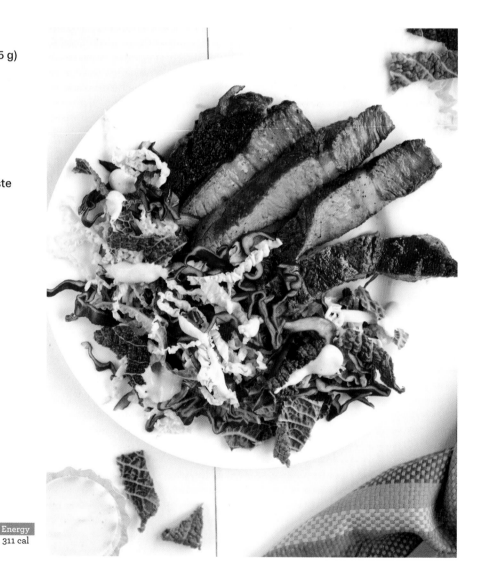

MACRONUTRIENTS (per serving)				
Fat	Protein	Carbs	Fiber	Energy
25g	3g	10g	4g	311 cal
81%	4%	15%		

Creamy Keto Slaw

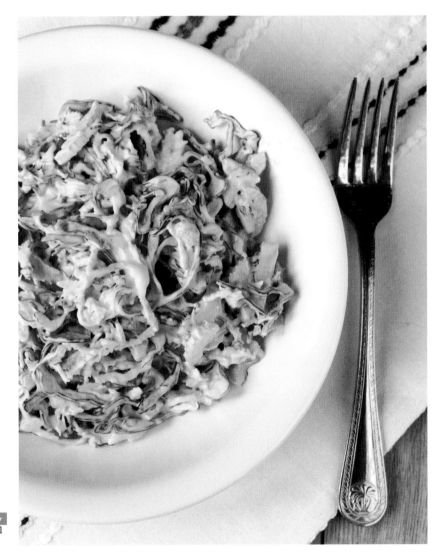

DAIRY-FREE

EGG-FREE

NUT-FREE

Prep Time: 10 minutes
Yield: **6 servings**

This delicious slaw has very little protein, so pair it with a nice protein, such as pork, steak, chicken, or fish. Pulled Pork (page 311) and slaw is a tried-and-true pairing.

2 cups (8 ounces/225 g) shredded green cabbage

1 cup (4 ounces/115 g) shredded red cabbage

4 stalks celery, thinly sliced

¼ cup (¼ ounce/7 g) coarsely chopped fresh parsley

DRESSING:

1 cup (8 ounces/225 g) mayonnaise

1 teaspoon prepared no-sugar-added horseradish

¼ cup (2 ounces/55 g) sour cream

1 tablespoon prepared yellow mustard

¼ teaspoon garlic powder

¼ teaspoon onion powder

¼ teaspoon fine sea salt

2 to 4 drops liquid stevia, to taste

1. In a medium bowl, mix together the green and red cabbage, celery, and parsley.

2. In a small bowl, combine the ingredients for the dressing and blend well. Add to the slaw, mixing thoroughly.

3. Serve chilled or at room temperature.

MACRONUTRIENTS
(per serving)

Fat	Protein	Carbs	Fiber	Energy
44.3g	0.5g	6.8g	1.5g	428 cal
93%	1%	7%		

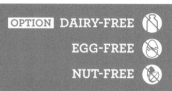

OPTION DAIRY-FREE

EGG-FREE

NUT-FREE

Braised Red Cabbage

Prep Time: 10 minutes | **Cook Time: 20 minutes**
Yield: 5 servings

Serve this tasty and tangy side with a poultry dish, such as fried or confit duck, or on its own.

¼ cup (2 ounces/55 g) coconut oil or butter, melted

4 cups (1 pound/455 g) shredded red cabbage

½ teaspoon onion powder

½ cup (4 fluid ounces/120 ml) filtered water

¼ cup (2 fluid ounces/60 ml) apple cider vinegar

3 drops to ½ teaspoon liquid stevia, to taste (optional)

½ cup (2 ounces/55 g) crumbled fresh (soft) goat cheese (optional)

1. Heat the coconut oil in a large sauté pan or wok over medium heat. Add the cabbage and onion powder and stir well.

2. Add the water, vinegar, and stevia, if using; reduce the heat to low. Simmer for 15 to 20 minutes, until the cabbage is nicely braised.

3. Serve topped with the goat cheese, if desired.

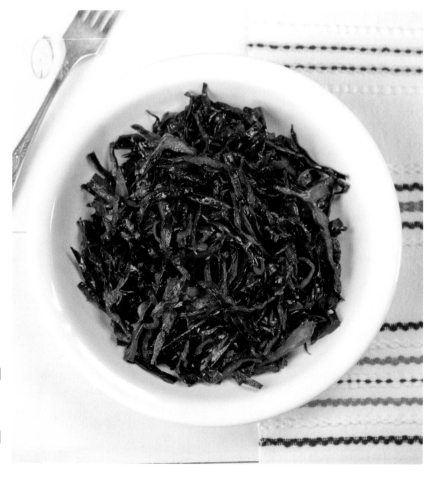

MACRONUTRIENTS
(cabbage only)

Fat	Protein	Carbs	Fiber	Energy
11.4g	1g	5.2g	1.4g	126 cal
81%	3%	16%		

MACRONUTRIENTS
(cabbage with goat cheese)

Fat	Protein	Carbs	Fiber	Energy
13.8g	3g	6.4g	1.4g	158 cal
77%	7%	16%		

Creamed Spinach

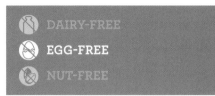

DAIRY-FREE

EGG-FREE

NUT-FREE

Prep Time: **5 minutes** | Cook Time: **10 minutes**
Yield: **3 servings**

This high-fat creamed spinach is one of the best sides to pair with steak or chicken—or to eat on its own as a snack.

9 cups fresh baby spinach (9 ounces/255 g), or 1 (10-ounce/ 285-g) package frozen spinach, thawed

¼ cup plus 2 tablespoons (3 ounces/85 g) butter

2 cloves garlic, minced

4 ounces (115 g) cream cheese

½ cup (4 fluid ounces/120 ml) almond milk

½ teaspoon fine sea salt

¼ teaspoon onion powder

Ground black pepper

1. If using fresh spinach, bring a pot of salted water to a boil. Add the spinach and turn off the heat, leaving the pot on the burner. Let sit for 1 to 2 minutes, then drain and press out the excess moisture. If using frozen spinach, rinse and drain it.

2. Transfer the spinach to a cutting board and chop it into 1-inch (2.5-cm) pieces.

3. In a medium saucepan over medium heat, melt the butter. Add the garlic and cook for 1 to 2 minutes, taking care not to burn the garlic. Add the cream cheese, milk, salt, onion powder, and pepper to taste; whisk until well blended.

4. Add the chopped spinach and mix well. Cook for 4 to 5 minutes, until heated through and ready to serve.

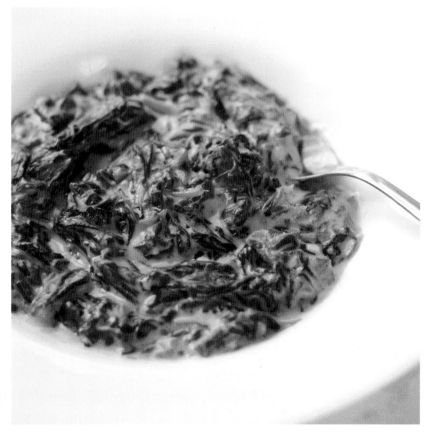

MACRONUTRIENTS (per serving)				
Fat	Protein	Carbs	Fiber	Energy
35.6g	5.3g	5.3g	2.3g	366 cal
88%	6%	6%		

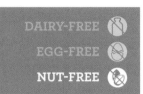

DAIRY-FREE

EGG-FREE

NUT-FREE

Loaded Cauliflower Bake

Prep Time: **15 minutes** | Cook Time: **40 minutes**
Yield: **3 servings**

4 cups (15 ounces/425 g) cauliflower florets (about 1 medium head), cut into bite-sized pieces

½ cup (4 ounces/115 g) sour cream

½ cup (4 ounces/115 g) mayonnaise

4 ounces (115 g) cream cheese, softened

¼ cup (2 ounces/55 g) butter or butter-flavored coconut oil

2 tablespoons nutritional yeast

½ teaspoon fine sea salt

¼ teaspoon garlic powder

Ground black pepper

¼ cup (1 ounce/28 g) shredded cheddar cheese

2 tablespoons grated Parmesan cheese

8 thick-cut slices bacon, cooked and chopped, for garnish

Snipped fresh chives, for garnish

1. Preheat the oven to 350°F (177°C). Grease a 9-inch (13-cm) square or oval baking dish.

2. Bring a saucepan of water to a boil over high heat. Add the cauliflower florets and turn off the heat, leaving the pan on the burner. Let the cauliflower sit in the hot water for 9 to 10 minutes, until crisp-tender.

3. Meanwhile, in a food processor, combine the sour cream, mayonnaise, cream cheese, butter, nutritional yeast, salt, garlic powder, and pepper to taste.

4. Drain the cauliflower and pat dry. In a mixing bowl, combine the cream cheese mixture with the cauliflower until well mixed.

5. Pour into the prepared baking dish and top with the cheeses. Bake for 25 to 30 minutes, until the cauliflower is soft and the top is golden brown.

6. Remove from the oven and top with the bacon and chives before serving.

MACRONUTRIENTS
(per serving)

Fat	Protein	Carbs	Fiber	Energy
56g	17.7g	11.7g	4g	632 cal
81%	11%	8%		

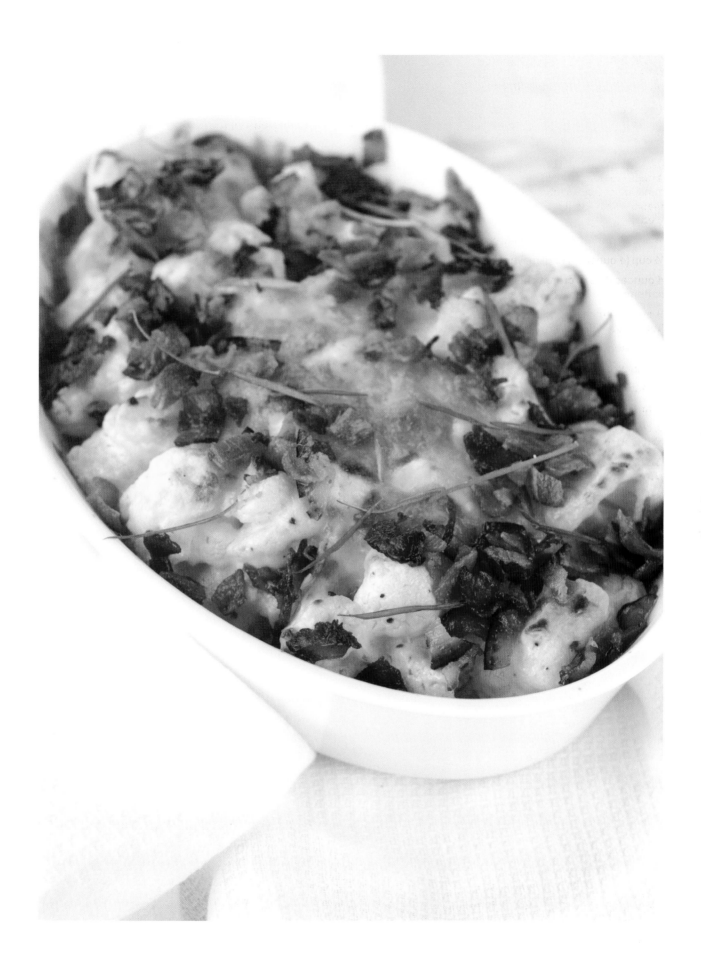

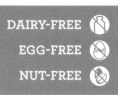

DAIRY-FREE

EGG-FREE

NUT-FREE

Avocado Fries

Prep Time: **15 minutes** | Cook Time: **6 minutes**
Yield: **3 servings**

If you have never been fond of avocados, you should try these fries. The texture of the avocado is completely different when fried than when eaten raw. And if you love avocados, you will adore these!

¼ cup (2 ounces/55 g) refined coconut oil, for frying (see note)

2 medium avocados, peeled and sliced

Sea salt and ground black pepper

note

I always use lard or coconut oil for frying, but you need to watch coconut oil carefully. It has a lower smoke point than other oils, so it can catch fire if left unattended.

1. Heat the coconut oil in a deep skillet over medium heat to 375°F (190°C).

2. Carefully place the avocado slices in the hot oil and fry for 2 to 3 minutes on each side.

3. Remove the avocado slices from the skillet to a paper towel–lined plate for 1 to 2 minutes to cool slightly. Season to taste with salt and pepper before serving.

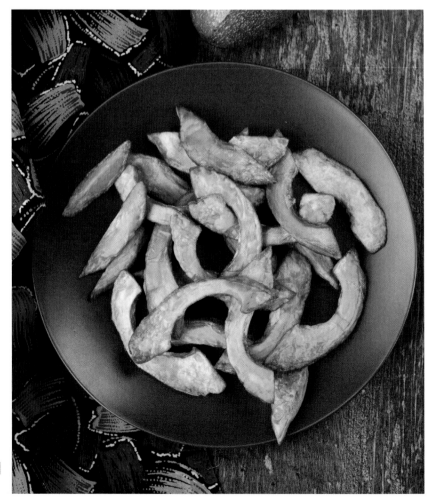

MACRONUTRIENTS
(per serving)

Fat	Protein	Carbs	Fiber	Energy
30.6g	0g	8g	5.3g	306 cal
90%	0%	10%		

Broccoli Stem Fries

DAIRY-FREE

EGG-FREE

NUT-FREE

Prep Time: **15 minutes** | Cook Time: **6 minutes**
Yield: **2 servings**

Why do we always throw out the broccoli stem when it is so nutritious? I found a great way to use the stem and enjoy this amazing superfood. My husband loves these fries! Cooking them twice in a deep-fryer (the double fry) gives them the perfect crunchy texture.

Stems from 2 large heads broccoli, trimmed

Refined coconut oil or lard, for frying (see note, opposite)

Sea salt and ground black pepper

1. Cut the broccoli stems lengthwise into slices that resemble french fries. Heat the coconut oil in a deep-fryer to 338°F (170°C).

2. Fry the broccoli stems for 2 to 3 minutes.

3. Remove the fries to a paper towel–lined plate. Increase the oil temperature in the deep-fryer to 375°F (190°C), then fry the stems for another 2 to 3 minutes. Set the fries on the paper towel–lined plate to drain and cool for a couple of minutes. Season with salt and pepper before serving.

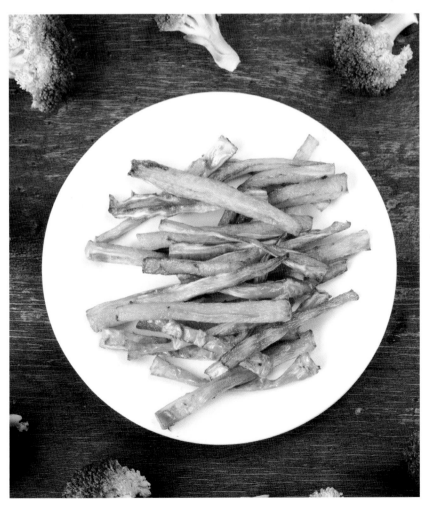

MACRONUTRIENTS
(per serving)

Fat	Protein	Carbs	Fiber	Energy
42g	4g	6g	5g	418 cal
90%	4%	6%		

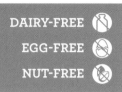

DAIRY-FREE

EGG-FREE

NUT-FREE

Toasted Coconut Chips

Prep Time: **5 minutes** | Cook Time: **7 minutes**
Yield: **4 servings**

I love to snack on coconut chips (aka coconut flakes), and I particularly enjoy them toasted. Toasting the coconut makes for a crunchy snack full of energy and flavor to take with you on the go.

2 cups (18 ounces/500 g) unsweetened coconut flakes

1 to 2 teaspoons powdered stevia, to taste

Pinch of sea salt

Pinch of ground Ceylon cinnamon or regular cinnamon (optional)

1. Preheat the broiler to medium-high. Spray a rimmed baking sheet with coconut oil spray.

2. Place the coconut flakes in a bowl. Sprinkle with the stevia, salt, and cinnamon, if using, and toss to combine well.

3. Spread the coconut chips on the prepared baking sheet and spray them with coconut oil spray.

4. Broil the chips for 3 to 5 minutes, until golden brown, watching carefully so the chips do not burn. Remove from the oven, use a spatula to flip the chips over, and broil for another 1 to 2 minutes.

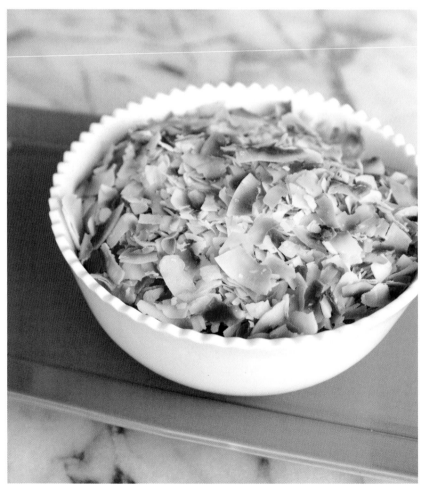

MACRONUTRIENTS
(per serving)

Fat	Protein	Carbs	Fiber	Energy
18.5g	1.5g	6g	4.5g	183 cal
85%	3%	12%		

Broccoli Mash

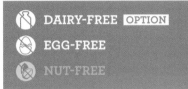

DAIRY-FREE OPTION

EGG-FREE

NUT-FREE

Prep Time: **10 minutes** | Cook Time: **8 minutes**
Yield: **2 servings**

Nothing is more nourishing to our healthy gut bacteria than cabbage and cruciferous vegetables such as cauliflower and broccoli. This broccoli mash is a great way to incorporate these superfoods into your regular menu rotation.

2 cups (12½ ounces/355 g) broccoli florets

¼ cup (2 ounces/55 g) butter or butter–flavored coconut oil, melted

2 tablespoons almond milk

Pinch of garlic powder

Sea salt and ground black pepper

1. Bring a saucepan of water to a boil over high heat. Add the broccoli florets and turn off the heat, leaving the pot on the burner. Let the broccoli sit in the hot water for 5 to 8 minutes, until bright green. Drain.

2. Return the drained broccoli to the pot. Add the butter, milk, and garlic powder and season to taste with salt and pepper.

3. Using an immersion blender, blend until smooth.

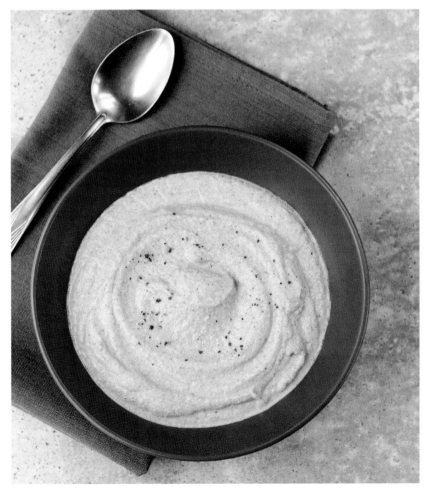

MACRONUTRIENTS
(per serving)

Fat	Protein	Carbs	Fiber	Energy
23.5g	2.5g	6g	2.5g	237 cal
86%	4%	10%		

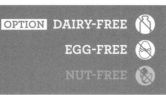

OPTION DAIRY-FREE

EGG-FREE

NUT-FREE

Cauliflower Mash

Prep Time: 10 minutes | **Cook Time: 8 minutes**
Yield: 2 servings

Traditional mashed potatoes are a staple of some of our most comforting childhood and special-occasion meals. Cauliflower mash incorporates the same wonderful buttery flavors, replacing the potatoes with a gut-nourishing food that everyone will enjoy just as much, all while enhancing their health!

2 cups (8 ounces/225 g) bite-sized cauliflower florets

¼ cup (2 ounces/55 g) butter or butter-flavored coconut oil, melted

2 tablespoons almond milk

Pinch of garlic powder

Sea salt and ground black pepper

1. Bring a saucepan of water to a boil over high heat. Add the cauliflower florets and turn off the heat, leaving the pan on the burner. Let the cauliflower sit in the hot water for 5 to 8 minutes, until cooked, then drain.

2. Return the cauliflower to the pan. Add the butter, milk, and garlic powder.

3. Using an immersion blender, blend until smooth. Season to taste with salt and pepper.

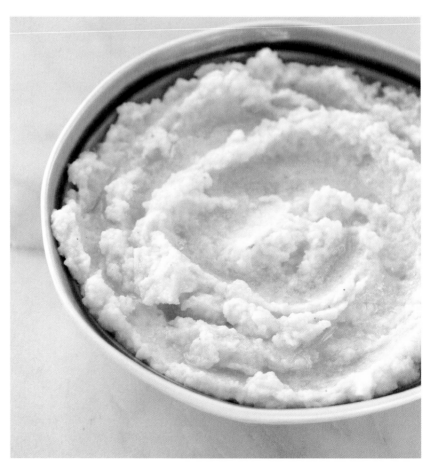

MACRONUTRIENTS
(per serving)

Fat	Protein	Carbs	Fiber	Energy
23.5g	2.5g	6g	2.5g	237 cal
86%	4%	10%		

Keto Bacon
"Potato" Salad

Prep Time: 10 minutes, plus 1 hour to chill | **Cook Time:** 25 minutes
Yield: 3 servings

Potato salad is one of those comfort foods that I missed on keto—especially at summer picnics and family-style meals—until I tried this potato-free version. I was thrilled by how much it resembles the original! Radishes are so versatile and taste very similar to potatoes when boiled or roasted. If you like, add some chopped unsweetened pickles.

20 large radishes, trimmed

6 slices bacon

6 eggs, hard-boiled, peeled and quartered

2 stalks celery, chopped

¼ cup sliced green onions

Several sprigs fresh dill, chopped

1 teaspoon fine sea salt

¼ teaspoon ground black pepper

¼ cup plus 2 tablespoons (3 ounces/85 g) mayonnaise

1 tablespoon Dijon or prepared yellow mustard

1 teaspoon apple cider vinegar

1. In a saucepan over high heat, boil the radishes whole for 20 to 25 minutes, until soft.

2. Meanwhile, fry the bacon in a skillet until cooked through and crispy, 6 to 7 minutes; remove from the pan and chop.

3. Drain and quarter the radishes. In a mixing bowl, combine the radishes, bacon, eggs, celery, onions, dill, salt, and pepper.

4. In a small bowl, combine the mayonnaise, mustard, and vinegar. Pour over the salad and gently toss until well coated. Cover and refrigerate for 1 to 2 hours or overnight. Serve chilled.

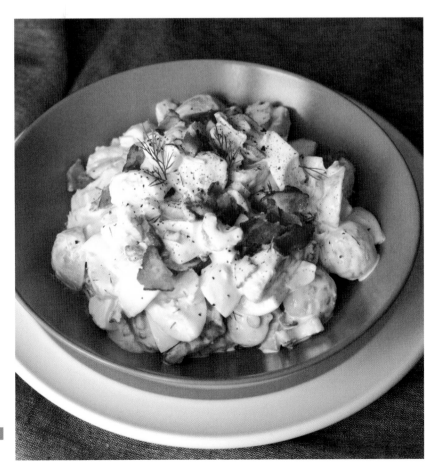

MACRONUTRIENTS
(per serving)

Fat	Protein	Carbs	Fiber	Energy
39g	18g	4.6g	1.7g	445 cal
80%	16%	4%		

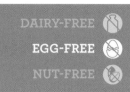

DAIRY-FREE

EGG-FREE

NUT-FREE

Roasted Eggplant
with Tahini-Almond Sauce

Prep Time: **20 minutes** | Cook Time: **35 minutes**
Yield: **3 servings**

A globe eggplant is generally 7 to 8 inches (18 to 20 cm) long and weighs about 1 pound (455 grams). Adjust accordingly if buying a different type of eggplant at the store. The Greek yogurt in this recipe should have at least 10 grams of fat per 100 grams; check the Nutrition Facts panel to be sure. To make this a full keto meal, add 4 ounces (115 grams) of protein, such as grilled chicken, beef, or pork, per person.

1 globe eggplant (1 pound/455 g), top removed, sliced lengthwise into 6 long wedges

1 teaspoon fine sea salt, divided

2 tablespoons olive oil or MCT oil

¼ cup (2 fluid ounces/60 ml) cold filtered water

¼ cup (2 fluid ounces/60 ml) MCT oil

2 tablespoons tahini

2 tablespoons unsweetened almond butter

1 tablespoon freshly squeezed lemon juice

½ teaspoon garlic powder

½ teaspoon paprika

¼ teaspoon turmeric powder

¼ teaspoon ground black pepper

1 teaspoon sesame seeds, for garnish

Coarsely chopped fresh mint or parsley, for garnish

½ cup (4 ounces/115 g) plain Greek yogurt, minimum 10% fat, for serving

1. Place the eggplant in a colander or on a bed of paper towels. Sprinkle on both sides with ½ teaspoon of the salt and let sit for 10 to 15 minutes. Wipe well with paper towels to dry the eggplant and remove the salt.

2. Preheat the oven to 350°F (177°C). Lay the eggplant slices on a rimmed baking sheet and brush or drizzle with the 2 tablespoons of olive oil. Bake for 30 to 35 minutes, until softened and fully cooked. Remove from the oven and set aside to cool.

3. In a food processor, combine the water, MCT oil, tahini, almond butter, lemon juice, garlic powder, paprika, turmeric, remaining ½ teaspoon of salt, and pepper. Blend until smooth.

4. Plate the eggplant and drizzle with the tahini sauce. Garnish with the sesame seeds and mint and serve with dollops of yogurt.

note

A quenelle is a decorative and pretty presentation of a thick substance formed with two spoons. To up your presentation game, use quenelles, not just dollops, of yogurt in Step 4. You can find some great tutorials showing you how to form quenelles on YouTube.

	MACRONUTRIENTS (per serving)			
Fat	Protein	Carbs	Fiber	Energy
59g	27g	12.5g	5.5g	684 cal
77%	16%	7%		

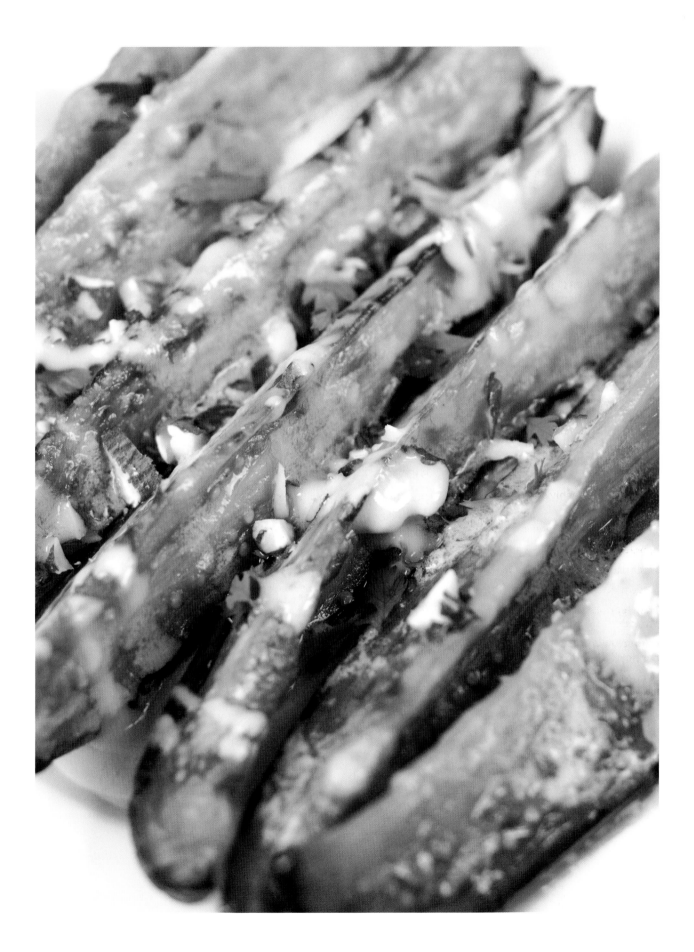

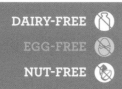

DAIRY-FREE

EGG-FREE

NUT-FREE

Deep-Fried Brussels Sprouts
with Tangy Sauce

Prep Time: **15 minutes** | Cook Time: **10 minutes**
Yield: **5 servings**

Deep-fried in coconut oil, these incredibly delicious Brussels sprouts with bacon make a perfect side for a holiday meal—or any meal! Not only that, but this dish has perfect keto macros. If you prefer, you can fry the sprouts in a skillet; I've included instructions for both cooking methods. The double fry is the trick to getting crispy—not soggy—sprouts.

Refined coconut oil, lard, or duck fat, for frying

15 slices bacon, cut into 1-inch (2.5–cm) pieces

1 pound (455 g) Brussels sprouts (about 20), cut in half

2 tablespoons capers

SAUCE:

3 tablespoons mayonnaise

1 tablespoon prepared yellow mustard

1 large clove garlic, minced, or ¼ teaspoon garlic powder

½ teaspoon hot sauce

¼ teaspoon fine sea salt

1 or 2 drops liquid stevia

notes

It is important to use fresh, not frozen, Brussels sprouts for this recipe. Frozen vegetables contain a lot of water, and water in a deep-fryer can lead to explosive results! While you could drain and dry frozen sprouts very well, it's easier and safer to use fresh. In addition, coconut oil can ignite during cooking, so use safety precautions.

The nutrition information assumes that the sprouts retain about 2 tablespoons of coconut oil per serving after frying.

1. If using a deep-fryer, heat the coconut oil in the fryer to 338°F (170°C). An air-fryer will work well here, too. If you are not using a deep-fryer or an air-fryer, heat enough oil to reach about 2 inches (5 cm) up the sides of a large, heavy pot to 338°F (170°C) over medium-high heat.

2. Meanwhile, in a skillet, fry the bacon over medium-high heat for 3 to 5 minutes, until cooked but still soft. Remove from the pan and set aside.

3. If using a deep-fryer, when the oil reaches temperature, use the frying basket to cook the sprouts for 2 to 3 minutes. Remove from the oil and let rest in the basket. Increase the heat to 375°F (190°C). When the oil reaches temperature, fry the sprouts a second time for 1 to 2 more minutes.

   If using an air-fryer, follow the manufacturer's instructions, frying the sprouts for 8 to 10 minutes.

   If pan-frying, when the oil reaches temperature, gently add the spouts and fry for 2 to 3 minutes. Remove from the oil and set on a plate. Increase the temperature to 375°F (190°C). When the oil reaches temperature, fry the sprouts a second time for 1 to 2 more minutes.

4. Meanwhile, whisk together all the ingredients for the sauce.

5. Place the fried sprouts in a serving bowl. Add the bacon and capers and drizzle with the sauce, lightly tossing the mixture together. Alternatively, divide the sauce between 5 small serving bowls and serve on the side as a dip.

MACRONUTRIENTS
(per serving)

Fat	Protein	Carbs	Fiber	Energy
18.6g	11.2g	10g	4.2g	230 cal
66%	18%	16%		

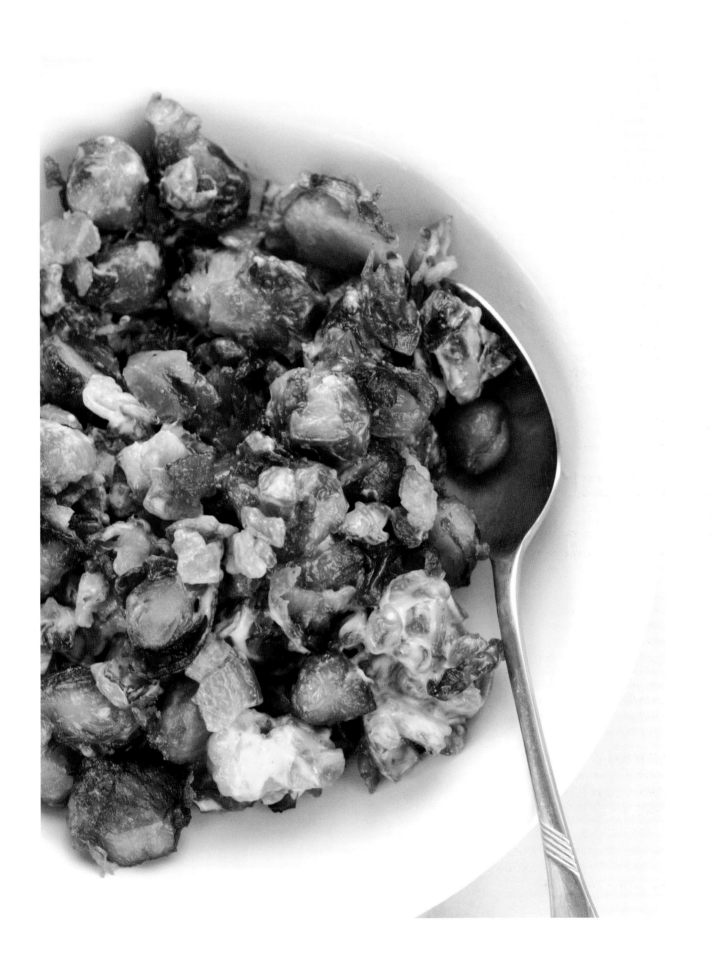

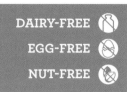

DAIRY-FREE

EGG-FREE

NUT-FREE

Duck Fat–Roasted Rosemary Radishes

Prep Time: **10 minutes** | Cook Time: **20 minutes**
Yield: **2 servings**

This is a wonderful low-carb side dish and an alternative to traditional rosemary potatoes! You'll love these savory radishes as a dinner side dish, but give them a try for breakfast, too.

¼ cup plus 2 tablespoons (3 ounces/85 g) duck fat, melted

1 tablespoon chopped fresh rosemary, or 1½ teaspoons dried rosemary

2 cups (8¾ ounces/245 g) halved or quartered radishes (depending on size)

½ teaspoon fine sea salt

¼ teaspoon ground black pepper

¼ teaspoon garlic powder

1. Preheat the oven to 450°F (232°C). Line a rimmed baking sheet with aluminum foil.

2. In a medium bowl, combine the duck fat and rosemary. Add the radishes and toss to coat. Season with the salt, pepper, and garlic powder.

3. Distribute the radishes across the prepared baking sheet. Bake for 20 minutes, until tender and lightly browned. Serve warm.

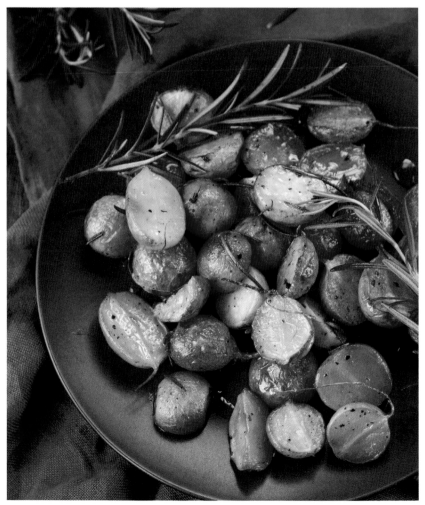

MACRONUTRIENTS
(per serving)

Fat	Protein	Carbs	Fiber	Energy
25.5g	1g	4g	2g	244 cal
92%	2%	6%		

Zucchini Chips

Prep Time: **10 minutes** | Cook Time: **15 minutes**
Yield: **2 servings**

These crispy, crunchy, cheesy snacks are great on their own or paired with a dip. They can also be packed up and taken on the go.

1 medium zucchini, ends trimmed, thinly sliced into rounds

¼ cup (2 ounces/60 ml) MCT oil

½ cup (2 ounces/55 g) grated Parmesan cheese

½ teaspoon garlic powder

½ teaspoon fine sea salt

¼ teaspoon ground black pepper

1. Preheat the oven to 350°F (177°C). Spray a rimmed baking sheet with coconut oil spray.

2. In a bowl, toss the zucchini slices with the MCT oil until well coated.

3. In another bowl, combine the Parmesan, garlic powder, salt, and pepper.

4. Spread the zucchini in a single layer on the prepared baking sheet. Sprinkle the Parmesan mixture evenly over the zucchini slices.

5. Bake for 13 to 15 minutes. If you prefer crispier chips, extend the baking time to 15 to 20 minutes, or broil on high for 1 to 2 minutes after baking.

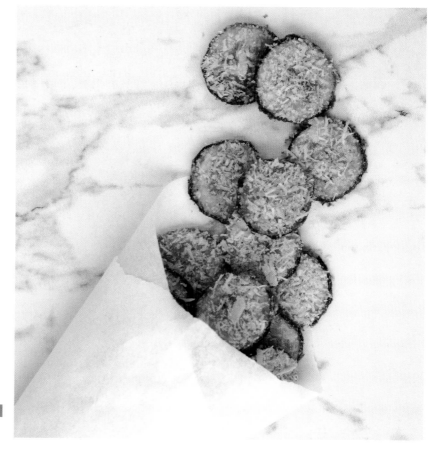

MACRONUTRIENTS
(per serving)

Fat	Protein	Carbs	Fiber	Energy
36g	11g	5g	1g	385 cal
84%	11%	5%		

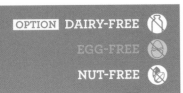

OPTION DAIRY-FREE
EGG-FREE
NUT-FREE

Cauliflower Sausage Herb
Stuffing

Prep Time: **30 minutes** | Cook Time: **1 hour 15 minutes**
Yield: **6 servings**

I was always a stuffing girl. Sure, the turkey is great at the holidays, as are all the other tasty sides, but to me, nothing was ever as delish as the stuffing! This holiday stuffing is so good, it beats the original that I grew up with. I have served it to non-keto friends and family, who rave about it. Make your next holiday meal completely keto by including this dish on your menu. I also love this stuffing for breakfast with eggs; see Eggs with Sausage Stuffing (page 126).

½ cup (4 ounces/115 g) butter or butter-flavored coconut oil, plus more for the dish

1 medium onion, chopped

2 stalks celery, chopped or thinly sliced

1 medium head cauliflower, cut into 1-inch (2.5-cm) cubes

1 cup (2½ ounces/75 g) white or brown mushrooms, sliced

1 clove garlic, minced

8 ounces (225 g) Italian sausage, removed from casings

4 ounces (115 g) ground beef

¼ cup (¼ ounce/7 g) chopped fresh parsley

2 tablespoons chopped fresh rosemary

1 tablespoon chopped fresh sage, or 1 teaspoon dried rubbed sage

½ cup (4 fluid ounces/120 ml) turkey bone broth

¼ teaspoon fine sea salt

¼ teaspoon ground black pepper

1 egg, lightly beaten

1. Preheat the oven to 350°F (177°C). Grease a 13 by 9-inch (33 by 23-cm) baking dish with butter.

2. In a large skillet over medium heat, melt the butter. Add the onion and celery; sauté for 5 to 6 minutes, until soft. Add the cauliflower, mushrooms, and garlic and cook for 3 to 4 minutes, stirring occasionally. Remove the vegetables from the skillet and place in a mixing bowl.

3. In the same skillet, cook the sausage and ground beef over medium heat for 4 to 5 minutes, breaking up the meat with a wooden spoon, until lightly browned.

4. Remove the meat from the skillet and add to the cauliflower mixture, along with the herbs and broth. Season with the salt and pepper.

5. Add the egg and blend gently.

6. Pour into the prepared baking dish and bake for 50 to 60 minutes, until deep brown and crisp.

MACRONUTRIENTS
(per serving)

Fat	Protein	Carbs	Fiber	Energy
23g	12g	8g	3g	281 cal
83%	11%	16%		

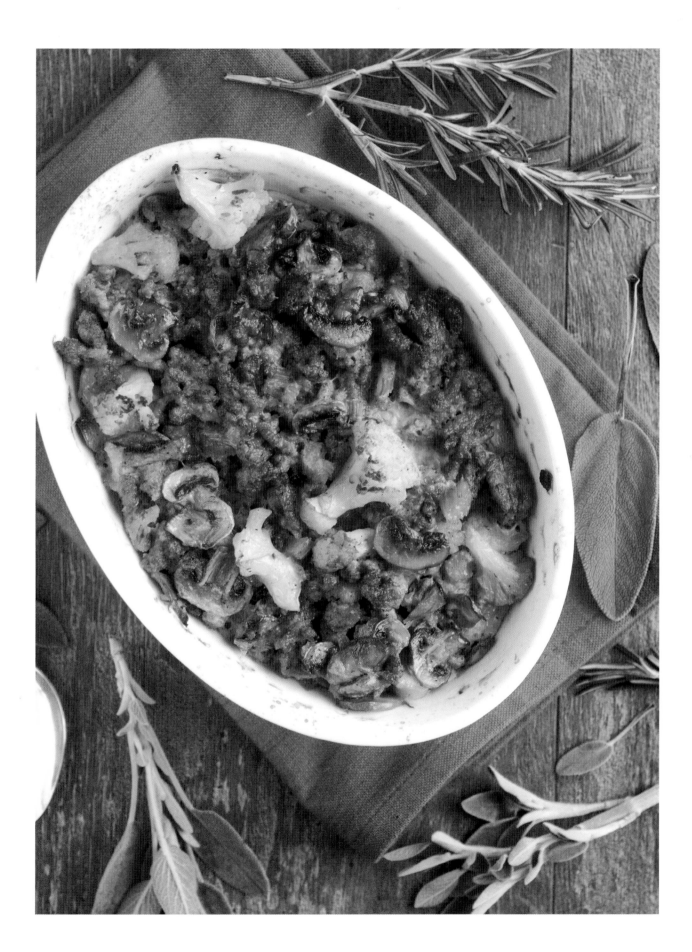

Poultry & Seafood

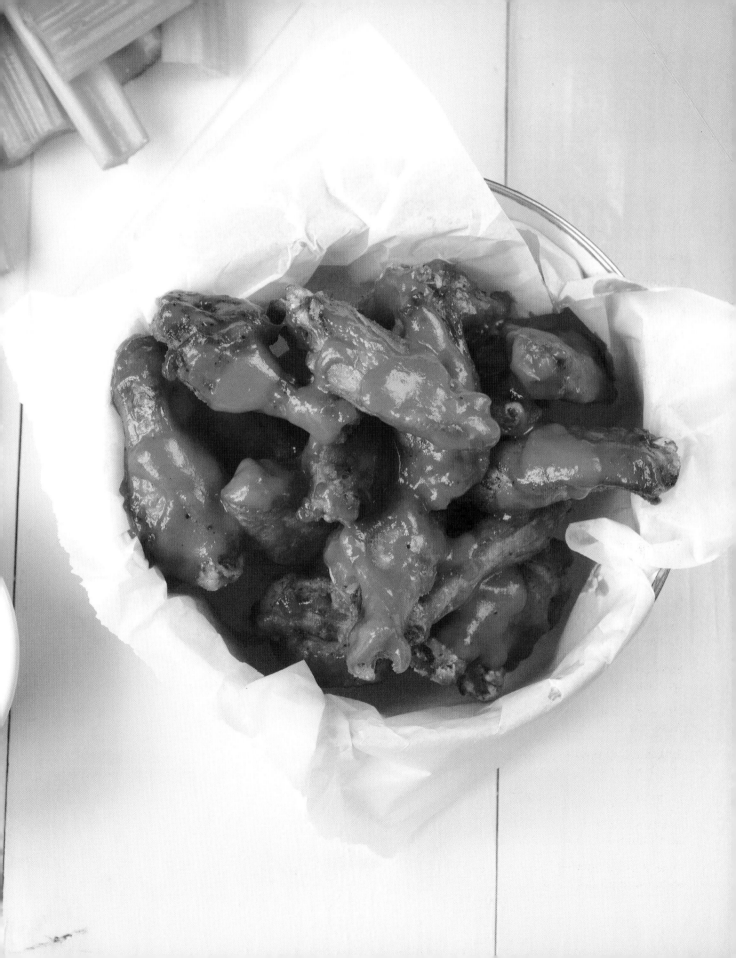

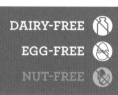

DAIRY-FREE

EGG-FREE

NUT-FREE

Thai Chicken Satay

Prep Time: **10 minutes** | Cook Time: **12 minutes**
Yield: **4 servings**

Satay sauce is traditionally made with peanut butter and sugar. I've replaced those ingredients here with almond butter and natural sweetener for all the flavor without the sugar. This recipe is cooked on skewers, and you can use metal or bamboo. If you use bamboo skewers, you will need to soak them in water for 30 minutes prior to grilling.

1 pound (455 g) boneless chicken breasts, preferably skin-on, cubed

2 tablespoons coconut oil, melted

2 cups (4 ounces/115 g) shredded iceberg lettuce

Lime wedges, for serving (optional)

SATAY SAUCE:

¾ cup (6 ounces/170 g) coconut cream (see note, page 108)

¼ cup (2 ounces/55 g) unsweetened almond butter

2 tablespoons crushed almonds

1 tablespoon apple cider vinegar

1 tablespoon fish sauce

1 tablespoon freshly squeezed lime juice

1 tablespoon red curry paste

1 tablespoon tamari

1 tablespoon erythritol, or
½ teaspoon liquid stevia (optional)

1. Divide the cubed chicken between 8 skewers. Use a brush to coat the chicken well with the coconut oil.

2. If using a grill, preheat the grill to medium heat. Grill the chicken skewers for 5 to 6 minutes, flip, and grill for another 5 to 6 minutes. Alternatively, you can use a stovetop grill pan over medium heat, cooking for 5 to 6 minutes on each side. The chicken will be white all the way through when finished.

3. Meanwhile, in a medium saucepan over low heat, stir together all the satay sauce ingredients until well blended, 3 to 4 minutes.

4. Place one-quarter of the lettuce on each of 4 plates. Divide the chicken skewers between the plates. Top the chicken with the satay sauce, or serve the sauce on the side as a dip. Serve with lime wedges, if desired.

MACRONUTRIENTS
(per serving)

Fat	Protein	Carbs	Fiber	Energy
42.5g	27g	5.5g	2.5g	511 cal
75%	21%	4%		

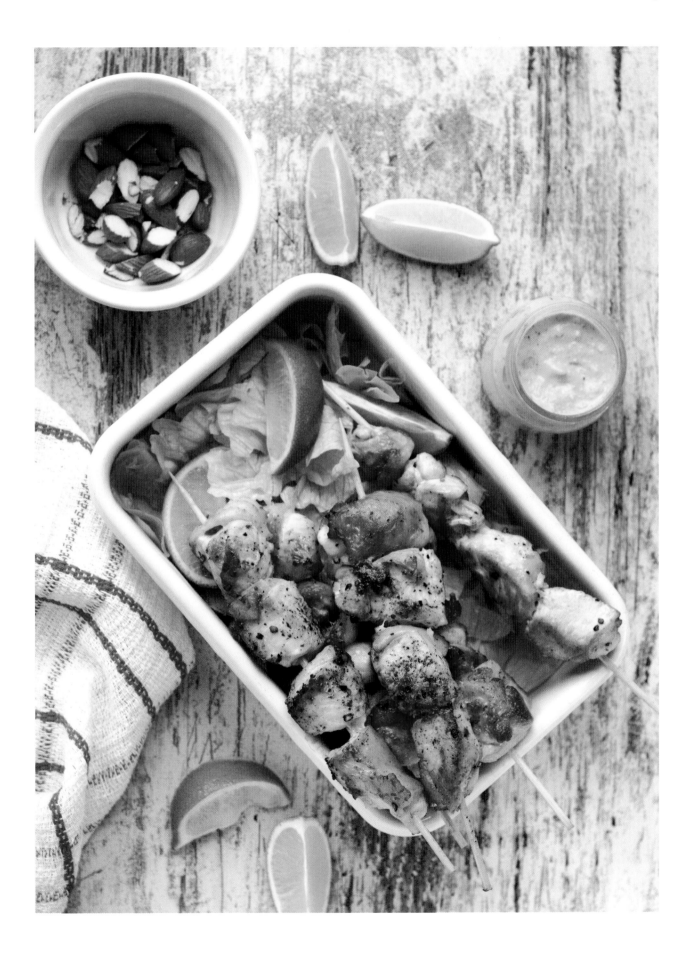

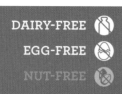

DAIRY-FREE

EGG-FREE

NUT-FREE

Pesto Chicken Skewers

Prep Time: 10 minutes | **Cook Time: 14 to 30 minutes, depending on method**
Yield: 2 servings

This is one of the easiest keto recipes for entertaining and summer grilling, but it is so tasty and satiating that I often make it in the winter, too. This is a super-keto recipe, with the MCT oil generating fat-burning ketones and providing all-day fuel. The chicken is cooked on skewers; you can use metal or bamboo. If you use bamboo skewers, you will need to soak them in water for 30 minutes prior to making the recipe.

8 ounces (225 g) boneless, skinless chicken breasts

1 batch Pesto (page 142)

1. If baking the chicken skewers, preheat the oven to 350°F (177°C). If grilling the skewers, preheat a grill to medium heat.

2. Cut the chicken into cubes. Place the pesto in a mixing bowl. Add the cubed chicken to the bowl and mix until all the pieces are well coated.

3. Slide the coated chicken breast cubes evenly onto 4 skewers.

4. If grilling the chicken, grill for 6 to 7 minutes, until the chicken lifts off the grill easily. Flip and grill for another 6 to 7 minutes, until white all the way through. If baking the chicken, bake for 25 to 30 minutes, until golden brown and white in the center.

tip

Serve this dish with a tasty green side dish or salad.

MACRONUTRIENTS
(per serving)

Fat	Protein	Carbs	Fiber	Energy
61g	33g	7g	2g	688 cal
78%	18%	4%		

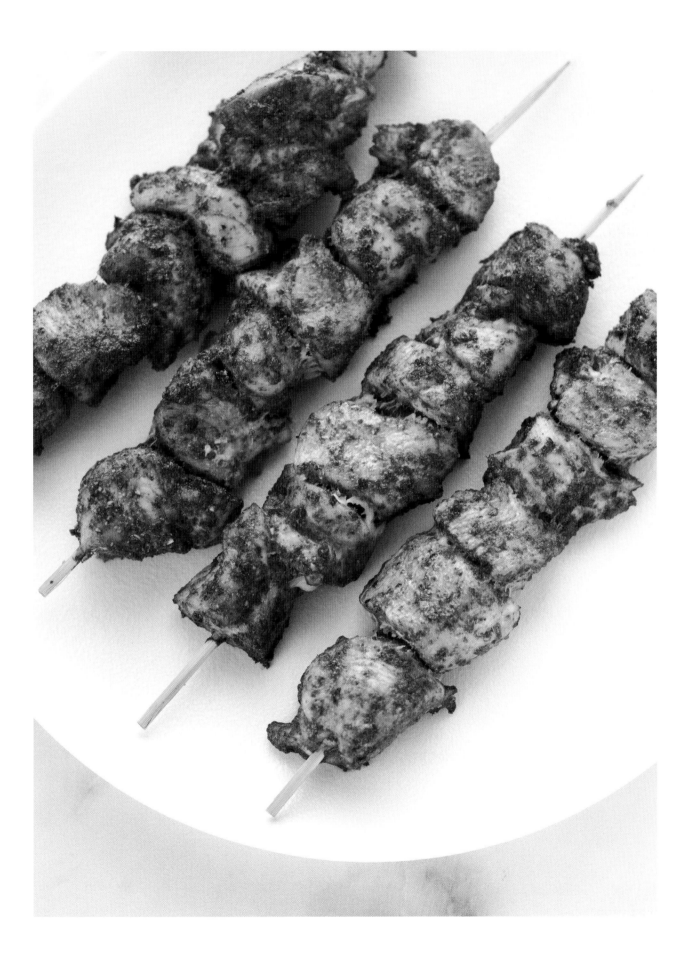

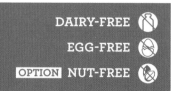

DAIRY-FREE
EGG-FREE
OPTION NUT-FREE

Lemon Chicken

Prep Time: **10 minutes** | Cook Time: **20 minutes**
Yield: **4 servings**

This is a dish that I ate often while growing up in China. I love anything with a tangy lemon flavor and enjoy it even more now that I'm keto. The lemon pairs so well with broccoli, cilantro, and cashews.

LEMON SAUCE:

⅛ tablespoon guar gum or xanthan gum

½ cup (4 fluid ounces/120 ml) filtered water

¼ cup (2 ounces/55 g) butter-flavored coconut oil

2 tablespoons freshly squeezed lemon juice

2 tablespoons erythritol (optional)

½ to 1 teaspoon liquid stevia, to taste

1 teaspoon tamari

¼ teaspoon fine sea salt

¼ cup (2 ounces/55 g) coconut oil

1 clove garlic, peeled and crushed (see note, page 108)

1 teaspoon thinly sliced fresh ginger

3 green onions, sliced

8 boneless chicken thighs, preferably skin-on

2 cups (13½ ounces/385 g) small broccoli florets

1 tablespoon chopped fresh cilantro

1 tablespoon crushed cashews (optional)

1. Start the sauce: In a small bowl, combine the guar gum and water; let rest for 10 to 15 minutes, until thickened.

2. Meanwhile, prepare the chicken: Heat the coconut oil in a large skillet over medium heat. Add the garlic, ginger, and onions; fry for 2 to 3 minutes, until fragrant.

3. Add the chicken to the skillet and increase the heat to medium-high. Fry for 5 to 6 minutes per side until nice and golden brown on both sides and cooked through in the center.

4. Complete the sauce: In a saucepan over low heat, melt the butter-flavored coconut oil. Add the lemon juice, erythritol (if using), stevia, tamari, and salt. Stir in the guar gum mixture. Increase the heat to high and bring the sauce to a boil, then reduce the heat to low and simmer the sauce until it thickens, 10 to 15 minutes.

5. Bring a saucepan of water to a boil. Add the broccoli florets and turn off the heat, leaving the pan on the burner. Let the broccoli sit in the hot water for 2 to 3 minutes, until very lightly cooked and still dark green. Drain.

6. Add the lemon sauce to the chicken in the skillet and mix until the chicken pieces are well coated.

7. Sprinkle the cilantro and cashews, if using, over the chicken and serve with the broccoli.

tip

For a nice Asian twist, place each serving of chicken and broccoli over ½ cup (2 ounces/55 g) of cauliflower rice or ½ cup (4 ounces/115 g) shirataki noodles or shirataki rice.

MACRONUTRIENTS (using liquid stevia only)				
Fat	Protein	Carbs	Fiber	Energy
49.8g	38.8g	5.7g	1.5g	631 cal
71%	25%	4%		

MACRONUTRIENTS (with erythritol)				
Fat	Protein	Carbs	Fiber	Energy
49.8g	38.8g	11.7g	7.5g	631 cal
69%	24%	7%		

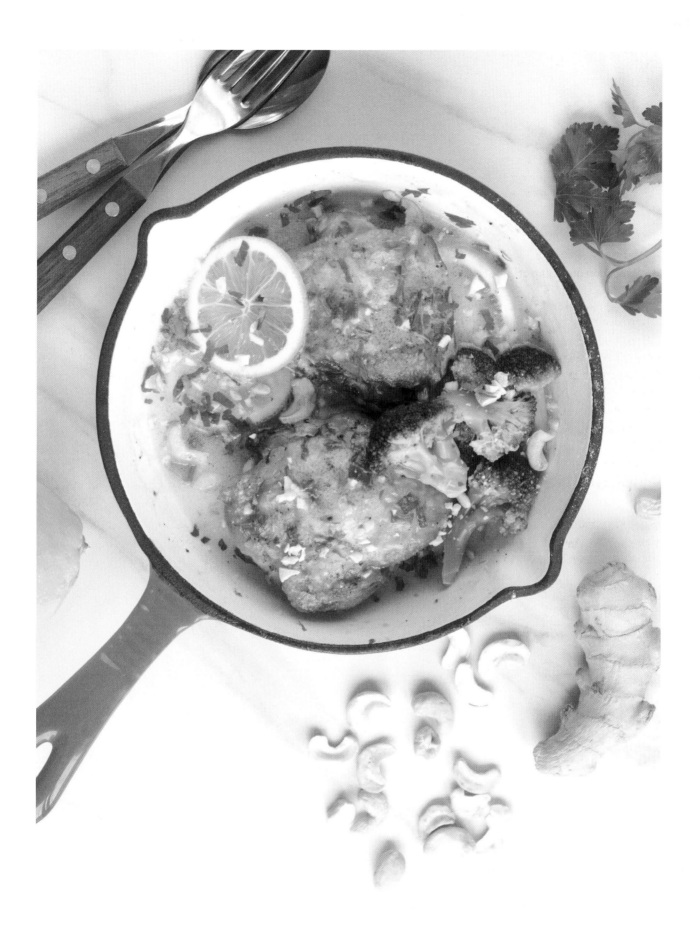

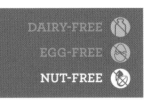

DAIRY-FREE

EGG-FREE

NUT-FREE

Chicken and Bacon Pâté

Prep Time: 20 minutes, plus time to chill | **Cook Time: 1 hour 40 minutes**
Yield: 6 servings

I love picnic-style food, and especially cold plates with meats, cheeses, and pâté. I enjoy finding pâté at local markets, but I've learned over the years that it's tricky to find this treat without added sugars. It was a total revelation to learn that I could make my own and that the process is relatively easy. Pâté does not require advanced cooking skills but has such a wow factor when you serve it.

Pâté is on the higher end of the nourishing foods spectrum, as it contains organ meat; it is also very ketogenic, portable, and delicious. If the word liver sends you running for the hills, I can relate. But give it a try. The bacon flavor is so rich in this recipe, you might not notice the liver!

¾ cup (6 ounces/170 g) unsalted butter, divided

1 pound (455 g) chicken livers, trimmed, rinsed, and patted dry

8 ounces (225 g) bacon, divided

2 egg yolks

½ cup (4 fluid ounces/120 ml) heavy whipping cream

½ onion, finely chopped

1 tablespoon chopped fresh parsley

1 teaspoon chopped fresh thyme, or ¼ teaspoon dried thyme leaves

½ teaspoon fine sea salt

¼ teaspoon ground black pepper

¼ teaspoon ground allspice

2 to 4 drops liquid stevia, or 1 teaspoon erythritol (optional)

note

I like to serve this pâté with seed crackers, cucumbers, or pork rinds.

1. Preheat the oven to 350°F (177°C).

2. Melt ½ cup (4 ounces/115 g) of the butter and pour it into a food processor. Add the chicken livers and three-quarters of the bacon and pulse until well blended. Add the egg yolks, cream, onion, parsley, thyme, salt, pepper, allspice, and stevia, if using, and blend well.

3. Line the bottom of a 2-quart (2-L) ceramic baking dish (or a 9 by 5-inch/23 by 13-cm glass or ceramic loaf pan) with the remaining bacon. Top with the pâté mixture. Press down and smooth the surface. Place the baking dish inside a large deep pan. Carefully pour enough hot water into the pan, surrounding the baking dish, to create a water bath halfway up the sides of the baking dish. Carefully move the pan to the oven and bake the pâté for 90 to 100 minutes, until it is set and a metal skewer inserted in the center comes out clean.

4. Let the pâté cool to room temperature in the water bath. Remove the baking dish from the water bath, cover with parchment paper, then place a small heavy plate that fits inside the baking dish over the parchment paper to press down on the pâté (or top with heavy cans). Transfer the pâté to the refrigerator and chill overnight. In the morning, drain any excess water.

5. Once cool, remove the parchment paper and weights. Melt the remaining ¼ cup (2 ounces/55 g) of butter and pour it over the top of the pâté. Return it to the fridge for 20 to 30 minutes, until solid, to create a butter seal. It will keep in the refrigerator for up to 4 days.

tip

If you prefer to not heat up the oven, try my easy No-Bake Chicken and Bacon Pâté (page 244). This baked version has a denser set, while the no-bake version has a creamier texture and a more vibrant taste with the fresh herbs.

MACRONUTRIENTS (per serving)				
Fat	Protein	Carbs	Fiber	Energy
44g	29g	2.2g	0.3g	530 cal
80%	19%	1%		

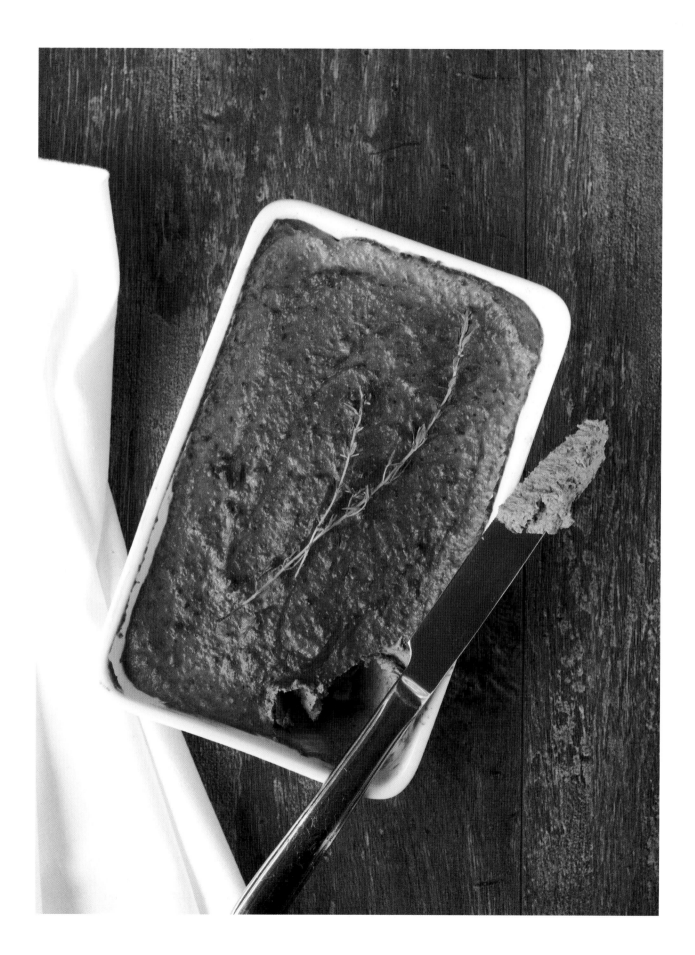

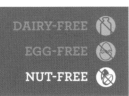

DAIRY-FREE

EGG-FREE

NUT-FREE

No-Bake
Chicken and Bacon Pâté

Prep Time: 20 minutes, plus time to chill | **Cook Time:** 15 minutes
Yield: 6 servings

Pâté is so rich, creamy, and decadent! I love it with pickle or cucumber slices or with flax-seed or chia seed crackers, which I find in health-food stores or make my own. (Search on the internet for flaxseed crackers *and you'll see how simple and quick they are to make.) Pork rinds are always a great option as well. If you prefer to make your pâté in the oven, check out my Chicken and Bacon Pâté (page 242).*

8 ounces (225 g) bacon

1 pound (455 g) chicken livers, trimmed, rinsed, and patted dry

¾ cup (6 ounces/170 g) unsalted butter, divided

½ onion, finely chopped

1 teaspoon fresh thyme, or ¼ teaspoon dried thyme leaves

1 tablespoon chopped fresh parsley

2 pasteurized egg yolks

½ cup (4 fluid ounces/115 g) heavy whipping cream

¼ teaspoon ground allspice

2 to 4 drops liquid stevia, or 1 teaspoon erythritol

½ teaspoon fine sea salt

Ground black pepper, to taste

1. Line a 2-quart ceramic baking dish or a glass or ceramic 9 by 5-inch (23 by 13-cm) loaf pan with parchment paper.

2. In a skillet over medium heat, fry the bacon for 4 to 5 minutes, until cooked and tender but not crisp. Remove from the pan and set aside, leaving the bacon fat in the pan. Fry the chicken livers in the bacon fat over medium heat until cooked through, 7 to 9 minutes.

3. Remove the chicken livers from the pan and slice each one into 4 to 6 segments. Melt ½ cup (4 ounces/115 g) of the butter in the skillet.

4. Using a food processor, blend the chicken livers and bacon with the melted butter, onion, herbs, egg yolks, cream, allspice, stevia, salt, and pepper until well mixed. For extra flavor, add the pan drippings to the food processor and pulse until combined.

5. Transfer the pâté to the prepared baking dish. Press down and smooth the surface.

6. Chill the pâté in the refrigerator for 1 to 2 hours. Once cool, melt the remaining ¼ cup (2 ounces/60 g) of butter and pour it over the top of the pâté. Return the pâté to the fridge for another 20 to 30 minutes, until solid, to create a butter seal. It will keep in the refrigerator for up to 4 days.

MACRONUTRIENTS
(per serving)

Fat	Protein	Carbs	Fiber	Energy
44g	29g	2.2g	0.3g	530 cal
80%	19%	1%		

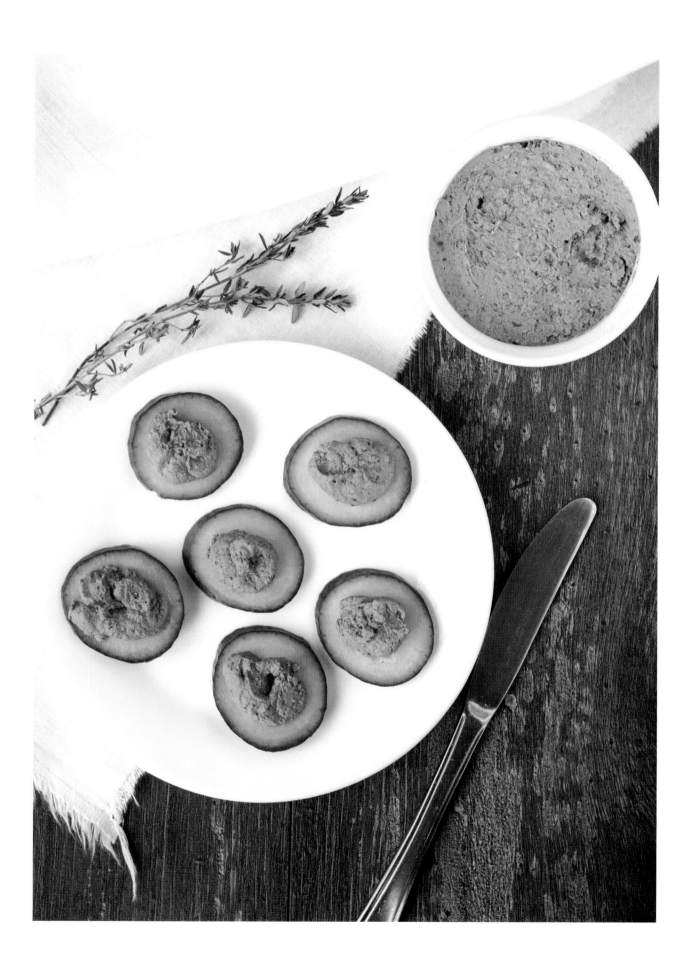

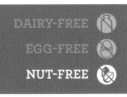

DAIRY-FREE

EGG-FREE

NUT-FREE

Hot Wings
with Blue Cheese and Celery

Prep Time: 20 minutes | **Cook Time:** 12 minutes
Yield: 3 servings

Chicken wings are a restaurant favorite and an excellent keto meal to make at home. Even without the usual batter and breading, these wings taste fantastic! Surprisingly, this is a super-keto and low-carb recipe, with only 1 percent carbohydrate.

½ cup (4 ounces/115 g) butter

½ cup (4 fluid ounces/120 ml) medium–hot hot sauce

1 tablespoon apple cider vinegar

Sea salt and ground black pepper

Refined coconut oil or lard, for frying

1 pound (455 g) chicken wings, cut into wingettes and drumettes

6 medium stalks celery, chopped into 4 segments each

2 tablespoons Blue Cheese Dressing (page 357)

1. In a medium saucepan over low heat, melt the butter. Add the hot sauce, vinegar, and salt and pepper to taste.

2. If using a deep-fryer, heat the coconut oil in the deep-fryer to 338°F (170°C). Alternatively, heat 2 inches (5 cm) of coconut oil in a deep heavy skillet over medium-high heat to 375°F (190°C). Pat the wings dry and season with a bit of salt and pepper.

3. If using a deep-fryer, fry for 8 to 10 minutes, then remove to a plate lined with paper towels and let cool. Increase the oil temperature to 375°F (190°C) and fry the wings again for 30 seconds to 1 minute.

   If cooking the wings on the stovetop, fry until crispy and cooked through, about 10 minutes.

4. Remove the wings from the oil and coat with the hot sauce mixture.

5. Divide the wings between 3 plates and serve each with 8 celery segments and 1 tablespoon of the blue cheese dressing.

tip

When I make these succulent wings in a deep-fryer, I like to fry them twice. The first fry is at the near-highest setting. Then I remove the wings and let them cool. Then I fry them again for a few minutes at the highest setting. The result is crispy, not soggy, wings.

MACRONUTRIENTS
(per serving)

Fat	Protein	Carbs	Fiber	Energy
60g	28.3g	8.3g	1.3g	686 cal
79%	16%	4.5%		

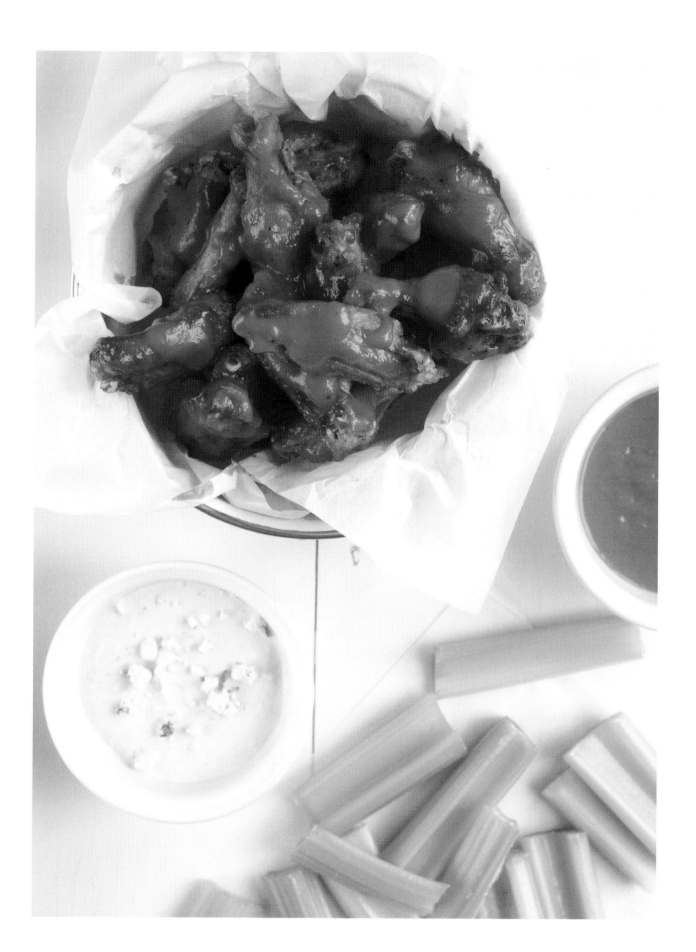

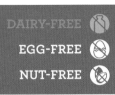

DAIRY-FREE

EGG-FREE

NUT-FREE

Spicy Chicken Fajitas

Prep Time: 5 minutes | **Cook Time:** 25 minutes
Yield: 4 servings

One of the most keto-friendly culinary traditions is Mexican food! Mexican cuisine empha-sizes high-fat avocados, cream, cheese, and wonderful spices (which reduce the need for condiments, as they do in Thai and Indian cuisine). It also makes it easy to stick to keto when eating out or traveling in Mexico—if you hold the tortillas, rice, and beans and add guacamole, sour cream, and cheese, you can hit your keto macros easily.

8 tablespoons (4 ounces/115 g) butter or coconut oil, divided

4 ounces (115 g) boneless chicken thighs, preferably skin-on, or 8 ounces (225 g) bone-in, skin-on thighs

1 cup (3½ ounces/100 g) green bell pepper strips

1 cup (3½ ounces/100 g) red bell pepper strips

2 tablespoons thinly sliced green onions

1 clove garlic, minced

½ cup (4 fluid ounces/120 ml) filtered water

1 medium avocado

1 tablespoon freshly squeezed lime juice

¼ teaspoon cayenne pepper

¼ teaspoon garlic powder

¼ teaspoon onion powder

¼ teaspoon fine sea salt

½ head iceberg or butter lettuce, leaves separated

5 ounces (140 g) sour cream

½ cup (1¾ ounces/50 g) shredded cheddar cheese

FAJITA SPICE MIX:

1 teaspoon paprika

½ teaspoon cayenne pepper

½ teaspoon ground cumin

½ teaspoon garlic powder

½ teaspoon onion powder

½ teaspoon turmeric powder

½ teaspoon fine sea salt

1. In a medium skillet over medium heat, melt 2 tablespoons of the butter. Add the chicken thighs and fry until nicely browned and cooked through, about 7 minutes per side if boneless, or 14 minutes per side if bone-in. Remove from the heat and cut the meat into bite-sized pieces. Set aside.

2. In the same skillet over medium heat, melt 4 tablespoons of the butter. Add the bell peppers, onions, and garlic and cook for 2 to 3 minutes, until softened. Remove from the skillet and set aside.

3. Combine the spice mix ingredients in a small bowl.

4. In the same skillet over low heat, melt the remaining 2 tablespoons of butter. Return the chicken to the pan. Sprinkle the spice mix over the chicken. Pour in the water and stir well.

5. Increase the heat to medium and cook for 3 to 4 minutes, stirring occasionally, until the water has evaporated.

6. Cut the avocado in half and remove the pit. Scoop the flesh into a bowl. Add the lime juice, cayenne, garlic powder, onion powder, and salt and mix with a fork, mashing the avocado to the consistency of guacamole.

7. Serve the chicken in the lettuce leaves. Top with the sautéed vegetables, guacamole, sour cream, and shredded cheese.

MACRONUTRIENTS (per serving)				
Fat	Protein	Carbs	Fiber	Energy
48g	24.8g	8g	2.8g	557 cal
77%	17%	6%		

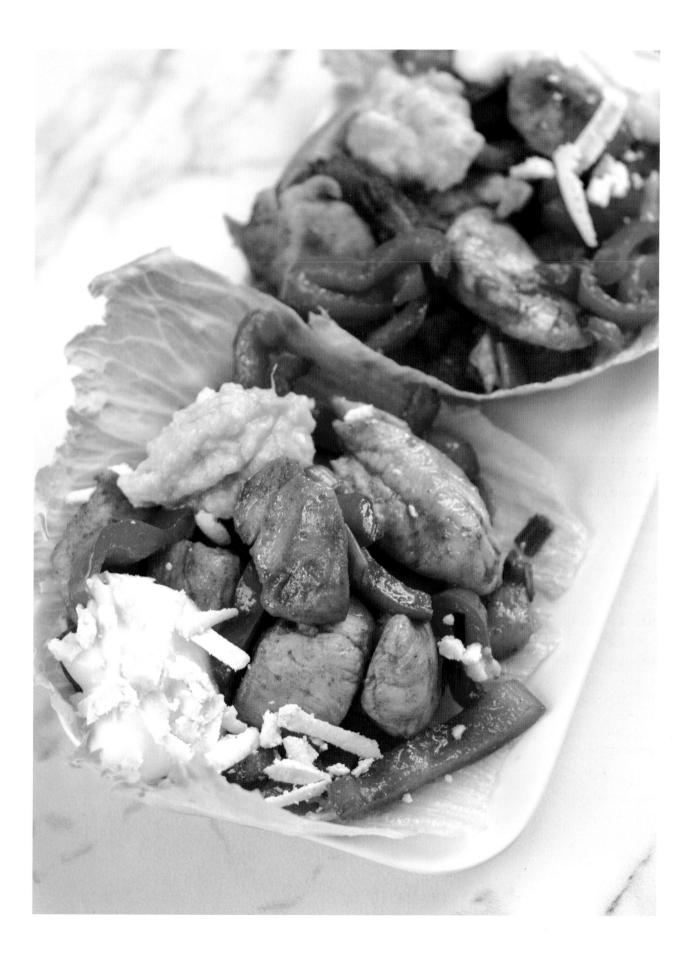

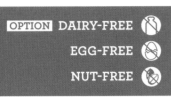

OPTION **DAIRY-FREE**

EGG-FREE

NUT-FREE

Teriyaki Chicken

Prep Time: 10 minutes | **Cook Time: 30 minutes**
Yield: 2 servings

My mom likes to say that her teriyaki chicken wings were how she got my father to marry her. Of course, we know it was all of her many incredible talents and qualities, although her cooking and entertaining skills are unmatched. This dish is based on a family recipe that she has perfected over the years and that I continue to enjoy keto-style.

5 tablespoons (2½ ounces/70 g) coconut oil or butter, divided

4 bone-in, skin-on chicken thighs (about 1 pound/455 g)

3 cups (12 ounces/340 g) shredded green cabbage

3 tablespoons apple cider vinegar

3 tablespoons tamari

1 tablespoon erythritol (optional)

½ to 1 teaspoon liquid stevia, to taste

1 tablespoon chopped fresh cilantro, for garnish

Sesame seeds, for garnish

1. In a skillet over medium heat, melt 2 tablespoons of the coconut oil. Add the chicken thighs, skin side down, and fry for 14 minutes on each side, until nicely browned and crispy and cooked through in the center.

2. Meanwhile, in a separate skillet over medium heat, melt the remaining 3 tablespoons of coconut oil. Add the cabbage and fry for 6 to 8 minutes, stirring constantly, until slightly translucent.

3. In a small saucepan over high heat, bring the vinegar, tamari, erythritol (if using), and stevia to a boil. The mixture will start to bubble up and caramelize.

4. Add the sauce to the skillet with the chicken and cook over medium-low heat until bubbling and thick, about 2 minutes, turning the chicken in the sticky sauce until nicely coated.

5. Serve the chicken over the cabbage, garnished with the chopped cilantro and sesame seeds.

MACRONUTRIENTS
(per serving)

Fat	Protein	Carbs	Fiber	Energy
60g	40.5g	11.5g	8g	721 cal
72%	22%	6%		

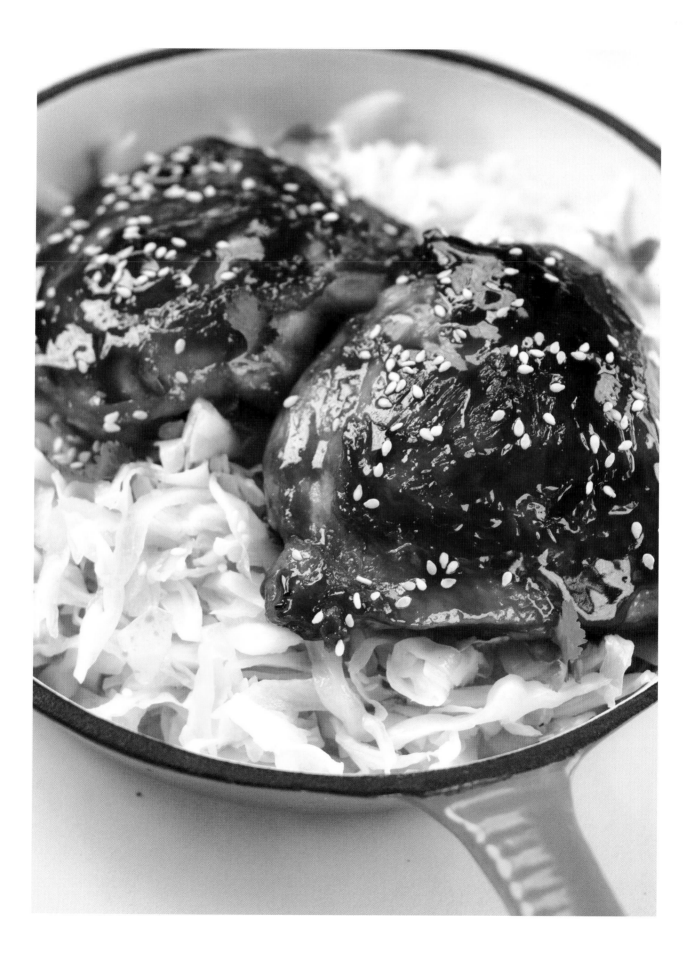

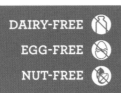

DAIRY-FREE

EGG-FREE

NUT-FREE

Duck Rillettes

Prep Time: 20 minutes, plus 1 hour to chill | **Cook Time: 2 hours**
Yield: 6 servings

This is an amazing "dip" or pâté-like dish! I love it with fermented pickles, sauerkraut, or my Sugar-Free Cranberry Sauce (page 346). This treat is very keto, with 80 percent fat and only 1 percent total carb.

4 duck legs

½ cup (4 ounces/115 g) duck fat, melted

3 cloves garlic, minced

1 tablespoon chopped fresh thyme

1 bay leaf

½ teaspoon fine sea salt

¼ teaspoon ground black pepper

2 tablespoons apple cider vinegar

¾ cup (6 fluid ounces/180 ml) duck fat from cooking

2 tablespoons thinly sliced green onions

⅛ teaspoon ground cloves

⅛ teaspoon ground Ceylon cinnamon or regular cinnamon

⅛ teaspoon ground nutmeg

1 tablespoon grated orange zest

½ teaspoon ginger juice, or 1 teaspoon grated fresh ginger

2 to 4 drops liquid stevia, or 1 teaspoon erythritol

1. Preheat the oven to 300°F (150°C).

2. Place the duck legs in a roasting pan. Rub the melted duck fat, garlic, thyme, bay leaf, salt, and pepper into the skin of the duck.

3. Add the vinegar to the pan. Cover with aluminum foil and bake for about 2 hours, until the meat is tender and falling off the bone.

4. Let cool, then pull the meat and skin from the bones with a fork. Remove ¾ cup (6 ounces/180 ml) of duck fat from the roasting pan and place it in a mixing bowl.

5. To the bowl with the duck fat, add the shredded meat and skin, along with the remaining ingredients. Toss everything together to combine. Divide between six ½-cup (4-ounce/115-g) ramekins and refrigerate for 1 hour or until the fat has solidified.

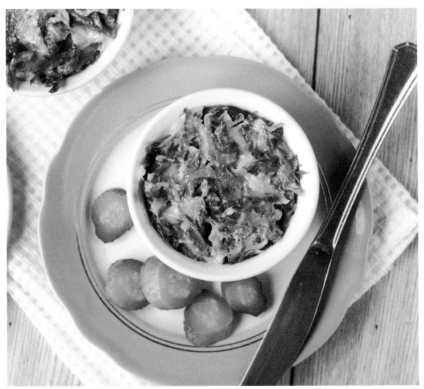

MACRONUTRIENTS
(per serving)

Fat	Protein	Carbs	Fiber	Energy
40g	23g	1.3g	0.3g	457 cal
80%	19%	1%		

Ceviche
with Spicy Mayo

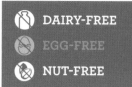

DAIRY-FREE

EGG-FREE

NUT-FREE

Prep Time: 15 minutes, plus 5 hours to marinate
Yield: 2 main-dish servings or 4 appetizer servings

Ceviche is one of my favorite foods and enjoying it with MCT oil and mayo takes it to the next level of delicious. This recipe makes four appetizers or two main courses.

12 ounces (340 g) halibut or other white fish fillets, chopped into ½-inch (1.25-cm) cubes

3 green onions, green parts only, thinly sliced

1 cup (8 fluid ounces/240 ml) freshly squeezed lime juice, plus more if needed

1 medium-sized ripe avocado, peeled and cut into ½-inch (1.25-cm) cubes

2 to 3 green jalapeño peppers or serrano chilies, finely chopped

¼ cup (¼ ounce/7 g) finely chopped fresh cilantro

¼ cup (2 fluid ounces/60 ml) MCT oil or olive oil

¼ teaspoon fine sea salt

¼ cup (2 ounces/55 g) mayonnaise

1 teaspoon hot sauce

1. Arrange the fish in a single layer in an 8-inch (20-cm) square baking dish or glass bowl. Sprinkle with the onions and pour the lime juice over the top, making sure the fish is fully covered in the juice; if it isn't, add more juice. Cover and place in the refrigerator for 4 to 5 hours to marinate.

2. Remove the fish from the refrigerator and verify that it is thoroughly "cooked"; it should be opaque in the center. Return it to the refrigerator to marinate longer, if needed.

3. Drain and transfer the fish to a bowl. Add the avocado, jalapeño, cilantro, oil, and salt; stir gently to combine.

4. Make the spicy mayo: In another bowl, combine the mayonnaise and hot sauce.

5. Serve the fish immediately, accompanied by the spicy mayo.

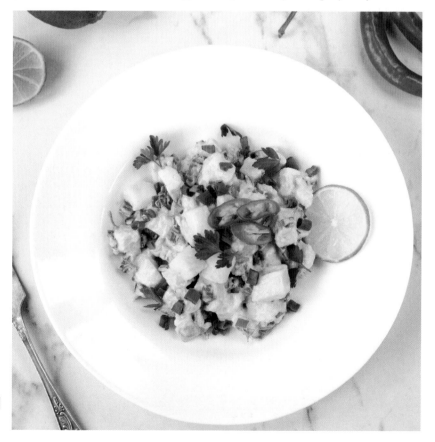

MACRONUTRIENTS (per serving)				
Fat	Protein	Carbs	Fiber	Energy
36.3g	18.3g	4.5g	2.5g	417 cal
78%	18%	4%		

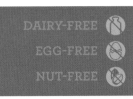

DAIRY-FREE

EGG-FREE

NUT-FREE

Crab Cakes
with Garlic–Dill Cream

Prep Time: 5 minutes | **Cook Time:** 15 minutes
Yield: 3 servings

I always used to avoid this classic French dish because it is so decadent. Without the bread-crumbs, however, crab cakes can be a perfect, nutritious keto meal, and it's a fast and easy meal to pull together. Blue crabmeat is wonderful in this dish.

CRAB CAKES:

8 ounces (225 g) fresh or canned crabmeat

¼ cup (2 ounces/55 g) mayonnaise

¼ cup (2 ounces/55 g) sour cream

2 tablespoons finely chopped green onions

1 tablespoon finely chopped fresh cilantro

1 teaspoon freshly squeezed lime juice

¼ cup (1 ounce/28 g) almond flour

1 tablespoon coconut flour

1 egg

2 tablespoons unsalted butter, for the pan

GARLIC-DILL CREAM:

3 tablespoons mayonnaise

3 tablespoons sour cream

1 teaspoon finely chopped fresh dill

¼ teaspoon garlic powder

1 or 2 drops liquid stevia, to taste

Sliced green onions, for garnish

Lime or lemon wedges, for serving (optional)

1. Place all the ingredients for the crab cakes, except the egg and butter, in a bowl. Blend with a fork. Add the egg and use the fork to fully incorporate it into the other ingredients.

2. Form the crab cake mixture into 6 small or 3 large cakes. Place in the refrigerator to chill for 10 minutes.

3. In another bowl, combine the ingredients for the garlic-dill cream. Place in the refrigerator to chill while you fry the crab cakes.

4. In a large skillet over medium heat, melt the butter. Working in batches, fry the crab cakes until golden brown, 3 to 4 minutes on each side.

5. Serve the crab cakes with the garlic-dill cream. Garnish with sliced green onions and serve with lime or lemon wedges, if desired.

MACRONUTRIENTS
(per serving)

Fat	Protein	Carbs	Fiber	Energy
52g	18g	4.3g	2g	557 cal
84%	13%	3%		

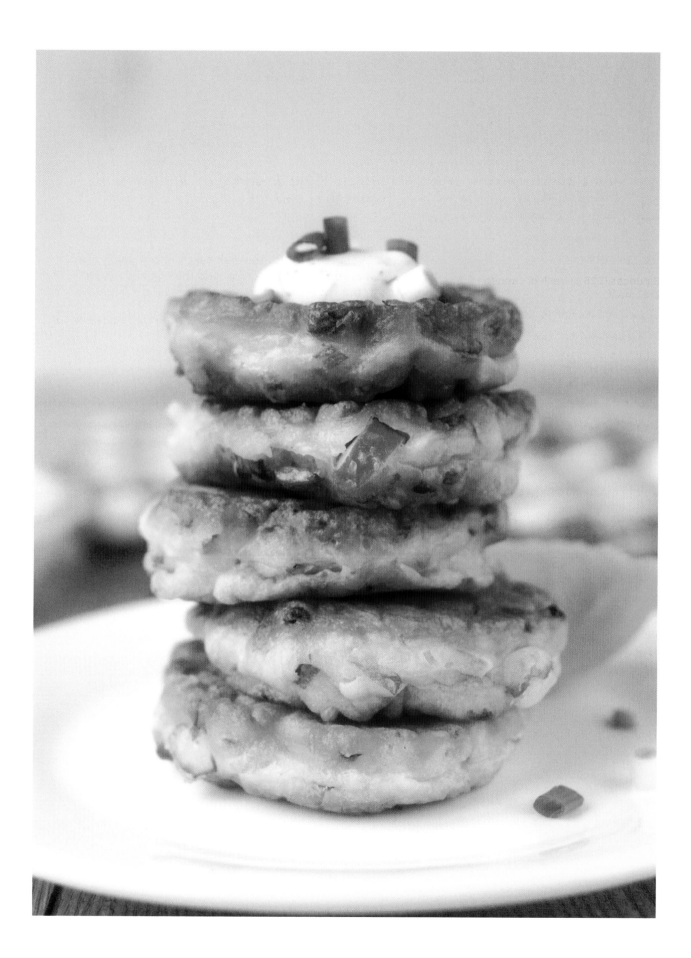

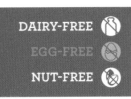

DAIRY-FREE

EGG-FREE

NUT-FREE

Spicy Shrimp Cocktail

Prep Time: 15 minutes, plus time to chill shrimp | **Cook Time:** 4 minutes
Yield: 4 servings

This alternative to traditional shrimp cocktail made with a ketchup-based cocktail sauce is an easy meal! It is extremely ketogenic at 89 percent fat, 8 percent protein, and 3 percent carbohydrate.

8 ounces (225 g) shrimp, thawed if frozen, peeled and deveined

2 ounces (55 g) canned hearts of palm, drained and sliced

½ cup (2½ ounces/70 g) grape tomatoes, chopped

2 medium stalks celery, chopped

½ medium cucumber, peeled and chopped

1 cup (8 ounces/225 g) mayonnaise

1 teaspoon freshly squeezed lemon juice

1 teaspoon hot sauce (optional)

½ teaspoon fine sea salt

Pinch of cayenne pepper

4 butter lettuce leaves

Chopped fresh dill or other herbs, for garnish (optional)

1. Bring a saucepan of water to a boil. Add the shrimp and lightly boil for 3 to 4 minutes, until bright pink and cooked through. Drain and set aside.

2. In a mixing bowl, combine the shrimp, hearts of palm, tomatoes, celery, cucumber, mayonnaise, lemon juice, hot sauce (if using), salt, and cayenne. Refrigerate for 10 to 20 minutes.

3. Place a lettuce leaf in the bottom and up the side of each of 4 serving bowls or glasses. Distribute the shrimp mixture between the bowls; garnish with dill, if desired. Serve cold.

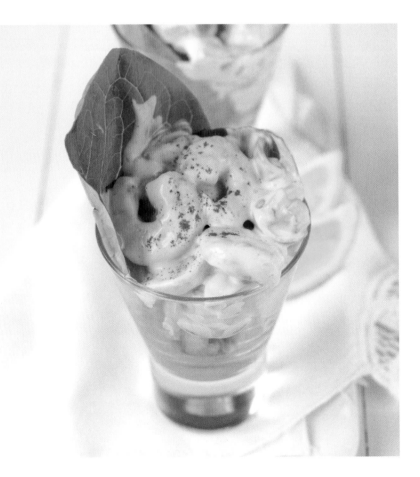

MACRONUTRIENTS
(per serving)

Fat	Protein	Carbs	Fiber	Energy
44g	9g	3.3g	0.8g	450 cal
89%	8%	3%		

Shrimp Hollandaise
Avocado Stacks

Prep Time: **10 minutes** | Cook Time: **4 minutes**
Yield: **2 servings**

This recipe uses chilled hollandaise, which is nice and thick. You can also substitute mayonnaise flavored with a little garlic powder, onion powder, and sea salt.

24 large shrimp, thawed if frozen, peeled and deveined

½ medium-sized ripe avocado, peeled and chopped into ¼-inch (6-mm) cubes

¼ cup plus 3 tablespoons (3½ ounces/100 g) Hollandaise (page 354), chilled

1 tablespoon sliced green onions

1 tablespoon chopped fresh cilantro

¼ teaspoon fine sea salt

2 thick slices tomato (from 1 medium tomato)

Fresh herbs of choice, for garnish (optional)

Ground black pepper, for garnish (optional)

1. Bring a medium saucepan of water to a gentle boil over medium-high heat; add the shrimp and lightly boil for 3 to 4 minutes until bright pink, being careful not to overcook them.

2. Drain the shrimp. When cool enough to handle, slice each into 3 or 4 pieces; place in the refrigerator to cool.

3. Remove the cooled shrimp from the refrigerator and mix with the hollandaise to coat. Add the green onions, cilantro, and salt and stir to combine.

4. Place a tomato slice on the bottom of a food shaper or molding ring. Scoop half of the shrimp mixture onto the tomato, then top with half of the avocado. Remove the mold and repeat with the rest of the ingredients. Garnish with fresh herbs and pepper, if desired.

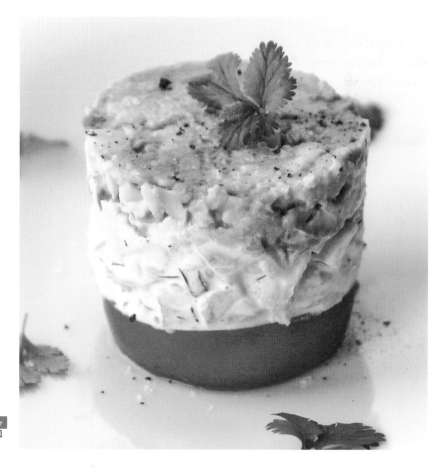

MACRONUTRIENTS
(per serving)

Fat	Protein	Carbs	Fiber	Energy
31.5g	13.5g	4.5g	2.5g	345 cal
79%	16%	5%		

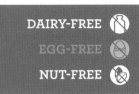

DAIRY-FREE

EGG-FREE

NUT-FREE

Crispy Calamari
with Aioli

Prep Time: 15 minutes | **Cook Time: 5 minutes**
Yield: 4 servings

Calamari used to be one of my go-to indulgences when eating out. In Vancouver, I discovered the restaurant Sandbar in Granville Island, which serves gluten-free calamari, and I always looked forward to their delicious calamari with spicy aioli. When I went keto, however, the corn flour used in that dish was no longer ideal for me. I tried making my own keto calamari, and it is delicious! This recipe is fairly simple to prepare, and you likely have all or most of the ingredients other than the calamari on hand. If you love calamari like I do, give this one a go and let me know how you and your loved ones enjoy it.

8 ounces (225 g) cleaned squid bodies, thawed if frozen, sliced into ¼-inch (6-mm) rings

2 eggs, lightly whisked

¼ cup (1 ounce/28 g) coconut flour

¼ teaspoon cayenne pepper

½ teaspoon fine sea salt

½ teaspoon ground black pepper

Lard, refined coconut oil, or duck fat, for frying

¼ onion, minced, for garnish

¼ cup (2 ounces/55 g) Aioli (page 352), for serving

Lemon wedges, for serving (optional)

1. Place the squid rings in a bowl with the whisked eggs so that the squid is well covered.

2. In a mixing bowl, combine the coconut flour, cayenne, salt, and black pepper.

3. One at a time, dredge the squid rings in the flour mixture.

4. Line a plate with paper towels. Heat the oil to 338°F (170°C) in a deep-fryer. Alternatively, heat about 4 inches (10 cm) of oil (but not more than halfway up the pot) in a heavy deep-sided pot to 375°F (190°C) over medium-high heat.

5. If using a deep-fryer, drop the squid rings into the frying basket and fry for 3 to 4 minutes to the desired color and crispness.

   If using a pot on the stovetop, fry the squid in the oil until golden brown and crisp, about 5 minutes. Don't overcrowd the pan or you will lower the oil temperature, which might make the calamari less crisp.

6. Remove the calamari from the oil and set on the paper towel–lined plate.

7. If using a deep-fryer, increase the oil temperature to 375°F (190°C). Fry the calamari for 1 to 2 more minutes, until golden-brown and crisp. Remove from the oil and set on the paper towels.

8. To serve, stack the calamari on a plate or place in a bowl and garnish with minced onion. Serve the aioli on the side. If desired, squeeze a lemon wedge over the calamari.

MACRONUTRIENTS
(per serving)

Fat	Protein	Carbs	Fiber	Energy
32g	13g	6g	3g	358 cal
80%	14%	6%		

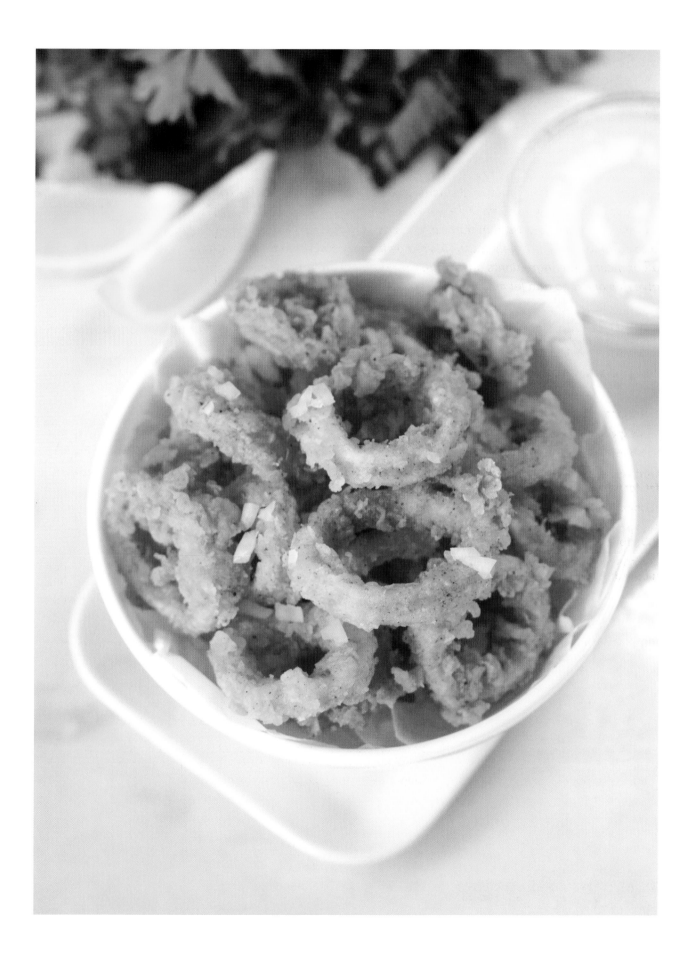

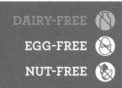

DAIRY-FREE

EGG-FREE

NUT-FREE

Keto Moules "Frites"
(Mussels and "Fries")

Prep Time: 15 minutes | Cook Time: 40 minutes
Yield: 4 servings

Moules frites is another quintessential French dish that my husband and I shared on one of our first dates. He is a mussel lover, and he quickly made me a believer in this light but flavor-packed dish. I have always been partial to the original version made with white wine, and you could add a bit of dry white wine to this dish. I have made it here without the wine, using white wine vinegar in its place and pairing the jus *with fragrant fresh herbs. Serve with the keto "fries" for a meal that tastes very indulgent but is as nourishing as it is delectable.*

FRIES:

2 tablespoons duck fat or coconut oil, melted

2 pounds (910 g) yellow wax beans, trimmed

¼ teaspoon fine sea salt

MUSSELS:

2 pounds (910 g) fresh mussels

½ cup (4 ounces/115 g) salted butter

3 cloves garlic, minced

1 shallot, finely chopped

¼ teaspoon red pepper flakes (optional)

¼ cup (2 fluid ounces/60 ml) white wine vinegar

1 cup (8 fluid ounces/240 ml) fish, clam, or chicken bone broth

1 cup (8 fluid ounces/240 ml) heavy whipping cream

½ teaspoon fine sea salt

¼ teaspoon ground black pepper

¼ cup (¼ ounce/7 g) finely chopped fresh parsley

1 teaspoon fresh thyme leaves

1. Preheat the oven to 338°F (170°C). Grease a rimmed baking sheet with a bit of the duck fat.

2. Make the fries: Toss the wax beans with the remaining duck fat and place on the prepared baking sheet in an even layer. Bake until the beans are lightly browned, 30 to 40 minutes.

3. When the fries are about halfway done, prepare the mussels: Sort through the mussels, discarding any that are open. Rinse, scrub, and debeard (if necessary) the mussels. Set aside.

4. In a Dutch oven over medium-low heat, melt the butter. Add the garlic, shallot, and red pepper flakes, if using, and cook until the shallot is translucent, about 5 minutes.

5. Increase the heat to medium; add the vinegar and simmer for 1 minute.

6. Stir in the broth, cream, salt, and black pepper and bring to a simmer. Add the mussels, cover with a tight-fitting lid, and cook until the mussels open, 2 to 5 minutes. Stir in the parsley and thyme. Discard any mussels that remain closed. Serve with the fries.

note

Alternatively, you can fry the beans in a deep-fryer for 5 to 7 minutes at 338°F (170°C), then for 2 additional minutes at 375°F (190°C). You can also fry the beans in an air-fryer, according to the manufacturer's instructions.

MACRONUTRIENTS
(per serving)

Fat	Protein	Carbs	Fiber	Energy
49g	32g	23.2g	3.8g	671 cal
67%	19%	14%		

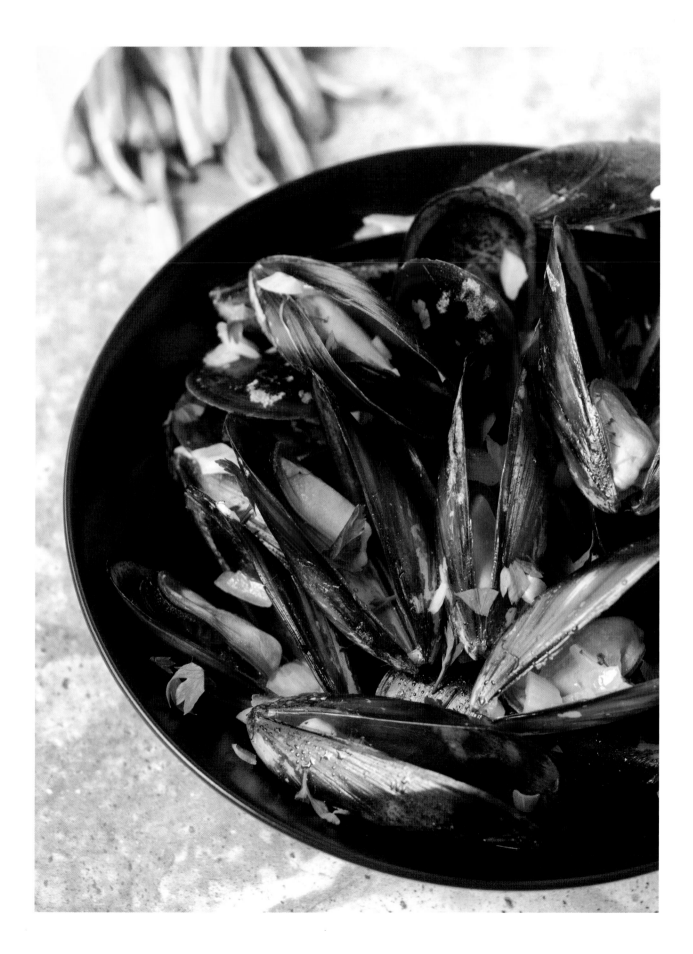

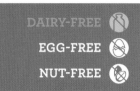

DAIRY-FREE

EGG-FREE

NUT-FREE

Easy Baked Lobster Tails
with Herb Butter

Prep Time: **5 minutes** | Cook Time: **10 minutes**
Yield: **4 servings**

To boost the total fat and nutrients of this decadent dish, serve it with a high-fat green side such as Creamed Spinach (page 217), one of the salads on pages 164 to 178, or some diced avocado.

1 cup (8 ounces/225 g) unsalted butter, melted

1 teaspoon freshly squeezed lemon juice

1 tablespoon chopped fresh parsley, or 1 teaspoon dried parsley

¼ teaspoon paprika

¼ teaspoon garlic powder

¼ teaspoon fine sea salt

¼ teaspoon ground black pepper

4 (5-ounce/150-g) lobster tails, thawed if frozen

1. Preheat the oven to broil.

2. In a bowl, whisk together the melted butter, lemon juice, parsley, paprika, garlic powder, salt, and pepper.

3. Shell the lobster. You can either slice the tails in half and remove the meat or, for a beautiful presentation, pull out and expose the meat on the top of the shell. To do so, use scissors to cut through the top of the shell lengthwise and pull apart carefully. Flip over and break the ribs of the shell. Flip over again and gently lift the meat in one piece out through the cut you made, then set the meat on top of the shell so that most of the meat is sitting outside the shell. Place the prepared tails on a rimmed baking sheet.

4. Pour 1 tablespoon of the butter mixture over each lobster tail.

5. Broil the lobster until the shells (if still attached) are lightly browned and the flesh turns an opaque white and is cooked through, about 10 minutes.

6. Divide the lobster between 4 plates and drizzle 1 tablespoon of the butter mixture over each tail. Give each person 2 tablespoons of the remaining herb butter as a dipping sauce.

MACRONUTRIENTS
(per serving)

Fat	Protein	Carbs	Fiber	Energy
47g	29.5g	2g	0g	542 cal
77%	21%	2%		

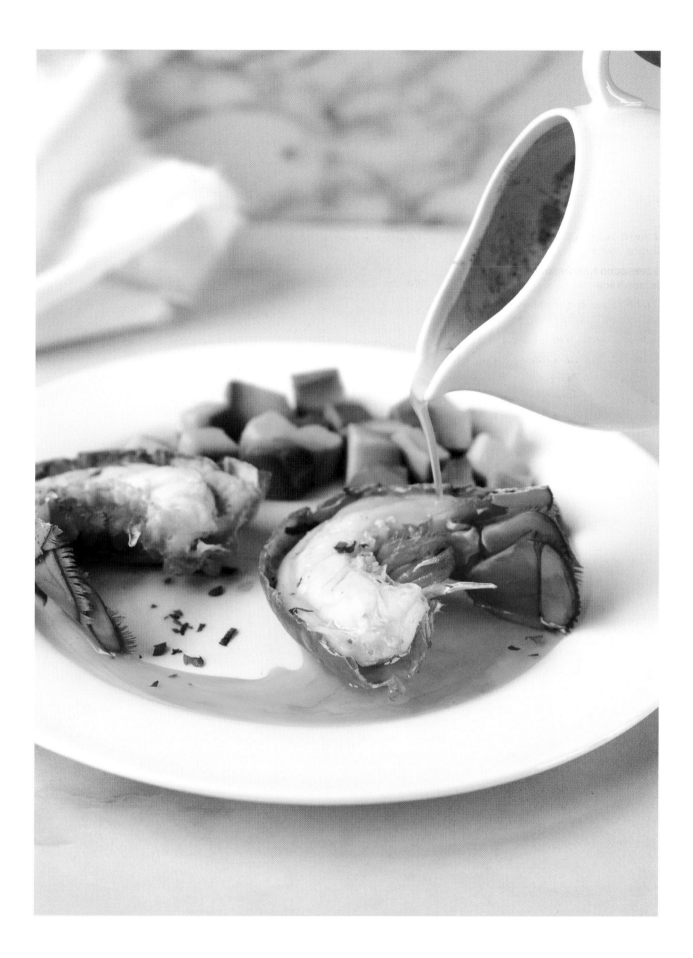

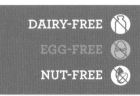

DAIRY-FREE

EGG-FREE

NUT-FREE

One-Pan Salmon
with Duck Fat–Roasted Rosemary Radishes and Asparagus

Prep Time: 10 minutes | **Cook Time: 20 minutes**
Yield: 4 servings

This super-easy weeknight dinner is delicious and healthy, with plenty of omega-3 fatty acids from the salmon.

3 ounces (85 g) duck fat, melted

1 tablespoon chopped fresh rosemary, or 1 teaspoon dried rosemary leaves

2 cups (8¾ ounces/245 g) halved or quartered radishes, depending on size

¼ teaspoon garlic powder

½ teaspoon fine sea salt

¼ teaspoon ground black pepper

½ cup (4 ounces/115 g) mayonnaise

1 tablespoon finely chopped fresh dill

2 cloves garlic, crushed in a garlic press

1 teaspoon Dijon mustard

4 (4-ounce/115-g) salmon fillets

16 asparagus spears, woody ends trimmed

1. Preheat the oven to 450°F (232°C). Line a rimmed baking sheet with aluminum foil.

2. In a bowl, combine the duck fat and rosemary.

3. In another bowl, toss the radishes with half of the duck fat mixture. Add the garlic powder, salt, and pepper and toss to distribute the seasonings. Spread the radishes across the prepared baking sheet.

4. In a small bowl, mix together the mayonnaise, dill, crushed garlic, and mustard. Place the salmon fillets on the pan with the radishes and top the salmon evenly with the mayonnaise mixture.

5. Coat the asparagus with the remaining half of the duck fat mixture; add to the baking sheet with the salmon and radishes.

6. Roast for 20 minutes, until the fish is opaque in the center and the vegetables are crisp-tender. Serve warm.

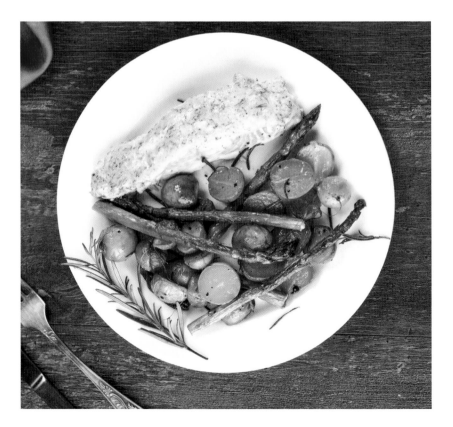

MACRONUTRIENTS
(per serving)

Fat	Protein	Carbs	Fiber	Energy
63.5g	35g	4.5g	2.3g	731 cal
78%	19%	3%		

Smoked Salmon Blini
with Dill Cream

Prep Time: 10 minutes | **Cook Time: 10 minutes**
Yield: 2 servings

	DAIRY-FREE OPTION
	EGG-FREE
	NUT-FREE

I first tried this traditional Eastern European dish while traveling with friends in Europe. It was so tasty that I just had to make a healthy keto version of it. I enjoyed coming up with the dill cream for it as well—caviar and fresh dill truly delight the senses!

BLINI:

2 eggs

2 tablespoons cream cheese or coconut cream (see note, page 108)

2 tablespoons almond milk

1 tablespoon coconut flour

3 or 4 drops liquid stevia, to taste

¼ teaspoon chopped fresh chives

¼ teaspoon onion powder

¼ teaspoon coarse or fine sea salt

3 tablespoons unsalted butter or coconut oil, for the pan

6 ounces (170 g) no-sugar-added smoked salmon

1 tablespoon black caviar (optional)

DILL CREAM:

3 tablespoons mayonnaise

3 tablespoons sour cream, or 3 tablespoons coconut cream mixed with 1 teaspoon apple cider vinegar

1 teaspoon finely chopped fresh dill, plus extra for garnish

½ teaspoon freshly squeezed lemon juice

¼ teaspoon fine sea salt

1 or 2 drops liquid stevia, to taste

1. In a medium bowl, combine the eggs, cream cheese, milk, flour, stevia, chives, onion powder, and salt. Beat with an electric mixer until smooth.

2. In a large skillet over medium-high heat, melt the butter.

3. Drop the batter into the pan to make small round blini, using 2 tablespoons to ¼ cup (2 ounces/55 g) of batter for each one. When cooked on one side (1 to 2 minutes), flip and cook on the other side. When cooked on the second side, remove and keep warm. Repeat with the remaining batter.

4. Meanwhile, combine all the dill cream ingredients in a bowl and mix thoroughly.

5. Divide the blini between 2 plates. Top with the smoked salmon, dill cream, and caviar, if using, and garnish with fresh dill, if desired. Serve at room temperature.

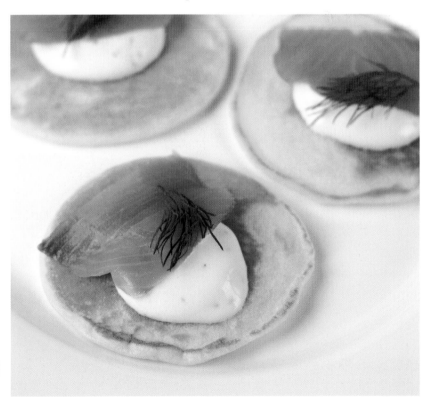

MACRONUTRIENTS
(per serving, with caviar)

Fat	Protein	Carbs	Fiber	Energy
57.5g	25.5g	4g	1.5g	648 cal
82%	16%	2%		

DAIRY-FREE 🚫

EGG-FREE 🚫

NUT-FREE 🚫

Salmon Avocado Poke

Prep Time: 10 minutes
Yield: **2 servings**

I love a poke bowl! Most of the ones sold commercially have a lot of added sugars, so making healthier keto poke bowls at home is a much better way to go. Sashimi- or sushi-grade salmon is flash-frozen to ensure that it is protected from bacteria and parasites. The best places to find it are at seafood markets or health-food stores that sell sushi or sashimi. Because you will be eating it raw, it's important to ensure that the salmon is safe for consumption.

DRESSING:

3 tablespoons light sesame oil

2 tablespoons apple cider vinegar

2 tablespoons tamari

1 teaspoon ginger juice, or 1 (1-inch/2.5-cm) piece fresh ginger, peeled and grated

1 teaspoon freshly squeezed lime juice

½ teaspoon hot sauce

½ teaspoon red pepper flakes

3 or 4 drops liquid stevia, to taste

8 ounces (225 g) sushi-grade salmon

½ ounce (15 g) dried wakame seaweed

1 cup (8 fluid ounces/240 ml) filtered water

1 avocado, peeled and cut into ¾-inch (2-cm) cubes

¼ cup thinly sliced green onions, plus more for garnish

2 tablespoons finely chopped cilantro

1 tablespoon sesame seeds, for garnish

Red pepper flakes, for garnish

1. In a medium bowl, thoroughly mix all the dressing ingredients.

2. Cut the salmon into ¾-inch (2-cm) cubes; add to the bowl of dressing and mix together. Refrigerate while you prepare the rest of the ingredients.

3. Place the seaweed and water in a bowl; let soak for 15 minutes to reconstitute. Drain completely and set aside.

4. Place the seaweed in a serving bowl and top with the salmon and dressing, avocado, green onions, and cilantro. Garnish with additional green onions, sesame seeds, and red pepper flakes.

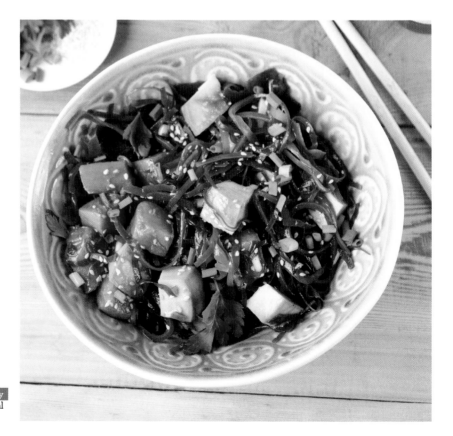

MACRONUTRIENTS
(per serving)

Fat	Protein	Carbs	Fiber	Energy
46.5g	29g	10.5g	7g	570 cal
73%	20%	7%		

Salmon Rillettes
on Cucumber Rounds

Prep Time: 10 minutes, plus time to chill | **Cook Time:** 8 minutes
Yield: 3 servings

DAIRY-FREE

EGG-FREE

NUT-FREE

This amazing pâté-like dish is a real crowd-pleaser. The cooling crispness of the cucumbers pairs so well with the delicious and buttery salmon. The butter preserves the rillettes well in the fridge for a couple of days, or you can store them in the freezer for up to 1 month.

1 pound (455 g) wild salmon fillets

1 cup (8 fluid ounces/240 ml) filtered water

¼ cup plus 2 tablespoons (3 ounces/85 g) unsalted butter, melted

5 tablespoons (2½ ounces/70 g) mayonnaise

1½ tablespoons freshly squeezed lemon juice

2 tablespoons finely chopped fresh chives

2 tablespoons thinly sliced green onions

1 tablespoon finely chopped fresh cilantro

6 ounces (170 g) no–sugar–added smoked salmon, sliced

½ teaspoon fine sea salt

¼ teaspoon onion powder

¼ teaspoon paprika

Pinch of cayenne pepper

½ English cucumber, sliced on the diagonal into ovals, for serving

1. In a medium pot over medium-low heat, bring the salmon and water to a gentle simmer. Cook for 6 to 8 minutes, until the salmon is cooked through (it will be opaque in the center). Drain, then use a fork to flake the fish apart.

2. In a small bowl, combine the cooked salmon with the rest of the ingredients, except the cucumbers. Mix well.

3. Divide the mixture between three 4-ounce (120-ml) ramekins or jars. Use a spoon or fork to press the mixture into each ramekin, then cover with plastic wrap. Refrigerate for 8 hours or overnight.

4. Serve with the cucumbers on the side, or scoop the rillettes mixture onto the cucumber "crackers."

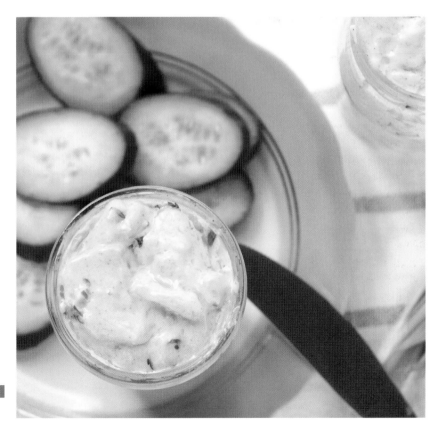

MACRONUTRIENTS (per serving)				
Fat	Protein	Carbs	Fiber	Energy
47g	23.7g	2.7g	0.3g	541 cal
80%	18%	2%		

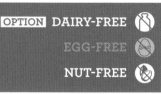

OPTION DAIRY-FREE
EGG-FREE
NUT-FREE

One-Pan Cod
with Broccolini and Mint Hollandaise

Prep Time: 15 minutes | **Cook Time: 15 minutes**
Yield: 4 servings

This delicious sauce has so many tasty applications. It is fantastic with white fish and broccolini, as in this recipe, or paired with short ribs or other grilled meats. It is important to use pasteurized eggs for the hollandaise, as the egg yolks are not thoroughly cooked in the hot butter.

4 (4-ounce/115-g) cod or halibut fillets

6 ounces (170 g) broccolini, larger stalks cut in half lengthwise

MINT HOLLANDAISE:

6 egg yolks from pasteurized eggs

¾ cup (6 ounces/170 g) butter, melted, or room-temperature MCT oil

1 tablespoon Dijon mustard

1 tablespoon freshly squeezed lemon juice

1 to 3 drops liquid stevia, to taste

½ teaspoon fine sea salt

Ground black pepper, to taste

2 tablespoons thinly sliced fresh mint

1. Preheat the oven to 400°F (205°C). Line a rimmed baking sheet with aluminum foil and spray the foil with coconut oil spray.

2. Arrange the fish fillets and broccolini on the prepared baking sheet and spray with coconut oil spray. Bake for 15 minutes, until cooked through.

3. Meanwhile, make the mint hollandaise: Place the egg yolks in a tall immersion blender container or a wide and tall mason jar. Add the melted butter, mustard, lemon juice, stevia, salt, and pepper. Insert the immersion blender so that it is at the bottom of the container. Turn on the blender and don't move it for 15 to 30 seconds. Gradually start moving it up as the sauce becomes creamy and blended; the hot butter will cook the egg yolks as the hollandaise emulsifies. While continuing to blend, slowly pull the immersion blender up and out of the container. Add the mint to the hollandaise and stir to combine.

4. Drizzle each portion of fish with ¼ cup (2 ounces/55 g) of the mint hollandaise and serve with the broccolini.

tip

Leftover hollandaise can be stored in the fridge for up to 6 days. If it separates, mix in a tablespoon of ice-cold water. It works like magic to blend the hollandaise back together and revive the creamy texture!

note

This is my super-easy immersion blender method of making hollandaise. To see the method in detail, check out the video on my Ketogenic Girl YouTube channel.

MACRONUTRIENTS
(per serving)

Fat	Protein	Carbs	Fiber	Energy
45.3g	29.5g	5g	1g	545 cal
78%	19%	3%		

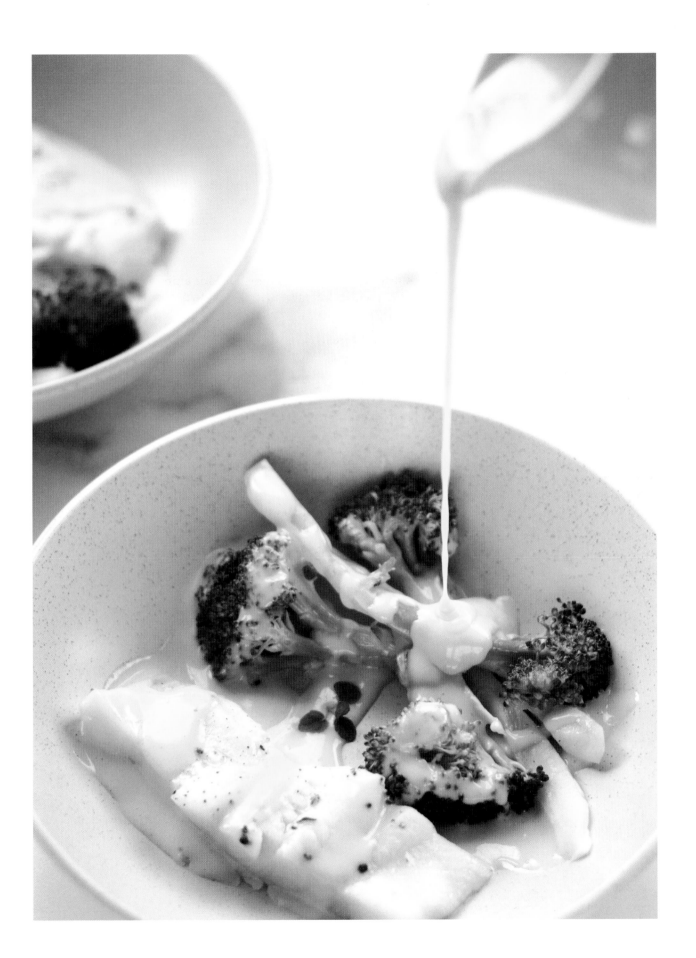

Chapter 13
Beef & Pork

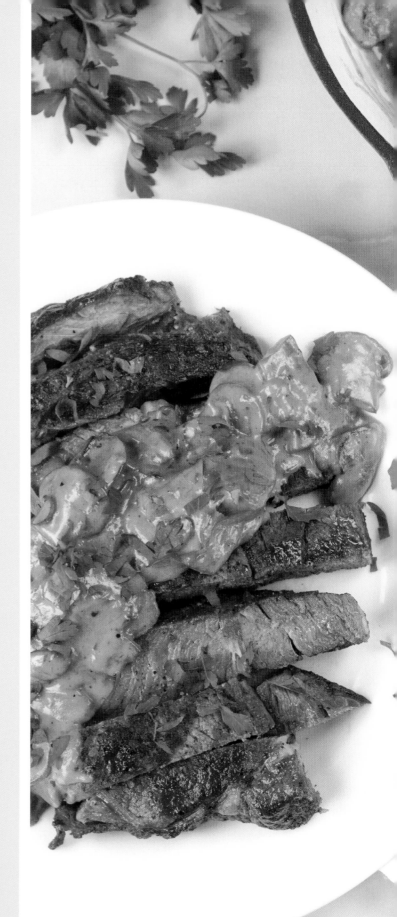

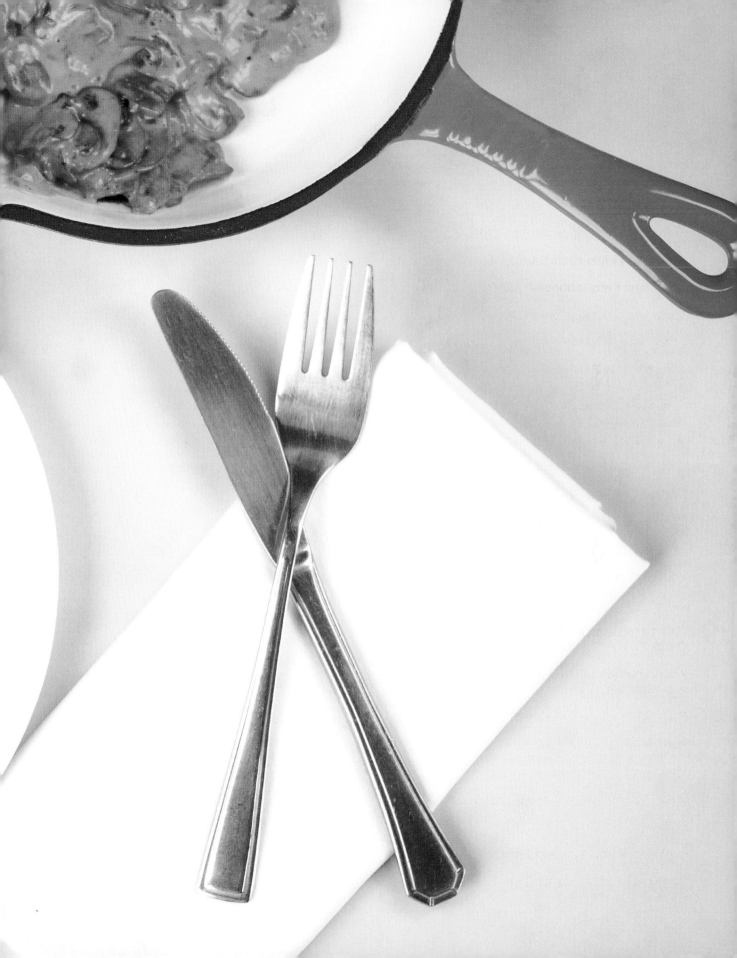

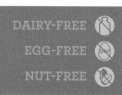

Easy Keto Meatloaf

Prep Time: 10 minutes | **Cook Time: 1 hour 15 minutes**
Yield: 6 servings

Meatloaf is traditionally made with quite a bit of ketchup and Worcestershire sauce. If you can find a healthy sugar-free ketchup, you can use it in this recipe along with my Homemade Worcestershire Sauce (page 356).

5 eggs

3 ounces (90 g) bacon

17 ounces (500 g) ground beef

17 ounces (500 g) ground pork

¼ cup plus 2 tablespoons (3 ounces/85 g) butter

½ cup (2½ ounces/70 g) chopped onions

1 clove garlic, minced

2 medium tomatoes, chopped

2 tablespoons Homemade Worcestershire Sauce (page 356)

¼ cup plus 2 tablespoons (1½ ounces/40 g) almond flour

2 tablespoons chopped fresh parsley, plus more for garnish

1. Preheat the oven to 350°F (177°C). Grease a 9 by 5-inch (23 by 13-cm) loaf pan.

2. Place 3 eggs in a saucepan of water and bring to a boil. Boil for 6 to 7 minutes, then remove the pan from the heat. Let the eggs sit in the hot water for an additional 10 minutes. Rinse under cold water until chilled, then peel. Set aside.

3. Meanwhile, in a skillet over medium heat, fry the bacon for 3 to 4 minutes, until cooked but not crispy. Remove from the pan, chop, and place in a bowl.

4. In the same skillet in which you cooked the bacon, brown the ground beef and pork until cooked through, breaking apart the meat with a wooden spoon, 6 to 8 minutes. Drain the excess fat, if needed.

5. In a large saucepan over low heat, melt the butter. Add the onions and garlic and cook for 2 to 3 minutes, until lightly cooked. Add the tomatoes and ground meat to the pan and mix well. Add the Worcestershire sauce and cook for about 2 more minutes, then transfer the mixture to a large mixing bowl and let cool slightly.

6. To the bowl with the ground meat mixture, add the bacon, flour, parsley, and 2 remaining eggs. Using your hands, mix the ingredients together, then place half of the mixture in the prepared loaf pan. Place the 3 hard-boiled eggs in a row on the meat mixture and top with the remaining meat mixture. Cook for 1 hour or until the meat is cooked through and reaches an internal temperature of 160°F (70°C). Garnish with chopped parsley before serving.

MACRONUTRIENTS
(per serving)

Fat	Protein	Carbs	Fiber	Energy
55g	40g	4.3g	1.2g	675 cal
74%	24%	2%		

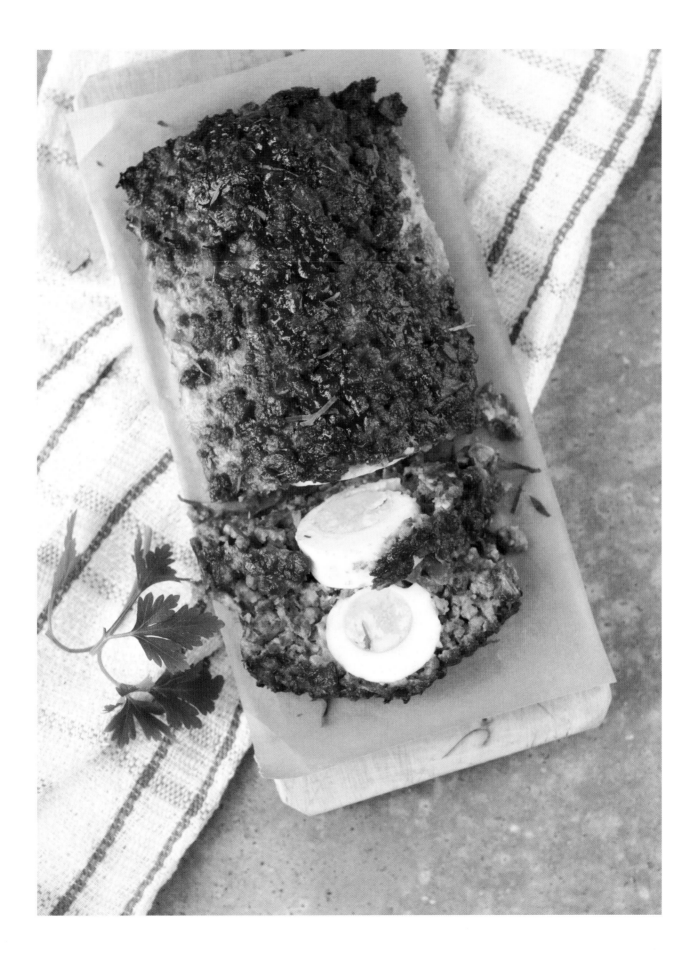

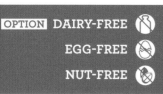

OPTION DAIRY-FREE

EGG-FREE

NUT-FREE

Keto Shepherd's Pie

Prep Time: 15 minutes | **Cook Time: 1 hour**
Yield: 4 servings

Shepherd's pie is one of my favorite comfort foods, but I gave it up long ago when I quit po-tatoes. This version has all the same delicious comforting flavors, but replaces the tradition-al potatoes, corn, peas, and carrots with low-carb veggies. Trust me; you won't miss them! Now shepherd's pie is a go-to meal in our home.

CAULIFLOWER MASH:

2 cups (8 ounces/225 g) chopped cauliflower

½ cup (4 ounces/115 g) butter or butter–flavored coconut oil

Sea salt and ground black pepper

MEAT FILLING:

¼ cup (2 ounces/55 g) butter, lard, or butter–flavored coconut oil

½ cup (2½ ounces/70 g) chopped onions

1 clove garlic, minced

2 stalks celery, chopped

1 cup (4 ounces/115 g) finely chopped radishes

1 green bell pepper, cored, seeds and ribs removed, and chopped

17 ounces (500 g) ground beef

6 small cherry tomatoes, chopped

½ teaspoon fine sea salt

½ teaspoon dried rosemary leaves

½ teaspoon dried thyme leaves

½ teaspoon garlic powder

½ teaspoon onion powder

½ teaspoon paprika

¼ teaspoon cayenne pepper (optional)

¼ teaspoon ground black pepper

1 tablespoon apple cider vinegar

1 tablespoon tamari

1 or 2 drops liquid stevia, to taste

¼ cup (2 fluid ounces/60 ml) beef bone broth

Chopped fresh parsley, for garnish

1. Preheat the oven to 350°F (177°C).

2. Make the cauliflower mash: In a medium saucepan of water over high heat, boil the cauliflower until soft. Drain and return the cauliflower to the pan. Add the butter and stir. Using an immersion blender, blend until smooth. Season with salt and pepper to taste. Set aside.

3. Make the meat filling: In a separate saucepan over medium heat, melt ¼ cup (2 ounces/55 g) of butter. Add the onions and garlic and sauté for 1 to 2 minutes, until fragrant. Add the celery and radishes and cook for 3 to 4 minutes, until softened, stirring occasionally. Add the bell pepper and cook for 3 to 4 more minutes, until softened. Remove from the heat.

4. In a large skillet over medium heat, lightly brown the ground beef, breaking up the meat while it cooks, 6 to 8 minutes. Add the tomatoes, salt, herbs, spices, vinegar, tamari, and stevia. Pour in the broth and stir well.

5. Add the vegetable mixture to the ground beef mixture and mix together.

6. Pour the beef and vegetable mixture into an 11 by 7-inch (28 by 18-cm) casserole dish. Top with the cauliflower mash and use a fork to trace decorative lines along the top. Bake for 20 to 30 minutes, until golden brown on top. Garnish with chopped parsley before serving.

MACRONUTRIENTS
(per serving)

Fat	Protein	Carbs	Fiber	Energy
47g	27.5g	12.5g	4.5g	577 cal
73%	19%	8%		

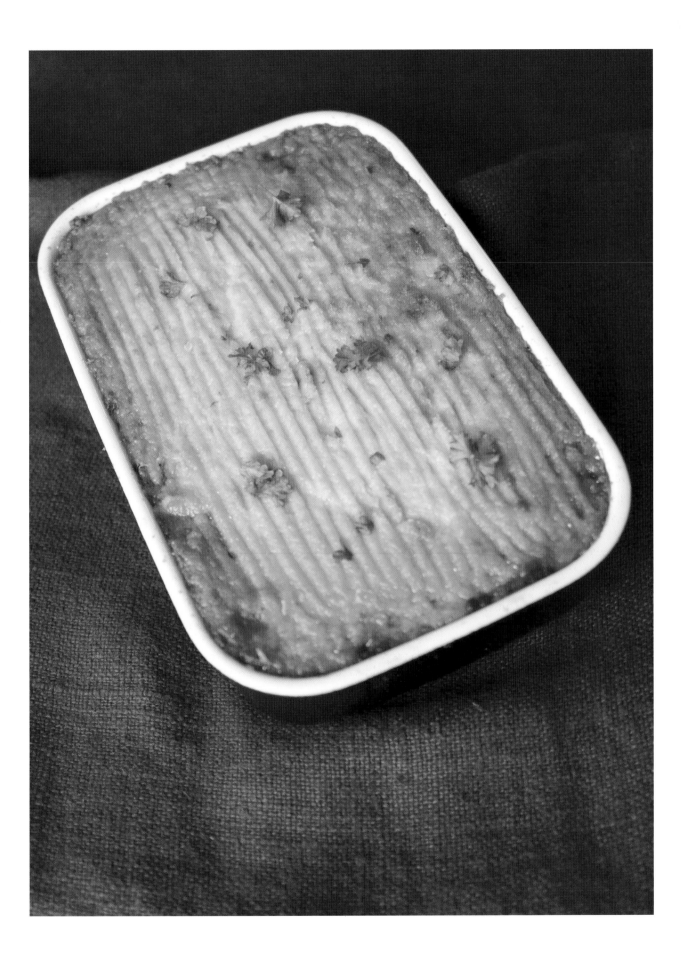

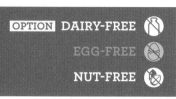

OPTION **DAIRY-FREE**

EGG-FREE

NUT-FREE

Steak with Béarnaise Sauce

Prep Time: **10 minutes** | Cook Time: **15 minutes**
Yield: **4 servings**

My recipe for béarnaise sauce makes about 1¼ cups, so you'll have a little extra. No worries! Béarnaise turns any meat dish into a heavenly preparation, so it's nice to have extra on hand. Store leftover sauce in the fridge for up to 6 days and revive it with 1 tablespoon of ice-cold water.

4 (6-ounce/170-g) boneless rib-eye steaks

Sea salt and ground black pepper

24 asparagus spears, woody ends trimmed

¾ cup plus 2 tablespoons (7 fluid ounces/210 ml) Béarnaise Sauce (page 354)

1. Preheat a grill to medium-high heat.

2. Prepare the steaks for grilling by seasoning them on both sides with salt and pepper. Grill the steaks for 4 to 5 minutes on each side for medium-done steaks, or to your desired level of doneness. Let rest for about 10 minutes.

3. In a wide, deep pan over high heat, bring 4 to 5 cups of water to a boil. Add the asparagus and turn off the heat, leaving the pan on the burner. Leave the asparagus in the hot water for 3 to 4 minutes, until bright green. Remove from the water and set aside to drain.

4. Serve each steak with 6 stalks of asparagus and 3½ tablespoons of the béarnaise sauce.

MACRONUTRIENTS
(per serving)

Fat	Protein	Carbs	Fiber	Energy
64.5g	36g	4g	4g	723 cal
79%	19%	2%		

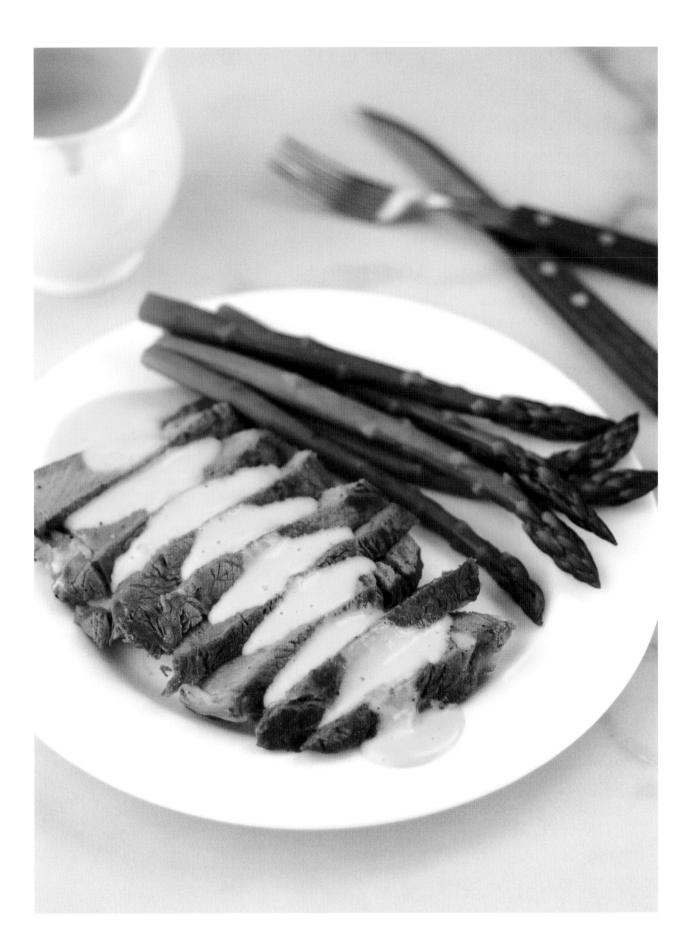

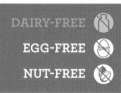

DAIRY-FREE

EGG-FREE

NUT-FREE

Steak with Mushroom Sauce

Prep Time: 10 minutes | **Cook Time: 30 minutes**
Yield: 4 servings

There's nothing like a steakhouse dinner, but grilling steak at home is much more budget-friendly than sitting down at a restaurant, which means that you can enjoy that steakhouse experience much more often! At times, home-grilled steak is even more satisfying, especially since it means you can fire up the barbecue.

4 (6-ounce/170-g) boneless rib-eye steaks

Sea salt and ground black pepper

MUSHROOM SAUCE:

¼ cup (2 ounces/55 g) butter

1 tablespoon minced shallots

1 clove garlic, minced

2 cups (5¼ ounces/150 g) sliced brown or white mushrooms

¾ cup (6 fluid ounces/180 ml) beef bone broth

1 teaspoon Dijon mustard

½ cup (4 fluid ounces/120 ml) heavy whipping cream

½ teaspoon fine sea salt

¼ teaspoon ground black pepper

2 tablespoons chopped fresh herbs, such as parsley, sage, or thyme, plus more for garnish (optional)

1. Preheat a grill to medium-high heat.

2. Prepare the steaks for grilling by seasoning them on both sides with salt and pepper. Grill the steaks for 4 to 5 minutes on each side for medium-done steaks, or to your desired level of doneness. Let rest for about 10 minutes.

3. Make the mushroom sauce: In a large saucepan over medium-low heat, melt the butter. Add the shallots and garlic and cook for 2 to 3 minutes, until lightly browned and fragrant. Add the mushrooms and cook for another 6 to 8 minutes, until nicely browned. Be careful not to burn the garlic or shallots, and try not to crowd the mushrooms.

4. Add the broth and mustard and stir to combine. Simmer for 10 minutes to reduce the sauce.

5. Add the cream, salt, pepper, and herbs, if using. Simmer, stirring often, for 6 to 8 more minutes, until the sauce is nice and thick.

6. Serve each steak with one-quarter of the sauce and garnish with more fresh herbs, if desired.

MACRONUTRIENTS
(per serving)

Fat	Protein	Carbs	Fiber	Energy
57g	28.5g	2.8g	0.5g	699 cal
80%	18%	2%		

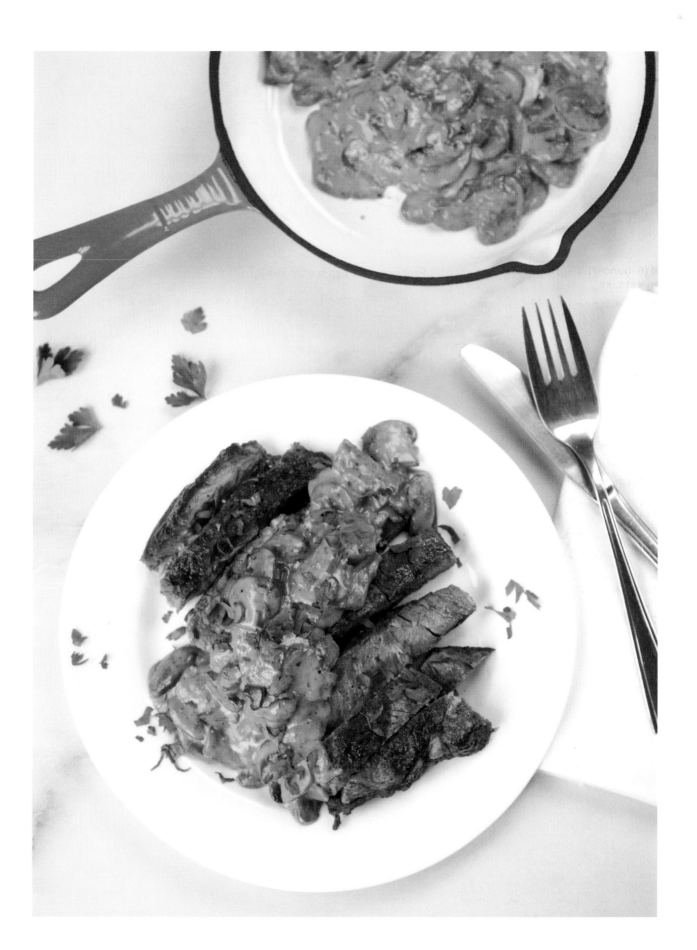

Steak and Keto Tabbouleh

Prep Time: 10 minutes | **Cook Time: 12 minutes**
Yield: 2 servings

This super-tasty dinner involves minimal prep work. The tabbouleh uses cauliflower rather than bulgur wheat as a base for a healthy, grain-free treat. Serve this dish with a little bit of melted butter or butter-flavored coconut oil on the steak to make it extra keto.

2 (5–ounce/170–g) boneless steaks (¾ inch/2 cm thick)

Sea salt and ground black pepper

KETO TABBOULEH:

2 cups (8 ounces/225 g) cauliflower florets

1 cup (1 ounce/28 g) finely chopped fresh parsley

2 tablespoons thinly sliced green onions

1 tablespoon finely chopped fresh mint

¼ cup (2 fluid ounces/60 ml) olive oil

Grated zest of 1 lemon

2 tablespoons freshly squeezed lemon juice

Pinch of cayenne pepper (optional)

Sea salt and ground black pepper

½ cup (2 ounces/55 g) crumbled fresh (soft) goat cheese (optional)

1. Prepare the steaks for grilling by seasoning them on both sides with salt and pepper.

2. Make the tabbouleh: Place the cauliflower in a food processor and pulse until chopped into small crumbles. Put the cauliflower, parsley, green onions, and mint in a bowl. Add the olive oil, lemon zest, lemon juice, cayenne (if using), and salt and pepper to taste. Mix together.

3. Heat a grill pan or heavy skillet (cast iron works well here) to medium-high heat. Sear the steaks for 5 to 6 minutes on each side for medium-done steaks, or to your desired level of doneness. Let rest for about 10 minutes.

4. Serve each steak with half of the tabbouleh, topped with goat cheese, if desired.

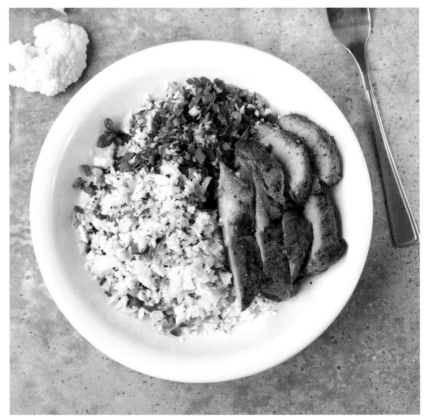

MACRONUTRIENTS (per serving)				
Fat	Protein	Carbs	Fiber	Energy
40g	29g	11g	3.5g	656 cal
69%	22%	9%		

Steak on "Honey"-Mustard Slaw

Prep Time: 10 minutes | Cook Time: 10 minutes
Yield: 2 servings

DAIRY-FREE
EGG-FREE
NUT-FREE

I love this yummy dish that pairs grilled steak with crunchy, slightly sweet slaw.

2 (4-ounce/115-g) boneless rib-eye steaks

Sea salt and ground black pepper

"HONEY"-MUSTARD DRESSING:

¼ cup plus 1 tablespoon (2½ ounces/70 g) mayonnaise

1 tablespoon prepared yellow mustard

¼ teaspoon garlic powder

¼ teaspoon onion powder

¼ teaspoon fine sea salt

2 to 4 drops liquid stevia, to taste

1½ cups (6 ounces/170 g) shredded green cabbage

½ cup (2 ounces/55 g) shredded red cabbage

1 cup (2¼ ounces/70 g) stemmed and chopped fresh kale

1 cup (3 ounces/85 g) broccoli slaw (thinly sliced broccoli stems)

1. Prepare the steaks for grilling by seasoning them on both sides with salt and pepper. Heat a grill pan or heavy skillet (cast iron works well here) to medium-high heat. Sear the steaks for 4 to 5 minutes on each side for medium-done steaks, or to your desired level of doneness. Let rest for about 10 minutes.

2. In a small bowl, whisk together all the dressing ingredients.

3. In a separate bowl, mix together the cabbage, kale, and broccoli slaw. Pour the dressing over the slaw and toss well to coat.

4. Divide the slaw between 2 plates. Slice the steak into strips and serve on top of the slaw.

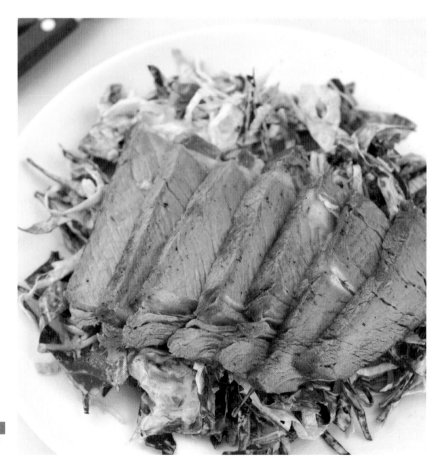

MACRONUTRIENTS (per serving)				
Fat	Protein	Carbs	Fiber	Energy
60.5g	24g	10.5g	4g	631 cal
80%	14%	6%		

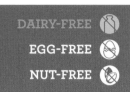

DAIRY-FREE

EGG-FREE

NUT-FREE

Steak
with Green Peppercorn Sauce

Prep Time: **2 minutes** | Cook Time: **15 minutes**
Yield: **2 servings**

I first had this dish in Italy and fell in love. The lush steak sauce in this dish makes any night of the week a special occasion! The recipe traditionally calls for brandy, but here I use apple cider vinegar as a replacement.

¼ cup (1¾ ounces/50 g) green peppercorns in brine, well drained

4 tablespoons (2 ounces/55 g) butter, divided

2 (5-ounce/140-g) boneless sirloin steaks (¾ inch/2 cm thick)

2 tablespoons minced shallots or green onions

½ cup (4 fluid ounces/120 ml) beef bone broth

¼ cup (2 fluid ounces/60 ml) apple cider vinegar

1 tablespoon tamari

½ cup (4 fluid ounces/120 ml) heavy whipping cream

¼ teaspoon fine sea salt

Fresh watercress, for garnish (optional)

1. Preheat the oven to 200°F (95°C).

2. In a mortar and pestle or using a food processor, crush the peppercorns to a paste.

3. In a skillet over medium-high heat, melt 2 tablespoons of the butter. Increase the heat to high and sear the steaks for 4 to 5 minutes on each side for medium-done steaks, or to your desired level of doneness. Remove from the pan and keep warm.

4. In the same skillet over medium heat, melt the remaining 2 tablespoons of butter. Add the shallots and peppercorn paste, scraping the pan to combine them with the steak drippings.

5. Pour in the broth, vinegar, and tamari and bring to a boil. Reduce the heat and simmer until the liquid has reduced by half, 5 to 6 minutes. Add the cream and salt and stir to combine.

6. Serve the sauce over the steaks and garnish with watercress, if desired.

MACRONUTRIENTS
(per serving)

Fat	Protein	Carbs	Fiber	Energy
57.5g	31g	4g	1.5g	667 cal
79%	19%	2%		

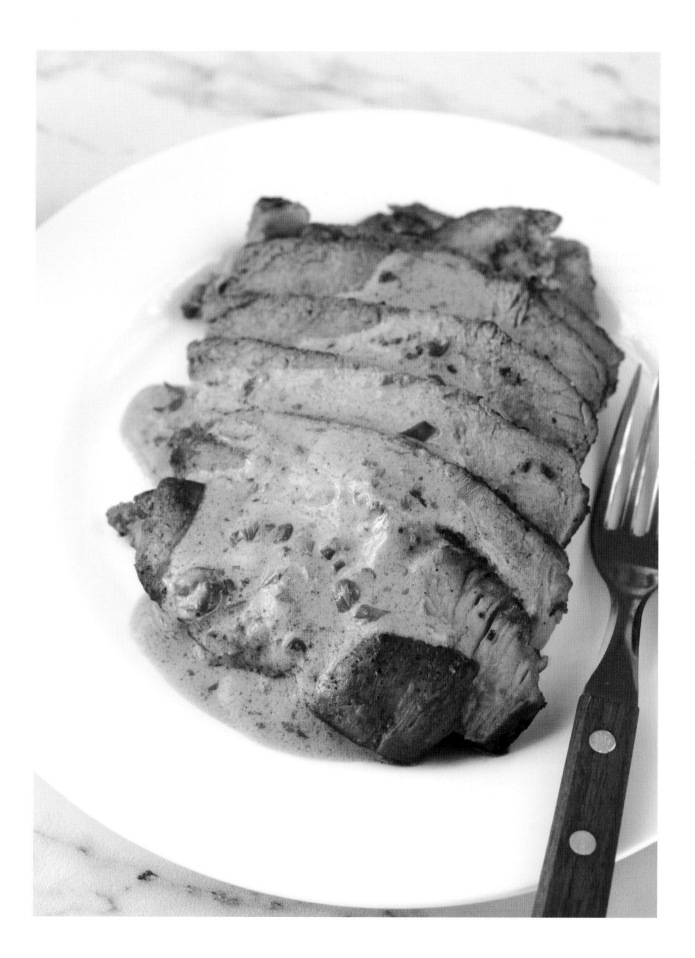

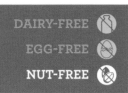

DAIRY-FREE

EGG-FREE

NUT-FREE

Trio of Beef Sliders

Prep Time: **20 minutes** | Cook Time: **15 minutes**
Yield: **4 servings**

Sliders are one of the most fun ways to enjoy burgers! I often make these for groups or parties, and everyone loves them. Depending on the type of gathering, I either set up a topping bar so that each person can select their own toppings, or assemble the trios of sliders so that everyone can try all three kinds.

1½ pounds (680 g) ground beef

½ medium onion, finely chopped

1 teaspoon cayenne pepper

1 teaspoon garlic powder

1 teaspoon paprika

1 or 2 drops liquid stevia, or
1 teaspoon erythritol

1 teaspoon fine sea salt

½ teaspoon ground black pepper

1 teaspoon maple flavoring, or
1 tablespoon sugar–free maple
syrup

TOPPINGS:

4 slices bacon

¼ cup (2 ounces/55 g) unsalted
butter

1 clove garlic, minced

½ cup (1¼ ounces/40 g) cremini or
white mushrooms, diced

2 ounces (55 g) blue cheese,
crumbled

1 avocado, peeled and pitted

1 teaspoon freshly squeezed lime
juice

¼ teaspoon garlic powder

Pinch of cayenne pepper

½ teaspoon fine sea salt

¼ cup (2 ounces/55 g) Special
Burger Sauce (page 363) or
mayonnaise

4 slices cheddar or Gouda cheese

2 unsweetened medium to large
dill pickles, sliced into rounds

12 butter lettuce leaves

1. In a bowl, mix together the ground beef, onion, cayenne, garlic powder, paprika, stevia, 1 teaspoon salt, and ½ teaspoon pepper.

2. Remove 8 ounces (225 g) of the meat mixture to a separate bowl and mix with the maple flavoring. Form four 2-ounce (55-g) sliders, each about 2 inches (5 cm) thick.

3. From the remaining meat mixture, make eight 2-ounce (55-g) sliders.

4. Heat a grill pan or heavy skillet (cast iron works well here) to medium-high heat. Grill the sliders for 4 to 5 minutes on each side for medium-done burgers, or to your desired level of doneness. Alternatively, you can grill the sliders on a gas or charcoal grill preheated to high heat for 5 to 6 minutes per side for medium-done burgers, or to your desired level of doneness. Set aside to rest.

5. Prepare the toppings: In a medium skillet over medium heat, fry the bacon for 3 to 4 minutes, until moderately crispy. Set aside.

6. In a saucepan over medium heat, melt the butter. Add the garlic and sauté for 1 to 2 minutes, until fragrant. Add the mushrooms and sauté for 3 to 4 minutes. Sprinkle with the blue cheese and allow it to melt while blending it into the mushrooms. Set aside.

7. Prepare guacamole by mashing together the avocado flesh, lime juice, garlic powder, cayenne, and ½ teaspoon salt.

8. Assemble the 3 types of sliders:

   Top each of the 4 maple sliders with 1 tablespoon of Special Burger Sauce, a slice of cheddar, a slice of bacon, and pickles.

   Top 4 more sliders with the guacamole.

   Top the last 4 sliders with the mushroom and blue cheese mixture.

9. Place each slider on a lettuce leaf and arrange one of each type of slider on each plate.

MACRONUTRIENTS
(per serving)

Fat	Protein	Carbs	Fiber	Energy
78.8g	42g	8g	5g	878 cal
78%	18%	4%		

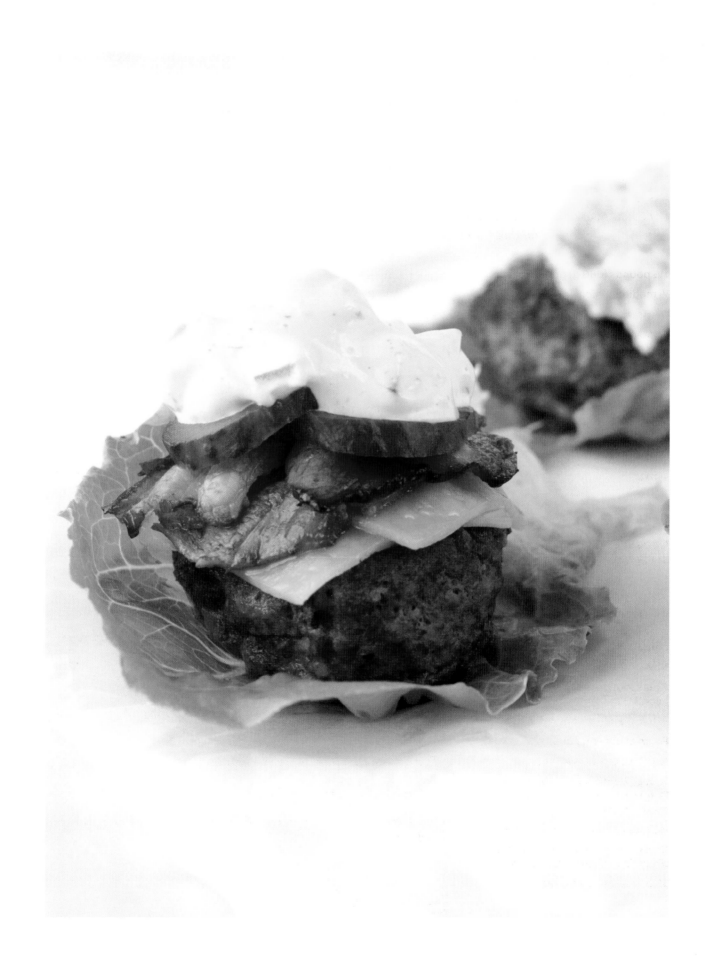

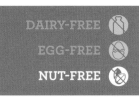

DAIRY-FREE
EGG-FREE
NUT-FREE

Zucchini Lasagna

Prep Time: **20 minutes** | Cook Time: **1 hour 10 minutes**
Yield: **6 servings**

A keto spin on a classic family dinner! In this dish, sliced zucchini replaces sheets of pasta.
It works best when as much water as possible is removed from the zucchini.

NOODLES:

2 medium to large zucchini, each sliced lengthwise into 6 long slices (a mandoline slicer works well)

1 to 2 tablespoons fine sea salt

½ cup (4 ounces/115 g) unsalted butter, divided

1 pound (455 g) ground beef

¼ cup (2 ounces/55 g) sliced green onions

1 clove garlic, minced

½ teaspoon red pepper flakes

12 cherry tomatoes, quartered

2 tablespoons finely chopped fresh basil, plus extra leaves for garnish

2 tablespoons finely chopped fresh oregano

½ teaspoon fine sea salt

¼ teaspoon ground black pepper

12 ounces (340 g) cream cheese, softened

½ cup plus 2 tablespoons (2½ ounces/70 g) grated Parmesan cheese, divided

½ cup (2 ounces/55 g) shredded mozzarella cheese

2 egg yolks

1. Preheat the oven to 375°F (190°C).

2. Salt the zucchini with 1 to 2 tablespoons of salt. Set the slices in a colander to drain for 10 to 15 minutes, then rinse the zucchini and wipe off the salt with paper towels. Meanwhile, prepare the rest of the ingredients for the lasagna.

3. In a large skillet over medium-low heat, melt ¼ cup (2 ounces/55 g) of the butter. Add the ground beef and cook until browned, breaking apart the meat as it cooks, 6 to 7 minutes.

4. In a medium saucepan over medium heat, melt the remaining ¼ cup (2 ounces/55 g) of butter. Add the green onions, garlic, and red pepper flakes and sauté for 1 to 2 minutes. Add the tomatoes and stir to combine.

5. Add the browned ground beef to the green onion mixture and stir together.

6. Stir in the basil, oregano, ½ teaspoon salt, and pepper, then slide the pan off the heat.

7. In a bowl, mix together the cream cheese, ½ cup (2 ounces/55 g) of the Parmesan, mozzarella, and egg yolks.

8. Have on hand a 10-inch (12.5-cm) to 12-inch (17.5-cm) ovenproof skillet. To layer the lasagna in the pan, spread half of the beef and tomato mixture over the bottom of the pan. Layer on 6 zucchini slices, trimming as necessary, then spread half the cheese mixture on top in an even layer. Repeat these layers once more. Top with the remaining 2 tablespoons of Parmesan.

9. Cover with aluminum foil and bake for 1 hour, removing the foil after 45 minutes. If desired, turn the oven to broil after 1 hour and broil for 1 to 2 minutes, until the top is brown and crispy. Garnish with fresh basil leaves.

MACRONUTRIENTS
(per serving)

Fat	Protein	Carbs	Fiber	Energy
50.5g	29g	6g	0.7g	586 cal
77%	19%	4%		

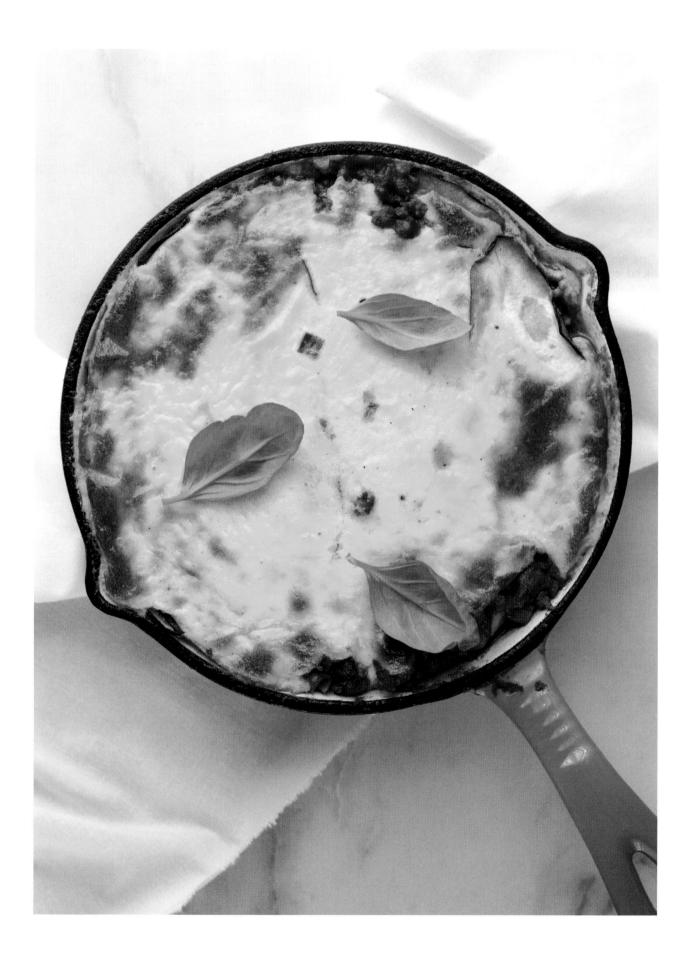

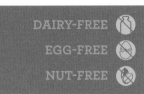

DAIRY-FREE

EGG-FREE

NUT-FREE

Feta-Stuffed Meatballs
with Greek Tomato Sauce

Prep Time: **20 minutes** | Cook Time: **30 minutes**
Yield: **4 servings**

I love meatloaf with warm, melty goat cheese in the center, so I decided to create a version with meatballs for a fun way to enjoy the same flavor profile in a different form. With feta, Kalamata olives, and tomato sauce, this recipe features a Mediterranean/Greek twist.

FETA-STUFFED MEATBALLS:

½ cup (2 ounces/55 g) almond flour

¼ cup (1 ounce/27 g) grated red onions

¼ cup (1¼ ounces/35 g) finely chopped Kalamata olives

2 tablespoons finely chopped fresh parsley

1 egg, lightly whisked

3 cloves garlic, minced

½ teaspoon fine sea salt

¼ teaspoon ground black pepper

¼ teaspoon ground nutmeg

1 pound (455 g) ground beef

6 ounces (170 g) firm feta cheese

GREEK TOMATO SAUCE:

2 cups (11 ounces/315 g) chopped plum tomatoes

⅓ cup (2¾ fluid ounces/80 ml) olive oil

1 teaspoon dried oregano leaves

1 teaspoon fine sea salt

¼ teaspoon red pepper flakes

¼ teaspoon ground black pepper

1. Preheat the oven to 400°F (205°C).

2. Make the meatballs: In a bowl, stir together the flour, onions, olives, parsley, egg, garlic, salt, pepper, and nutmeg. Crumble in the ground beef and mix with your hands until just combined. Divide into 20 equal portions and roll into 2-inch (5-cm) balls.

3. Cut the feta into twenty ½-inch (1.25-cm) cubes. Gently press a feta cube into the center of each meatball and close the meat around the cheese. Place the feta-filled meatballs in a 13 by 9-inch (33 by 23-cm) glass baking dish.

4. Make the tomato sauce: In a food processor or blender, pulse all the sauce ingredients until pureed. Pour the sauce over the meatballs.

5. Bake, uncovered, until the meatballs reach an internal temperature of 160°F (71°C), 25 to 30 minutes. The oils will rise to the top of the sauce. If desired, remove the meatballs from the dish and re-emulsify the sauce with an immersion blender. Serve the sauce over the meatballs.

MACRONUTRIENTS
(per serving)

Fat	Protein	Carbs	Fiber	Energy
50.5g	36.3g	8.3g	3g	621 cal
71.8%	23%	5.2%		

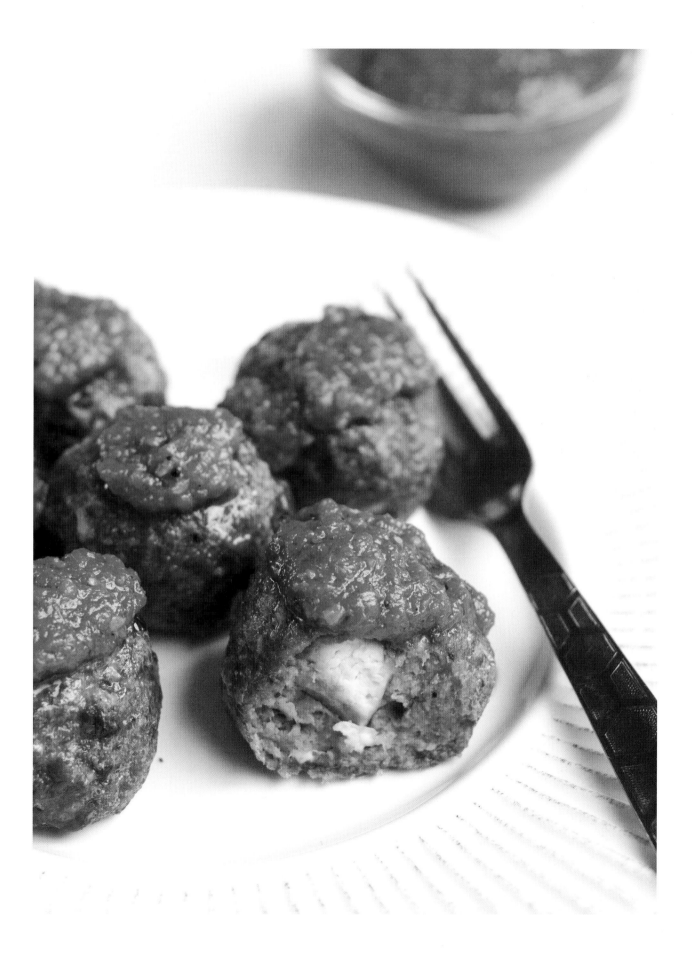

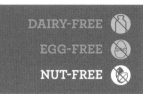

DAIRY-FREE

EGG-FREE

NUT-FREE

Keto Moussaka

Prep Time: **20 minutes** | Cook Time: **1 hour**
Yield: **6 servings**

When my husband and I were in Greece for our honeymoon, I ate the most delicious moussaka, and I knew that I had to make a version for this cookbook! Eggplant is such a delectable vegetable, and this combination of eggplant, spices, and white sauce is going to make for a family favorite.

MEAT SAUCE:

2 tablespoons olive oil

2 pounds (910 g) ground beef

2 teaspoons dried oregano leaves

1 teaspoon ground Ceylon cinnamon or regular cinnamon

½ teaspoon ground nutmeg

1 teaspoon fine sea salt

½ teaspoon ground black pepper

1 onion, diced

3 cloves garlic, minced

1 cup (5½ ounces/160 g) quartered grape tomatoes

1 cup (8 fluid ounces/240 ml) beef bone broth

EGGPLANT LAYER:

1 large eggplant (about 1 pound/ 455 g)

KETO WHITE SAUCE:

2 tablespoons butter

2 cups (16 fluid ounces/480 ml) heavy whipping cream

6 egg yolks

¼ teaspoon ground nutmeg

¼ teaspoon fine sea salt

¼ teaspoon ground black pepper

½ cup (2 ounces/55 g) grated Parmesan cheese, divided

1. Preheat the oven to 375°F (190°C).

2. Make the meat sauce: Heat the olive oil in a large skillet over medium heat. Add the ground beef, oregano, cinnamon, nutmeg, salt, and pepper; cook the meat, breaking it apart, until browned but not cooked through, about 5 minutes. Drain the excess moisture from the meat, leaving 1 tablespoon in the skillet, and remove the meat to a bowl.

3. Return the skillet to the stovetop. Add the onion and garlic and cook over medium heat until translucent, about 5 minutes. Stir in the cooked beef, tomatoes, and broth and simmer until thickened, about 10 minutes.

4. Cut the eggplant lengthwise into ⅛-inch (32-mm) slices.

5. Make the white sauce: In a heavy-bottomed pot over low heat, melt the butter. Whisk in the cream, egg yolks, nutmeg, salt, pepper, and half of the Parmesan cheese. Cook, while whisking, until thickened, about 10 minutes.

6. To assemble the moussaka: Ladle enough of the meat sauce into a 9-inch (23-cm) square baking dish to lightly cover the bottom. Top with half of the eggplant slices in an even layer, trimming as necessary to make the eggplant fit. Top with half of the remaining meat sauce, followed by the remaining eggplant slices, and then the remaining meat sauce. Pour the white sauce over the top, spreading it into an even layer. Sprinkle with the remaining Parmesan cheese.

7. Bake until bubbling and golden, 45 to 50 minutes. Tent with aluminum foil if the top starts to get too brown. Allow to sit for 10 minutes before slicing and serving.

MACRONUTRIENTS
(per serving)

Fat	Protein	Carbs	Fiber	Energy
60.6g 73%	37.5g 20%	13g 7%	3g	757 cal

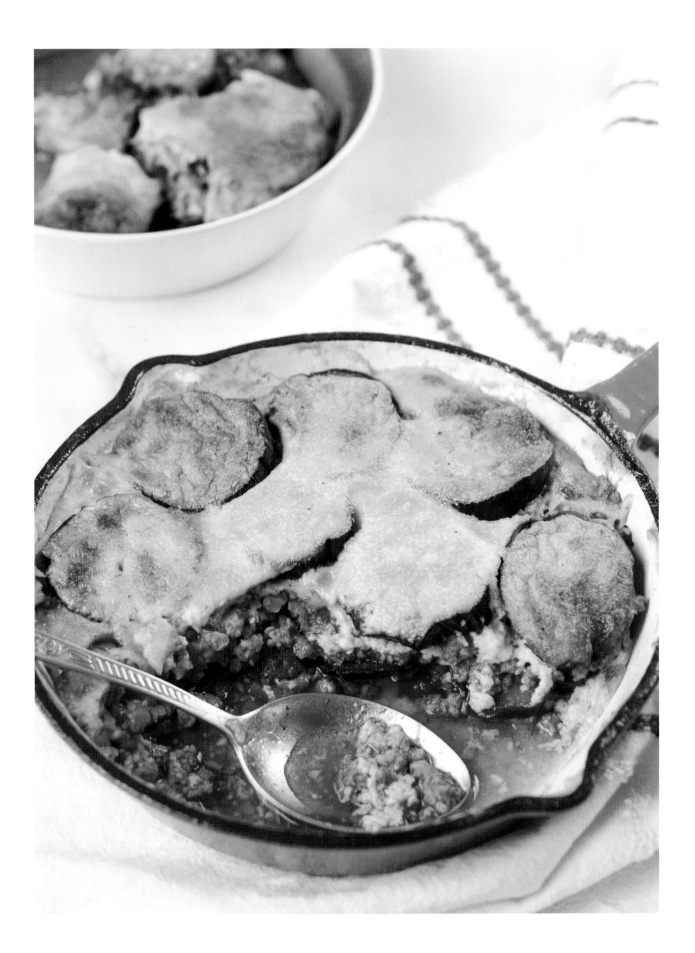

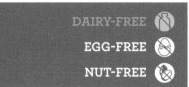

DAIRY-FREE

EGG-FREE

NUT-FREE

Stuffed Peppers

Prep Time: **10 minutes** | Cook Time: **1 hour**
Yield: **4 servings**

4 large green bell peppers

½ cup (4 ounces/115 g) butter

2 tablespoons thinly sliced green onions

1 clove garlic, minced

2 cups (8 ounces/225 g) riced cauliflower (see note)

½ cup (4 fluid ounces/120 ml) beef bone broth

8 ounces (225 g) ground beef

8 ounces (225 g) ground pork

1 medium tomato, chopped

1 tablespoon tamari

½ teaspoon fine sea salt

½ teaspoon garlic powder

½ teaspoon onion powder

½ teaspoon paprika

¼ teaspoon ground black pepper

3 ounces (85 g) mozzarella cheese, shredded

1. Preheat the oven to 350°F (177°C). Grease a 9-inch (23-cm) square baking dish.

2. Slice the top off of each bell pepper and trim the base to a flat edge so that the peppers will stand up. Carefully remove the core, seeds, and ribs, keeping the peppers intact. Arrange the peppers in the prepared baking dish.

3. In a deep skillet over low heat, melt the butter. Add the green onions and garlic and cook for 2 to 3 minutes, until softened.

4. Increase the heat to medium-low and add the riced cauliflower. Cook for 2 to 3 minutes, stirring often, until the cauliflower is lightly cooked and the butter is well mixed in.

5. Pour in the broth and increase the heat to medium. Simmer for 8 to 12 minutes, until the liquid is absorbed.

6. Meanwhile, in a separate large skillet over medium heat, cook the ground beef and pork until lightly browned, using a spatula to break apart the meat, 7 to 8 minutes. Drain any excess water, if needed. Add the tomato, tamari, salt, and spices and stir to combine.

7. Add the cauliflower mixture to the meat mixture; stir to combine. Spoon the meat and cauliflower mixture into the peppers and top with the mozzarella.

8. Bake for 25 to 30 minutes, until the tops are golden. If you want the tops extra brown, broil for an additional 1 to 2 minutes.

note

You can either purchase pre-riced cauliflower (often called cauliflower rice) or make it yourself. To make it, pulse cauliflower florets in a food processor for 30 seconds to 1 minute. Watch it closely; you want the cauliflower grated and approximately rice-sized, but not too fine. You can also use the large holes on a box grater to grate the cauliflower into ricelike pieces.

MACRONUTRIENTS
(per serving)

Fat	Protein	Carbs	Fiber	Energy
51.8g	23.3g	8.8g	3g	587 cal
78%	16%	6%		

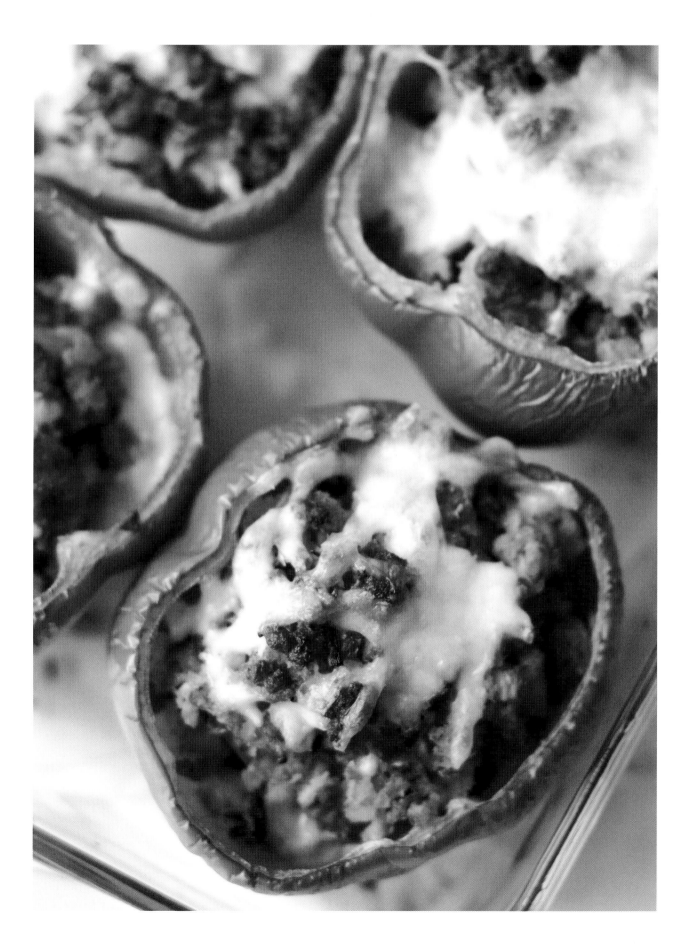

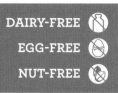

DAIRY-FREE

EGG-FREE

NUT-FREE

Ginger Beef

Prep Time: **10 minutes** | Cook Time: **15 minutes**
Yield: **4 servings**

My version of this tasty Chinese favorite is closer to the authentic recipe, which doesn't in-clude the battering and deep-frying involved in the typical North American interpretation.

¼ cup (2 ounces/55 g) coconut oil or lard

1 pound (455 g) boneless beefsteak, sliced

¼ cup (2 fluid ounces/60 ml) light sesame oil

½ onion, sliced into long segments

3 cloves garlic, minced

¼ cup (1 ounce/25 g) minced or grated fresh ginger

1 cup (7 ounces/195 g) coarsely chopped red bell peppers

1 cup (7 ounces/195 g) coarsely chopped green bell peppers

2 tablespoons apple cider vinegar

2 tablespoons tamari

1 small red chili pepper, sliced

½ teaspoon fine sea salt

½ teaspoon liquid stevia and/or 1 tablespoon granulated stevia, to taste

FOR GARNISH (OPTIONAL):

Sliced green onions

Chopped fresh cilantro

Sesame seeds

1. In a large skillet over medium-high heat, heat the coconut oil. Add the beef slices and sear for 3 to 4 minutes on each side, until cooked to your liking. Remove from the pan.

2. In the same skillet over medium-low heat, heat the sesame oil. Add the onion, garlic, and ginger and cook for 1 to 2 minutes, until fragrant. Add the bell peppers and brown for 2 to 3 minutes. Add the cooked beef and stir to combine.

3. In a bowl, mix the vinegar, tamari, chili pepper, salt, and stevia. Add the mixture to the beef and vegetables and cook together for 1 to 2 minutes.

4. Serve garnished with sliced green onions, chopped cilantro, and/or sesame seeds, if desired.

MACRONUTRIENTS
(per serving)

Fat	Protein	Carbs	Fiber	Energy
33.5g	23.5g	7.5g	2g	435 cal
71%	22%	7%		

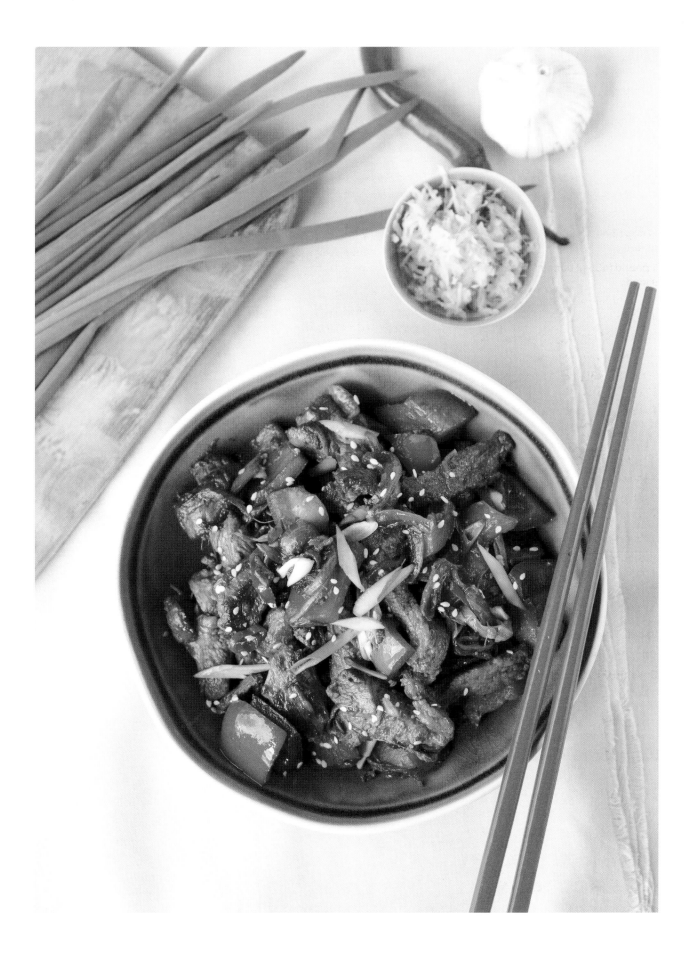

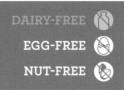

DAIRY-FREE

EGG-FREE

NUT-FREE

Easy Keto Casserole

Prep Time: **5 minutes** | Cook Time: **50 minutes**
Yield: **4 servings**

This is a great family-style casserole to add to your regular rotation. You can simplify the recipe by using all ground pork or all ground beef and only mozzarella or Parmesan.

½ cup (4 ounces/115 g) butter

2 tablespoons thinly sliced green onions

1 clove garlic, minced

2 cups (8 ounces/225 g) riced cauliflower (see note, page 292)

½ cup (4 fluid ounces/120 ml) beef bone broth

8 ounces (225 g) ground beef

8 ounces (225 g) ground pork

1 cup (7 ounces/195 g) chopped red and green bell peppers

1 medium tomato, chopped

1 tablespoon tamari

½ teaspoon fine sea salt

½ teaspoon garlic powder

½ teaspoon onion powder

½ teaspoon paprika

¼ teaspoon ground black pepper

4 ounces (115 g) cream cheese, softened

½ cup (2 ounces/55 g) shredded mozzarella cheese

½ cup (2 ounces/55 g) grated Parmesan cheese

1 tablespoon finely chopped fresh basil, for garnish (optional)

1. Preheat the oven to 350°F (177°C). Grease a 9-inch (23-cm) square baking dish or similar-sized casserole dish.

2. In a deep skillet over low heat, melt the butter. Add the green onions and garlic and sauté until crisp and lightly browned, 2 to 3 minutes.

3. Increase the heat to medium-low and add the cauliflower. Cook, stirring often, for 2 to 3 minutes, until the cauliflower is lightly cooked and the butter is mixed in well.

4. Pour in the broth and increase the heat to medium. Simmer for 5 to 7 minutes, until the liquid is absorbed.

5. Meanwhile, in a separate large skillet over medium heat, cook the ground beef and pork until lightly browned, using a spatula to break apart the meat, 6 to 7 minutes. Drain any excess liquid, if needed. Add the bell peppers, tomato, tamari, salt, and spices and cook for 4 to 5 minutes.

6. Add the cauliflower mixture to the beef mixture; stir to combine. Fold in the cream cheese, gently stirring to combine. Remove from the heat. Fold in the mozzarella. Pour into the prepared casserole dish and sprinkle with the Parmesan.

7. Bake for 25 minutes. Broil for an additional 1 to 2 minutes so that the Parmesan browns nicely. Sprinkle with the basil, if using, before serving.

MACRONUTRIENTS
(per serving)

Fat	Protein	Carbs	Fiber	Energy
53.8g	29.3g	7.3g	2.3g	631 cal
77%	18%	5%		

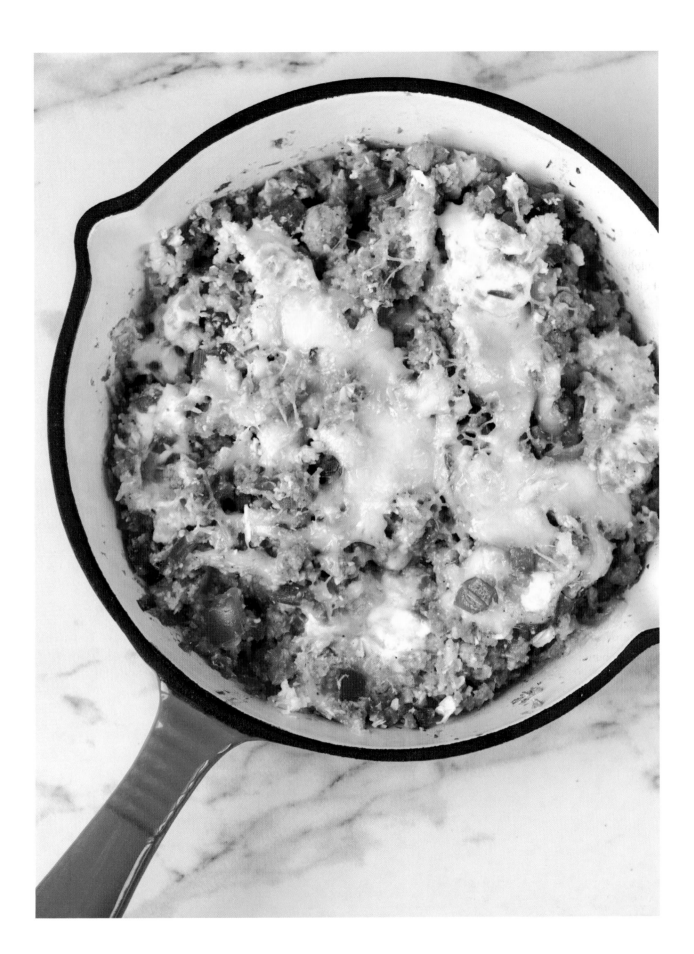

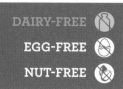

Bacon Poutine

Prep Time: **10 minutes** | Cook Time: **10 to 40 minutes, depending on cooking method**
Yield: **4 servings**

Here, this quintessential French-Canadian comfort food is transformed into a healthy keto-genic meal. Cheese curds are made from curdled cheese, and you can find them at specialty food markets and cheese shops. If cheese curds aren't available, substitute mozzarella cheese, preferably in small chunks that you can tear apart. You can bake or fry the wax beans in this recipe; I recommend frying for a texture more like french fries.

POUTINE:

1 pound (455 g) bacon

2 pounds (910 g) yellow wax beans, trimmed

Fat, for the fries (see Step 8 for type)

10 ounces (285 g) cheese curds

GRAVY:

½ cup (½ ounce/15 g) dried porcini mushrooms

¼ cup (2 fluid ounces/60 ml) filtered water

¼ cup (2 ounces/55 g) butter or butter–flavored coconut oil

1 clove garlic, minced

1 cup (8 fluid ounces/240 ml) beef bone broth

1 tablespoon coconut flour

2 tablespoons heavy whipping cream

1 teaspoon Dijon mustard

1 to 2 sprigs fresh thyme

1 teaspoon fine sea salt

Pinch of black or white peppercorns

1. In a medium skillet over medium-low heat, cook the bacon for 4 to 5 minutes, until lightly cooked. Remove the bacon, then chop it and set aside; reserve the fat for the gravy.

2. Begin to prepare the gravy: In a small bowl, soak the mushrooms in the water for about 10 minutes to rehydrate.

3. In a medium pan over low heat, melt the butter. Let simmer until lightly browned, swirling the pan to keep the butter from burning. (If using butter-flavored coconut oil, simply melt the oil in the pan, then proceed to the next step.)

4. Add the garlic and cook for 1 to 2 minutes, until fragrant.

5. Drain the mushrooms, then chop into small pieces. Add the mushrooms and reserved bacon fat to the pan with the garlic; stir until well combined.

6. Whisk in the broth, then the coconut flour, until well blended. Depending on how thick you like your gravy, simmer for 5 to 20 minutes on low heat. (I like to simmer mine for just 5 minutes.)

7. Remove from the heat and add the cream, mustard, thyme, salt, and peppercorns. Using an immersion blender, blend the gravy until it has a smooth, fine consistency; strain through a fine-mesh strainer. Return to the saucepan and set aside.

8. Prepare the wax beans. You have three options:

   To bake, melt 2 to 3 tablespoons of duck fat, lard, or coconut oil. Use some of it to grease a rimmed baking sheet. Place the beans on the pan and pour the remaining fat on top; toss to evenly coat. Bake in a preheated 350°F (177°C) oven for 20 to 30 minutes, until lightly browned.

   To deep-fry, heat 1 inch (2.5 cm) of duck fat or lard to 338°F (170°C) in a deep-fryer. Fry the beans for 4 to 5 minutes.

   To air-fry, fry the beans according to the manufacturer's directions, using 2 tablespoons of coconut oil or duck fat.

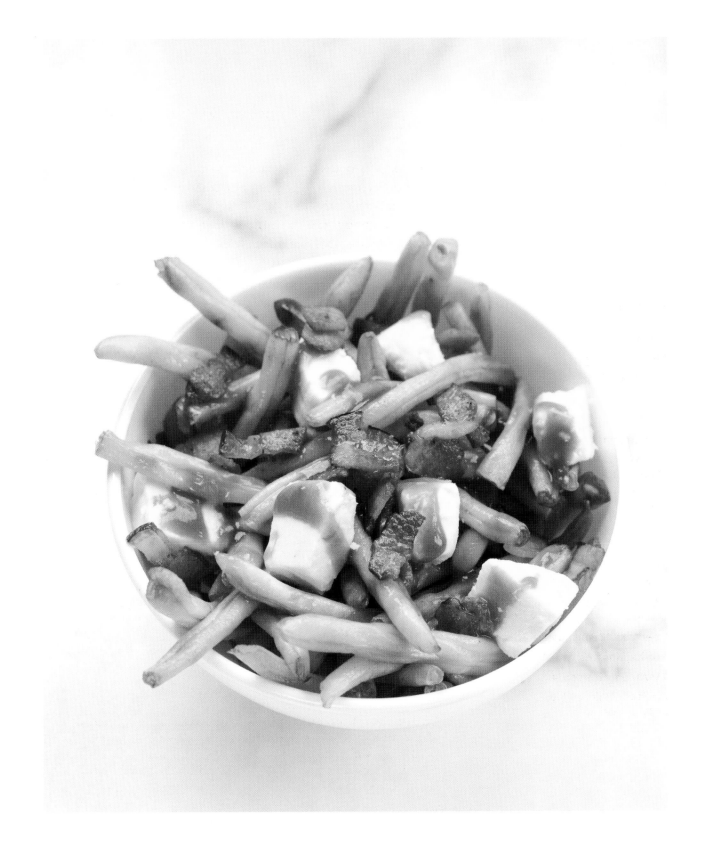

MACRONUTRIENTS
(per serving)

Fat	Protein	Carbs	Fiber	Energy
58g	28.8g	9.8g	4.5g	676 cal
77%	18%	5%		

9. Reheat the gravy to a nice simmer. Divide the wax bean fries between 4 bowls. Top each bowl evenly with the cheese curds and chopped bacon, then top with the gravy.

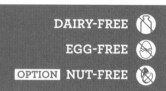

DAIRY-FREE

EGG-FREE

OPTION NUT-FREE

Green Thai Pork Curry

Prep Time: **10 minutes** | Cook Time: **35 minutes**
Yield: **2 servings**

Creamy Thai curries made with coconut milk are one of the best parts of eating keto! This recipe is very versatile. Depending on my carb intake for the day, I either make the pork curry and noodles alone or add veggies. If you are less strict with your carbs and would like to add more vegetables, fry up some green onions, red or green cabbage, green bell peppers, and sliced cucumbers for extra Thai curry flavor. For variety, you can serve this curry over shredded green cabbage fried in coconut oil or cauliflower rice.

1 cup (8 ounces/225 g) coconut cream (see note, page 108)

1 cup (8 fluid ounces/240 ml) filtered water

3 tablespoons coconut oil, divided

12 ounces (340 g) pork tenderloin, sliced or cubed

1 tablespoon green curry paste

1 teaspoon fish sauce

1 tablespoon tamari

1 tablespoon freshly squeezed lime or lemon juice

¼ teaspoon fine sea salt

3 or 4 drops liquid stevia, to taste

2 (7-ounce/200-g) packages angel hair–style zero-carb shirataki noodles

2 tablespoons thinly sliced green onions

1 clove garlic, minced

½ cup (2 ounces/55 g) cubed eggplant

½ cup (2 ounces/55 g) sliced zucchini

12 raw cashews (optional)

1 tablespoon chopped fresh cilantro (optional)

Sliced green chili peppers, for garnish (optional)

1. Mix the coconut cream with the water.

2. In a medium skillet over medium heat, melt 1 tablespoon of the coconut oil. When the oil is hot, add the pork. Cook for 10 to 12 minutes, flipping periodically, until the slices are slightly browned. Remove from the pan and set aside.

3. In a saucepan over low heat, heat 1 tablespoon of the coconut oil. Add the green curry paste and heat until fragrant, stirring often with a wooden spoon (be careful that it doesn't burn). Add the coconut cream and water mixture and bring to a simmer over medium heat.

4. Add the fish sauce, tamari, lime juice, salt, and stevia to the green curry mixture, reduce the heat to maintain a simmer, and cook for another 5 to 10 minutes.

5. Meanwhile, prepare the noodles: Rinse and drain the noodles. In a saucepan over high heat, boil the noodles in water for 1 to 2 minutes. Drain and set on paper towels to absorb the excess water.

6. In a skillet over medium heat, melt the remaining tablespoon of coconut oil. Add the green onions and garlic and cook for 1 to 2 minutes, until fragrant. Add the eggplant and cook for a few minutes, until soft. Add the zucchini and cook for an additional 5 to 6 minutes, until all the vegetables are cooked through.

7. Add the pork back to the pan and stir to combine. Add the green curry mixture and simmer for 1 to 2 minutes. Serve over the noodles. If desired, top with the cashews and cilantro and garnish with sliced green chilies.

MACRONUTRIENTS
(per serving)

Fat	Protein	Carbs	Fiber	Energy
45.5g	38g	10g	3.5g	608 cal
68%	25%	7%		

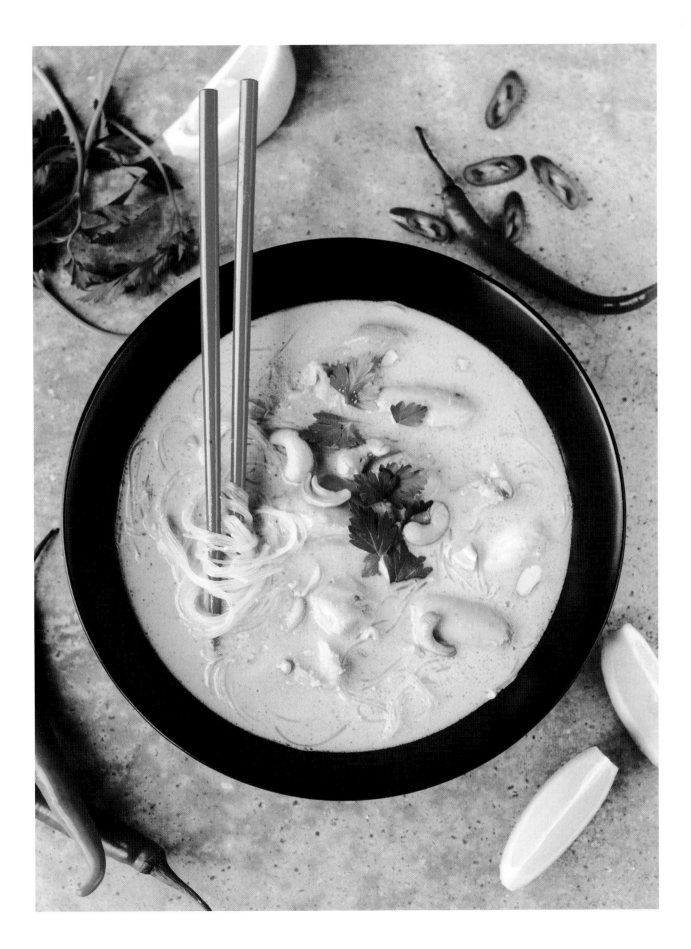

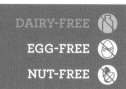

DAIRY-FREE

EGG-FREE

NUT-FREE

Pork Gyro Lettuce Wraps
with Quick Pickled Red Onions

Prep Time: 15 minutes, plus at least 30 minutes to marinate | **Cook Time:** 30 minutes
Yield: 4 servings (about 3 wraps per serving)

Gyros without the pita bread are a great ketogenic option for dining out, as there are limited restaurant options that provide fully compliant keto dishes. This dish and its restaurant counterparts are a little low in fat, although still low enough in protein and carbs. Make these lettuce wraps with pickled red onions and pair them with Tzatziki Dip (page 150) or Avocado Tzatziki Dip (page 151) for a restaurant-worthy keto dinner at home.

PORK GYROS:

¼ cup (2 fluid ounces/60 ml) freshly squeezed lemon juice

⅔ cup (5½ fluid ounces/160 ml) olive oil

3 cloves garlic, minced

2 teaspoons paprika

1 teaspoon dried oregano leaves

1 teaspoon ground coriander

1 teaspoon fine sea salt

½ teaspoon ground black pepper

2 pounds (910 g) pork tenderloin, cut into ½-inch (1.25-cm) slices

2 tablespoons salted butter

12 Bibb lettuce leaves, for serving

1½ cups Tzatziki Dip (page 150) or Avocado Tzatziki Dip (page 151), for serving (optional)

PICKLED ONIONS:

½ red onion, thinly sliced

1 tablespoon freshly squeezed lemon juice

1½ teaspoons red wine vinegar

¼ teaspoon dried oregano leaves

¼ teaspoon fine sea salt

1. Make the gyros: In a small bowl, whisk together the lemon juice, olive oil, garlic, paprika, oregano, coriander, salt, and pepper. Pour half of the mixture into a second, larger bowl and add the pork. Toss the pork in the marinade, cover, and refrigerate for 30 minutes or up to 1 day. Reserve the remaining marinade in the small bowl.

2. Preheat the oven to 450°F (232°C). Line a rimmed baking sheet with aluminum foil. Place the pork and the marinade in which it was soaking on the baking sheet. Dot the pork with the butter. (Don't worry about the amount of moisture; the pork will absorb all the liquid during cooking.) Bake, turning once, until the pork is starting to turn golden around the edges, 25 to 30 minutes. Remove the pork and toss it with the reserved marinade.

3. While the pork is cooking, make the pickled onions: Toss the onion slices with the lemon juice, vinegar, oregano, and salt. Allow to sit until the onions have turned bright purple and shrunk in size, 10 to 15 minutes.

4. Divide the pork among the lettuce leaves, using 2 or 3 slices per leaf. Garnish with the pickled onions and about 2 tablespoons of tzatziki per wrap, if desired.

MACRONUTRIENTS
(per serving, with tzatziki)

Fat	Protein	Carbs	Fiber	Energy
46.3g	52g	13.5g	1.5g	675 cal
62%	30%	8%		

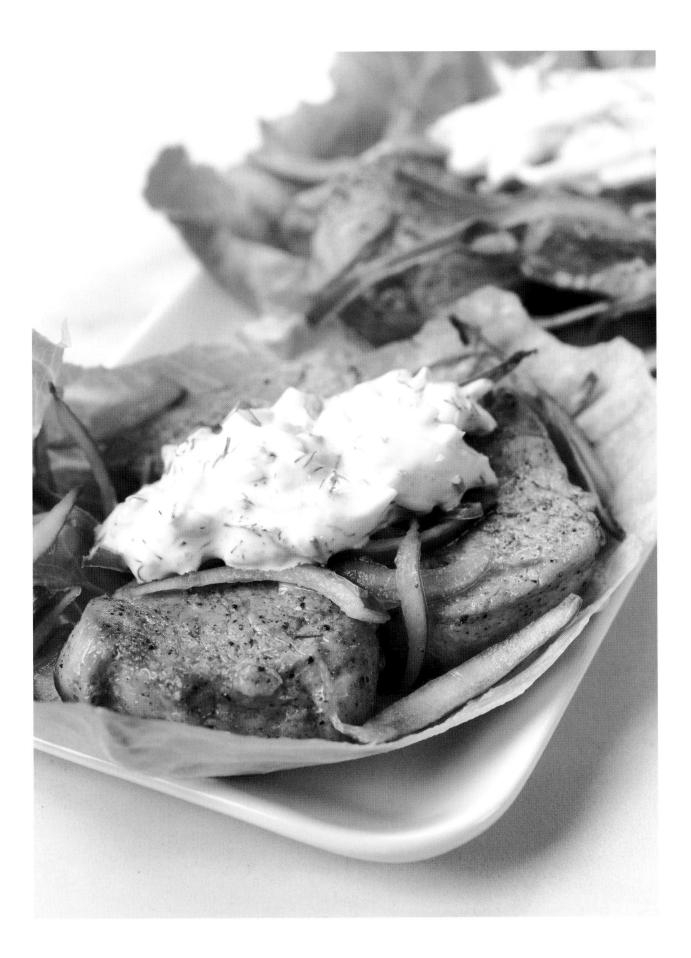

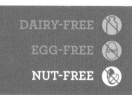

DAIRY-FREE

EGG-FREE

NUT-FREE

Asparagus
with Prosciutto and Hollandaise

Prep Time: 10 minutes | Cook Time: **15 minutes**
Yield: **2 servings**

I love white asparagus for this recipe. Although white or green will do, white is closer to the European version, and I find that it tastes sweeter than green. If you can't find fresh white asparagus, use green. Make sure to only lightly cook the asparagus so that it remains crisp-tender and does not get too soft.

18 spears white or green asparagus, woody ends trimmed

8 ounces (225 g) sliced prosciutto or Iberico ham

½ cup (4 ounces/120 ml) Hollandaise (page 354)

¼ cup (1 ounce/28 g) shaved Parmesan cheese

Chopped fresh dill, for garnish (optional)

Black or white truffle salt, for garnish (optional)

1. Bring a large, wide pot of water to a boil. Add the asparagus and remove from the heat. Allow to cook gently in the hot water for 10 to 15 minutes, until crisp-tender, then drain.

2. Divide the asparagus between 2 plates. Layer the prosciutto and ¼ cup (2 ounces/60 ml) of hollandaise on top of each plate. Finish with the shaved Parmesan. If desired, garnish each plate with fresh dill and, for a bonus rich flavor, some black or white truffle salt.

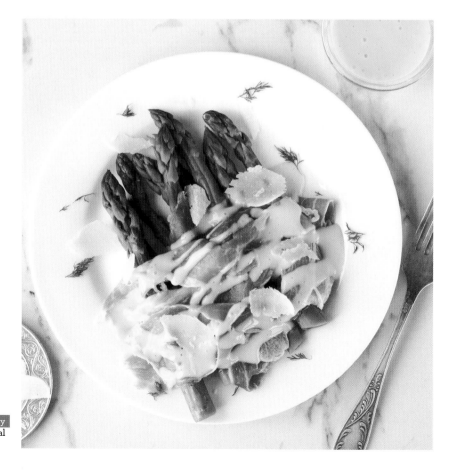

MACRONUTRIENTS
(per serving)

Fat	Protein	Carbs	Fiber	Energy
50g	33g	5.5g	2.5g	589 cal
74%	22%	4%		

Fully Loaded
Gourmet Hot Dogs

DAIRY-FREE OPTION
EGG-FREE
NUT-FREE

Prep Time: **10 minutes** | Cook Time: **6 to 8 minutes**
Yield: **4 servings**

This is a super-quick lunch or dinner! Everyone loves a hot dog from time to time. It's important to get organic hot dogs made from a humanely raised cows or pigs with no sugars added during the curing process. I like the Applegate brand; they are 100 percent grass-fed beef dogs that meet these criteria.

4 organic uncured beef or pork hot dogs

4 large romaine lettuce leaves, spines intact

¼ cup (1¼ ounces/35 g) sugar–free sauerkraut

1 tablespoon finely chopped onions

¼ cup (1 ounce/28 g) shredded Swiss cheese (optional)

½ cup (4 ounces/115 g) Special Burger Sauce (page 363)

TOPPING SUGGESTIONS:

Sliced green onions

Cooked and crumbled bacon

Sautéed sliced mushrooms

Diced avocado

Chopped fresh herbs

Crumbled blue cheese

1. Heat a grill or stovetop grill pan to medium heat. Grill the hot dogs for 6 to 8 minutes.

2. Lay out the lettuce leaves. Load each leaf with a hot dog. Divide the sauerkraut, onions, and cheese, if using, between the hot dogs. Top each hot dog with 2 tablespoons of the sauce.

3. If desired, top the hot dogs with green onions, bacon, mushrooms, avocado, fresh herbs, and/or blue cheese.

tip

If you like hot cheese, melt the Swiss cheese and pour it over the hot dogs.

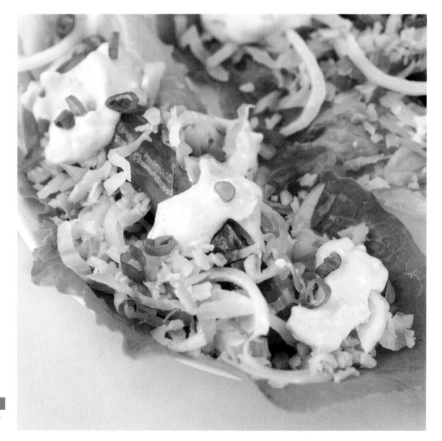

	MACRONUTRIENTS (per serving)			
Fat	Protein	Carbs	Fiber	Energy
35.8g	12.5g	3.8g	1g	390 cal
83%	13%	4%		

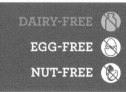

DAIRY-FREE

EGG-FREE

NUT-FREE

Pork Belly
with Caramelized Zucchini

Prep Time: 10 minutes, plus 15 minutes to rest | **Cook Time:** 2 hours 45 minutes
Yield: 5 servings

A mortar and pestle or a small food processor is great for making the fennel rub paste for this recipe.

FENNEL PASTE:

2 tablespoons fennel seeds

2 tablespoons coconut oil, lard, bacon fat, or avocado oil

1 teaspoon sea salt flakes or fine sea salt

2 cloves garlic, minced

1 pound (455 g) pork belly

2 tablespoons salted butter

3 zucchini, cut into ½-inch (1.25-cm) cubes (about 3 cups)

½ teaspoon liquid stevia (optional)

Pinch of ground Ceylon cinnamon or regular cinnamon

Pinch of sea salt

1. Preheat the oven to 350°F (177°C).

2. In a small skillet over low heat, toast the fennel seeds for a couple of minutes until they become fragrant, being careful not to burn them.

3. Remove the fennel seeds from the pan. Using a mortar and pestle or a small food processor, make a paste by grinding together the fennel seeds, coconut oil, salt, and garlic. Set the paste aside.

4. Using a sharp knife, score the skin of the pork belly with straight or diagonal lines, cutting about ⅛ inch (3 mm) into the meat. Lay the pork belly on a wire rack in a roasting pan, skin side up.

5. Rub the oil and fennel paste onto the top of the pork belly, which will enable the skin to crisp during cooking.

6. Bake for 2 hours, then increase the oven temperature to 400°F (205°C) and cook for another 30 to 40 minutes, until the top of the pork belly is nice and crisp.

7. Allow to rest for 15 minutes in a warming tray, or tent with aluminum foil and rest on the counter.

8. While the pork belly is resting, prepare the zucchini: In a saucepan over medium-high heat, melt the butter. Add the zucchini and stevia, if using, and sauté for 5 to 7 minutes, until the zucchini is lightly browned and caramelized. Season with the cinnamon and salt.

9. Slice the pork belly and serve with the caramelized zucchini.

MACRONUTRIENTS
(per serving)

Fat	Protein	Carbs	Fiber	Energy
60.4g	9g	3.4g	1.5g	598 cal
91%	7%	2%		

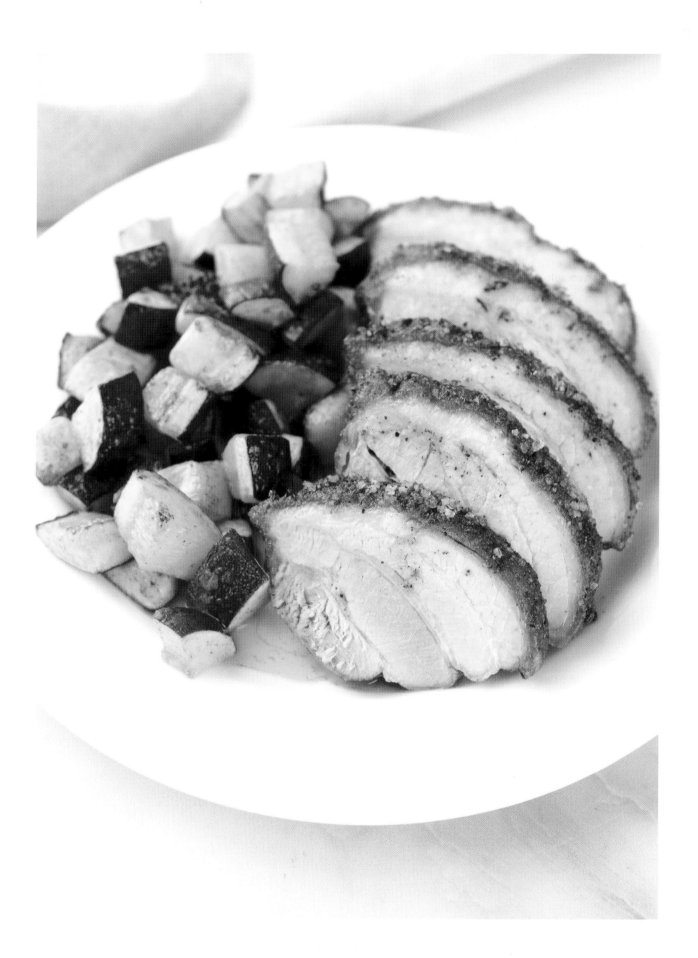

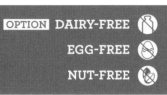

OPTION DAIRY-FREE

EGG-FREE

NUT-FREE

Pork Terrine

Prep Time: 20 minutes, plus time to chill overnight | **Cook Time:** 4 hours
Yield: 6 servings

This is a wonderful crowd-pleaser for entertaining! Serve this terrine with pork rinds or cucumber slices. The butter preserves the rillettes well in the fridge for a couple of days, or you can store them in the freezer for up to a month. At 93 percent fat, this terrine is like a savory fat bomb.

1 pound (455 g) pork belly, cubed

4 ounces (115 g) pork liver

½ teaspoon fine sea salt

¼ teaspoon ground black pepper

½ cup (4 fluid ounces/120 ml) filtered water

1 bay leaf

2 tablespoons chopped fresh parsley

1 tablespoon fresh thyme

¼ cup plus 2 tablespoons (3 ounces/85 g) butter or lard, melted

1. Preheat the oven to 250°F (120°C).

2. In a food processor, working in batches if necessary, pulse the pork belly, pork liver, salt, and pepper until smooth.

3. Transfer the pork mixture to a small (1-quart/1-L capacity) ovenproof ceramic baking dish. Pour the water on top and add the bay leaf. Bake for 3½ to 4 hours, stirring occasionally, until very soft.

4. Remove from the oven, pull out the bay leaf, and add the parsley and thyme. Use an immersion blender to mix thoroughly. Divide evenly between six 4-ounce (120-ml) ramekins, smoothing the tops. Cover each ramekin with the melted butter.

5. Refrigerate overnight before serving.

MACRONUTRIENTS
(per serving)

Fat	Protein	Carbs	Fiber	Energy
58g	10.5g	0g	0g	571 cal
93%	7%	0%		

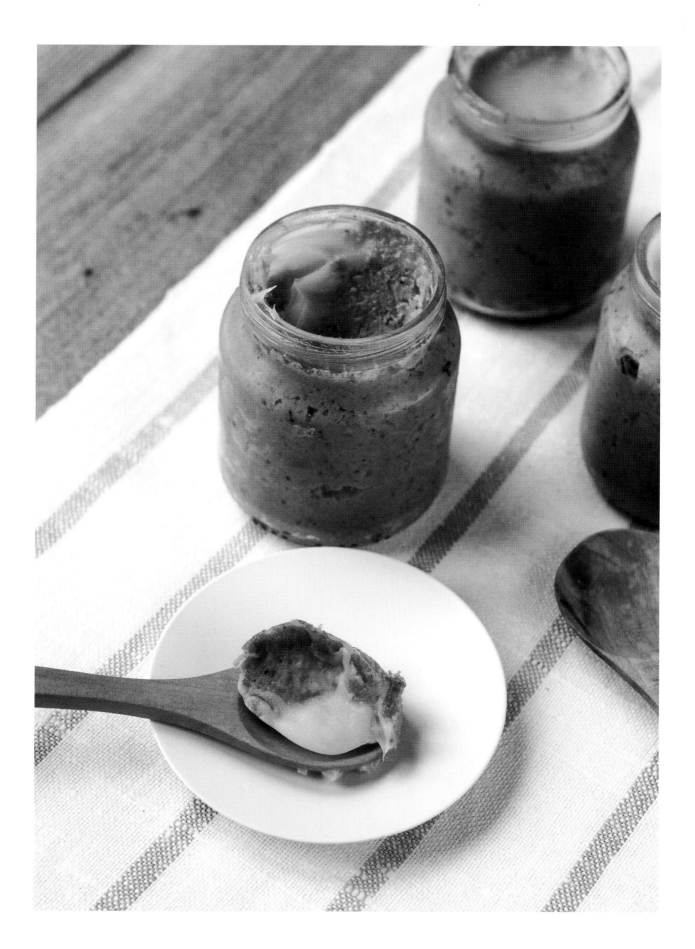

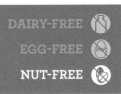

DAIRY-FREE

EGG-FREE

NUT-FREE

Spicy Pork Skewers
with Hollandaise

Prep Time: 15 minutes | **Cook Time: 15 minutes**
Yield: 3 servings

Rich and buttery hollandaise is the perfect foil to spicy paprika-tinged pork. This simple but complex-tasting dish has only 1 gram of carbs per serving! You'll need six skewers for this recipe. You can use either metal or bamboo skewers; if you use bamboo or wood skewers, soak them in water for thirty minutes before beginning the recipe.

¼ cup (2 fluid ounces/60 ml) olive oil or MCT oil

2 tablespoons paprika

1 teaspoon ground cumin

¼ teaspoon cayenne pepper

¼ teaspoon garlic powder

¼ teaspoon onion powder

¼ teaspoon ground black pepper

½ teaspoon fine sea salt

1 or 2 drops liquid stevia

1 pound (455 g) pork tenderloin, cubed

½ batch Hollandaise (page 354)

Chopped fresh parsley, for garnish (optional)

1. Preheat the oven to 350°F (177°C).

2. In a medium bowl, combine the oil, spices, salt, and stevia. Add the cubed pork and stir until all the pieces are well coated in the spice mixture.

3. Divide the pork evenly between 6 skewers. Roast for 10 to 15 minutes, until the pork is cooked through but still tender.

4. Remove from the oven and drizzle 3⅓ tablespoons of hollandaise over each skewer. Garnish with chopped parsley, if desired. Serve with extra hollandaise on the side.

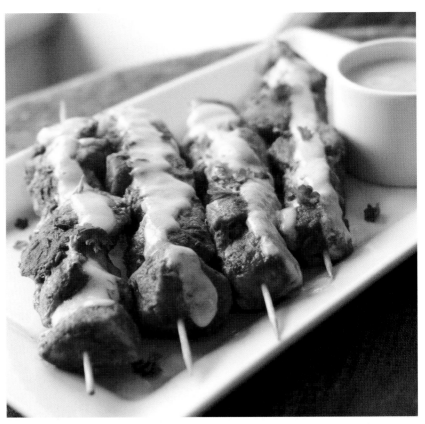

MACRONUTRIENTS
(per serving)

Fat	Protein	Carbs	Fiber	Energy
53g	33g	1g	0g	594 cal
78%	21%	1%		

Pulled Pork

Prep Time: 10 minutes | **Cook Time: 2 hours 20 minutes**
Yield: 3 servings

DAIRY-FREE

EGG-FREE

NUT-FREE OPTION

This dish is great on its own or as an outstanding basis for other recipes in this book, such as Pulled Pork and Avocado Boats (page 312) and Pulled Pork with Creamy Slaw (page 313). Pulled pork is an excellent staple to keep on hand for easy, tasty last-minute meals throughout the week. If you can't find a pork brisket or shoulder this small, just cut off the amount you need and freeze the rest.

1¼ pounds (565 g) boneless pork brisket or shoulder

Ground cumin

Sea salt

½ cup (4 fluid ounces/120 ml) filtered water

3 tablespoons butter

1 tablespoon almond flour, or ⅛ teaspoon guar gum or xanthan gum

Chopped fresh herbs, such as cilantro or parsley, for garnish (optional)

1. Preheat the oven to 350°F (177°C).

2. Rinse and pat dry the meat, sprinkle generously with cumin and salt, and place in a baking dish.

3. Pour the water into the baking dish and place in the oven. Bake for 1½ to 2 hours, until the pork shreds easily, occasionally basting and turning the pork.

4. Remove from the oven and pour the juices into a small saucepan. Whisk the butter and flour into the juices and bring to a boil over medium-high heat, then reduce the heat to low and simmer for 15 to 20 minutes, until the sauce has thickened.

5. Place the meat on a cutting board and use 2 forks to pull it apart. Serve with the sauce and garnish with chopped herbs, if desired.

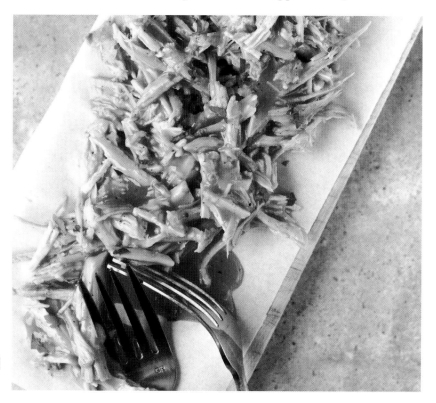

MACRONUTRIENTS (per serving)				
Fat	Protein	Carbs	Fiber	Energy
50g	47g	3.6g	1.6g	675 cal
69%	29%	2%		

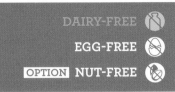

DAIRY-FREE

EGG-FREE

OPTION NUT-FREE

Pulled Pork and Avocado Boats

Prep Time: 10 minutes
Yield: 3 servings

What could be cuter than pulled pork served on little pork rind crackers? This attractive dish is great for entertaining. It's also a nice option for showing people how versatile and fun ketogenic eating can be. For this recipe, you'll make the Pulled Pork on page 311 and use about one-third of it for the boats. Save the rest to heat up for quick meals; for example, make a wrap by wrapping a lettuce leaf around a serving of pulled pork.

1 (1.7-ounce/50-g) bag pork rinds

1 avocado

⅓ batch Pulled Pork (page 311)

Chopped fresh cilantro or parsley, for garnish (optional)

1. Place the pork rinds on a plate. They will serve as little "boats" for the pulled pork. Peel and slice the avocado into ½-inch (1.25-cm) cubes.

2. Load each pork rind with some pulled pork and cubed avocado. Garnish with chopped cilantro or parsley, if desired.

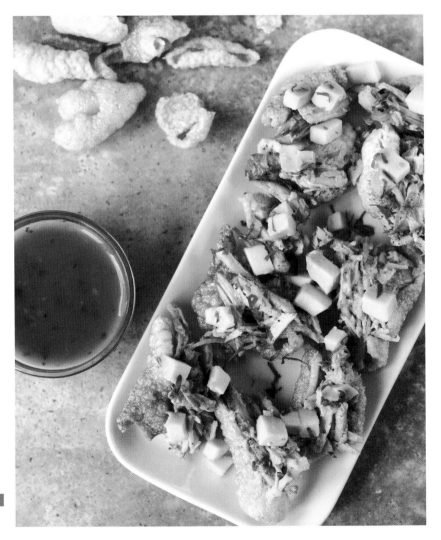

MACRONUTRIENTS (per serving)				
Fat	Protein	Carbs	Fiber	Energy
41g	28g	6g	4g	510 cal
73%	22%	5%		

Pulled Pork
with Creamy Slaw

Prep Time: 10 minutes
Yield: 6 servings

The combination of savory, juicy pulled pork and cool, crunchy slaw is a Southern comfort food for good reason. For a fun change, serve the pork between two slices of Keto Bread Loaf (page 156). You can serve the slaw on the side or directly on the sandwich for a tangy crunch.

1 batch Pulled Pork (page 311)

1 batch Creamy Keto Slaw (page 215)

Divide the pulled pork and slaw evenly between 6 plates and serve.

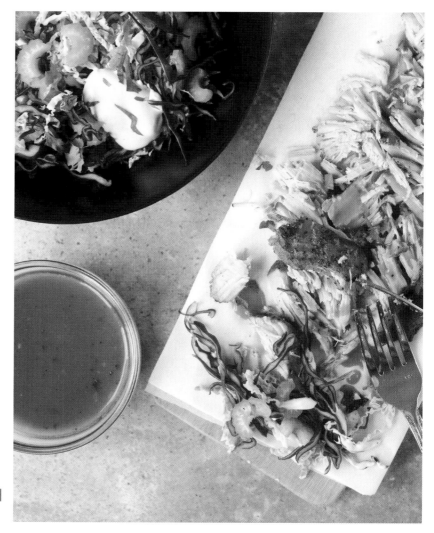

MACRONUTRIENTS (per serving)				
Fat	Protein	Carbs	Fiber	Energy
47.5g	24g	5.5g	1.8g	553 cal
78%	18%	4%		

Chapter 14
Desserts

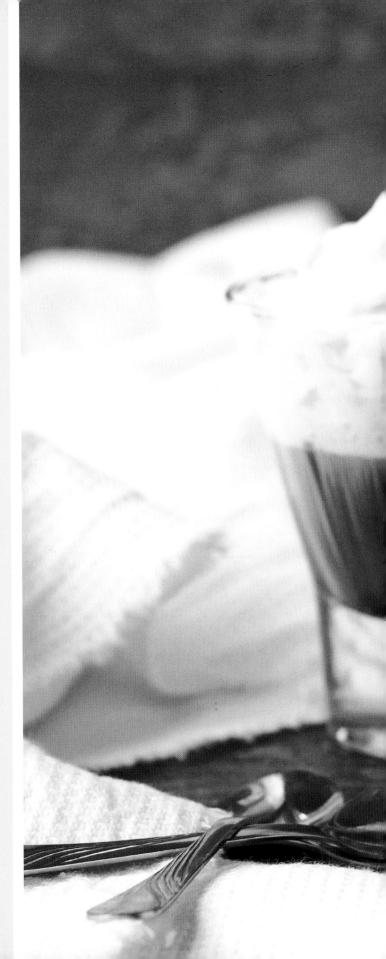

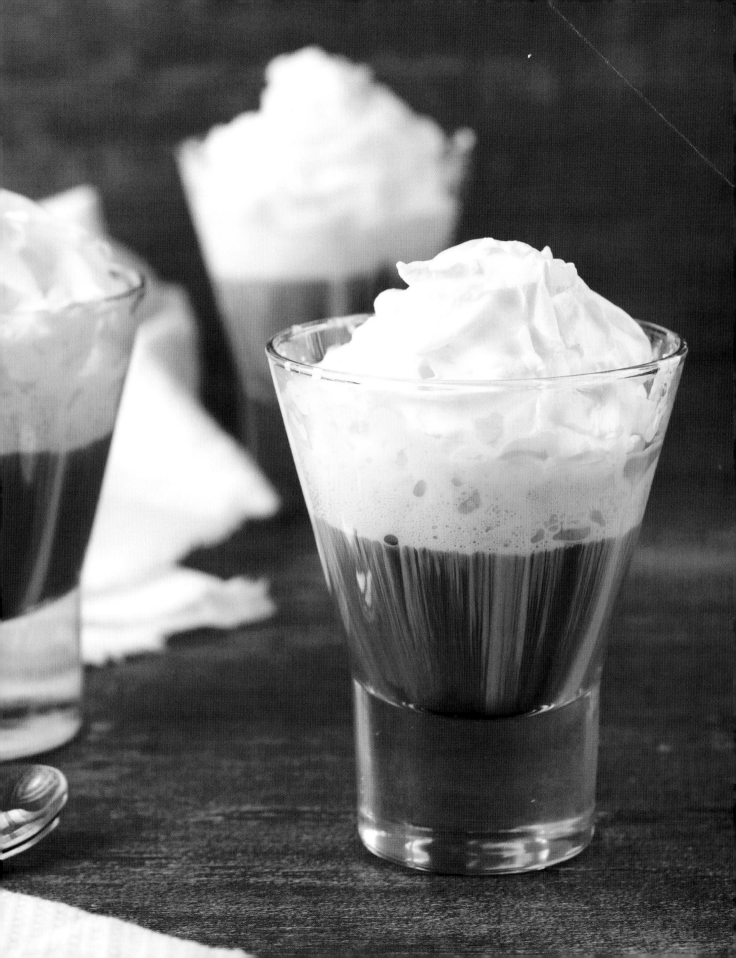

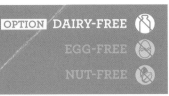

OPTION DAIRY-FREE

EGG-FREE

NUT-FREE

Crème Brûlée

Prep Time: 20 minutes, plus time to chill | **Cook Time:** 45 minutes
Yield: 4 servings

This is my go-to dessert recipe for entertaining. It's always a hit!

2 cups (16 fluid ounces/480 ml) heavy whipping cream, or 2 cups (16 ounces/455 g) coconut cream

¼ cup (2 fluid ounces/60 ml) almond milk

Seeds scraped from 1 vanilla bean, or 1 teaspoon vanilla extract

6 egg yolks

3 tablespoons erythritol, divided

1 teaspoon liquid stevia

1. Preheat the oven to 325°F (163°C).

2. In a medium saucepan over medium-high heat, bring the cream, milk, and vanilla to a boil. Remove from the heat and let cool for 15 to 20 minutes.

3. Meanwhile, whisk the egg yolks, 1 tablespoon of the erythritol, and stevia in a bowl until thickened and creamy. I like to do this with a hand mixer or with egg beaters, but you can also whisk it by hand for a few minutes.

4. Very slowly pour the cooled cream mixture into the egg yolk mixture, whisking or beating constantly.

5. Place four 4-ounce (120-ml) ramekins in a deep ovenproof baking dish. Divide the cream mixture between the ramekins. Pour boiling water into the baking dish so that it comes about halfway up the sides of the ramekins. Cover the baking pan loosely with aluminum foil so that the water steams the custard.

6. Bake for 40 to 45 minutes, until the custard is set but still a bit jellylike in the center.

7. Remove the custards from the water bath and place in the refrigerator to chill for 3 hours or up to overnight.

8. When ready to serve, remove the custards from the refrigerator and let sit on the counter for 20 to 30 minutes. Sprinkle the top of each with 1½ teaspoons of the remaining erythritol. Melt the sweetener either by placing the ramekins under the oven broiler for a couple of minutes (watch carefully!) or by using a kitchen torch. Let cool for a few minutes before serving.

note

For an extra-special presentation, garnish the Crème Brûlée with fresh mint and a few low-carb berries, such as blackberries.

MACRONUTRIENTS
(per serving)

Fat	Protein	Carbs	Fiber	Energy
23.8g	5g	10.1g	7.5g	252 cal
78%	7%	15%		

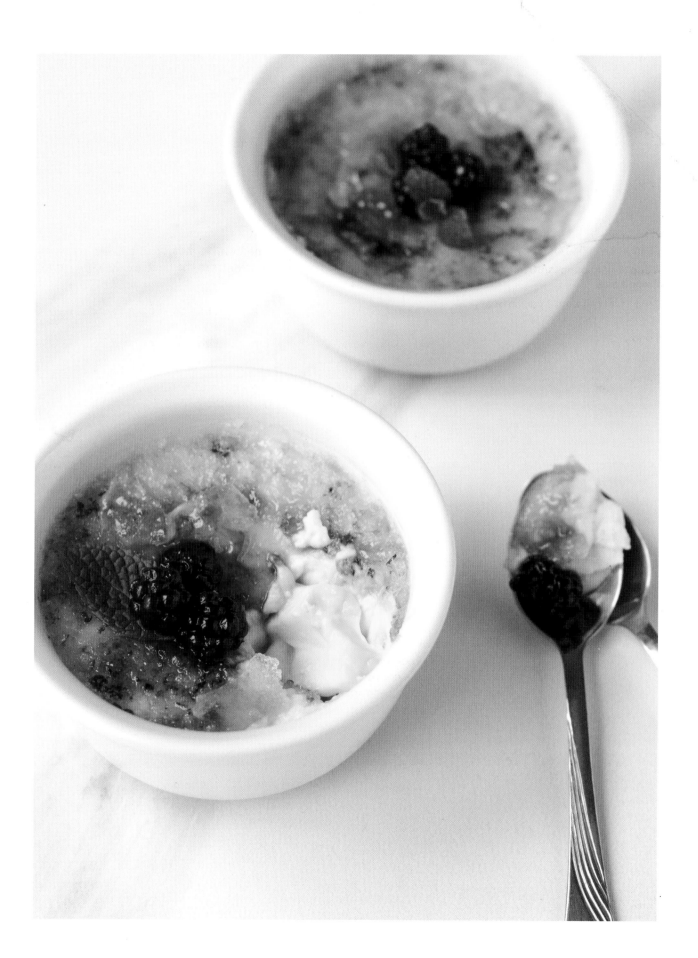

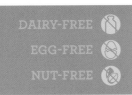

DAIRY-FREE

EGG-FREE

NUT-FREE

Vanilla Ice Cream

Prep Time: 5 minutes, plus time to churn
Yield: 2½ cups (15 ounces/430 g) (½ cup/3 ounces/85 g per serving)

Never in my life did I think that eating ice cream could a) be good for me or b) generate weight loss. The ketogenic diet truly is amazing! Enjoying my favorite flavor, vanilla, with MCT oil for fat-burning ketones, plus rich organic heavy cream, totally guilt-free is something I never imagined. Yet on the keto diet, it's real!

I use an ice cream maker for this recipe, but you don't need one. I have had success simply freezing this ice cream in a freezer-safe glass storage container, then letting it defrost a bit before serving. This method won't give you the same texture as an ice cream maker, but it's a great option. I have also used this recipe to make ice pops, freezing the ice cream in ice pop molds that I run under warm water before removing.

6 egg yolks from pasteurized eggs

1 cup (8 fluid ounces/240 ml) heavy whipping cream

1 cup (8 fluid ounces/240 ml) almond milk

¼ cup (2 ounces/57 g) erythritol

1 tablespoon coconut oil

1 tablespoon MCT oil

2 teaspoons almond extract

1 teaspoon vanilla paste, or 2 teaspoons vanilla extract

1 teaspoon liquid stevia

Pinch of sea salt

SPECIAL EQUIPMENT:

Ice cream maker (optional)

1. Place all the ingredients in a blender and blend on high for a few minutes.

2. If using an ice cream maker, remove the freezer bowl for the ice cream maker from the freezer. Pour the ice cream base into the ice cream maker and churn, following the manufacturer's instructions.

3. Eat right away or, if you prefer a more solid ice cream, freeze it for a bit longer in a freezer-safe glass container. I like to remove the ice cream from the freezer about 15 minutes before serving so that it softens a little.

4. If using a glass container to make the ice cream, pour the ice cream base into the container and place in the freezer. Remove from the freezer every 30 minutes and stir vigorously with a whisk or beat with an electric mixer until it has the texture of soft-serve ice cream, 2 to 3 hours. If a firmer texture is desired, freeze longer.

note

This recipe does not include the step of cooking the eggs, so it's important to use yolks from pasteurized, not raw, eggs. You can also temper the eggs and gently cook the mixture over very low heat, stirring constantly, and then chilling the mixture before freezing or churning it in an ice cream maker.

MACRONUTRIENTS
(per serving)

Fat	Protein	Carbs	Fiber	Energy
20.4g	3.8g	2.2g	2.6g	206 cal
88%	8%	4%		

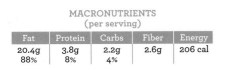

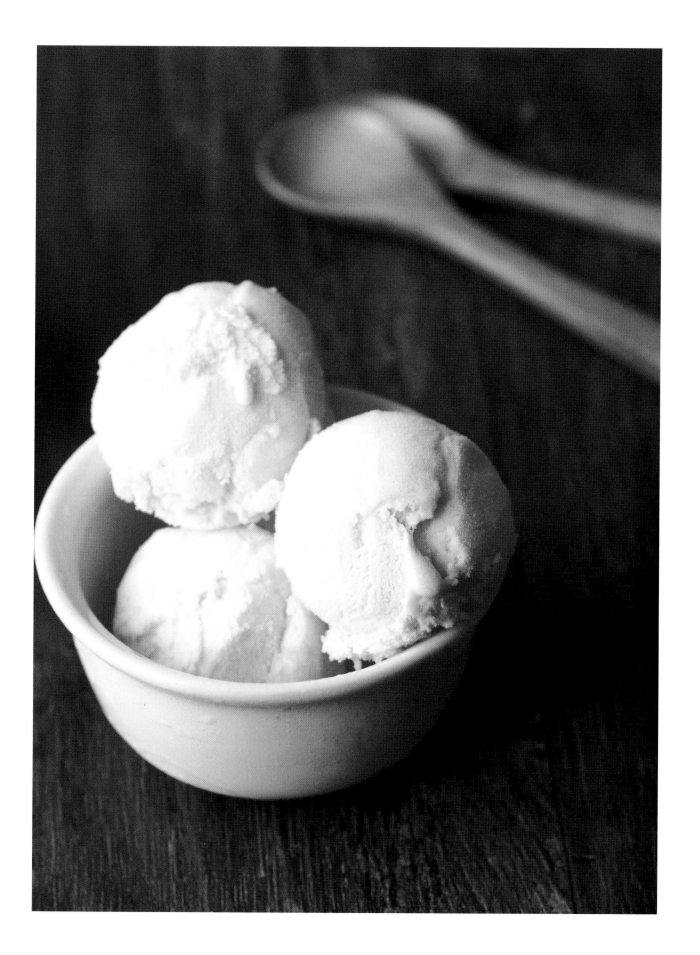

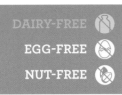

DAIRY-FREE

EGG-FREE

NUT-FREE

Cheesecake Fat Bombs

Prep Time: 5 minutes, plus time to chill
Yield: 4 servings

These are super-quick and easy fat bombs that you make using a stand mixer. With the added coconut oil, and at 91 percent fat and only 2 grams of carbs per serving, they are very ketogenic. Make sure to take the cream cheese and butter out of the fridge ahead of time.

1 (8-ounce/225-g) package cream cheese, softened

2 tablespoons butter, softened

2 tablespoons coconut oil, softened

1 teaspoon liquid stevia

1 teaspoon vanilla extract, or 1 tablespoon freshly squeezed lemon juice

Pinch of sea salt

Unsweetened coconut flakes, toasted, for garnish (optional)

1. Slice the cream cheese into 8 cubes; place in the bowl of a stand mixer or food processor. Add the butter and coconut oil and use the whisk attachment for the stand mixer to blend until smooth, or process in the food processor until smooth.

2. Stir in the stevia, vanilla, and salt.

3. Pour the cheesecake mixture into 4 regular-size or 8 mini paper muffin cups. Garnish with toasted coconut chips, if desired. Freeze for 5 minutes or place in the refrigerator for up to 1 hour to firm up.

note

For a different flavor, try blueberry, raspberry, or any other flavoring you love in place of the vanilla extract.

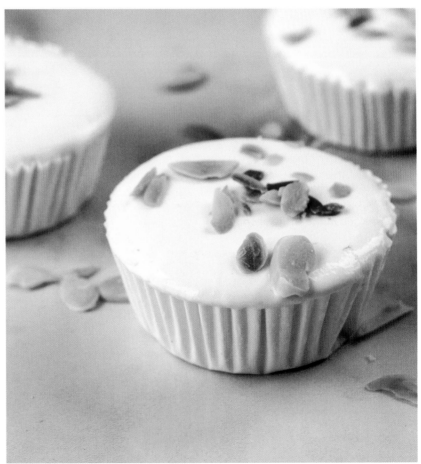

MACRONUTRIENTS
(per serving)

Fat	Protein	Carbs	Fiber	Energy
30.8g	4g	2g	0g	319 cal
91%	6%	3%		

Instant Chia Pudding

⊘ **DAIRY-FREE**

⊘ EGG-FREE

⊘ NUT-FREE

Prep Time: 5 minutes, plus time to chill
Yield: 4 servings

Chia pudding is a wonderful keto staple. This is one of the most popular recipes that I have created over the years for my meal plans and on KetogenicGirl.com. I recently revised the recipe to make it even richer and creamier!

1½ cups (12 ounces/340 g) coconut cream (see note, page 108)

1½ cups (12 fluid ounces/350 ml) almond milk

½ teaspoon liquid stevia

¼ teaspoon almond extract

¼ teaspoon vanilla extract

Pinch of sea salt

¼ cup (1½ ounces/38 g) chia seeds

Ground Ceylon cinnamon or regular cinnamon, for garnish

Raw pumpkin seeds, for garnish (optional)

note

If you forget to chill the cans of coconut milk ahead of time (allowing the cream to separate from the milk), you can use the same amount of room-temperature full-fat coconut milk. The pudding will have a slightly higher carb content when made with coconut milk.

1. In a blender, blend all the ingredients except the chia seeds and garnishes. Pour into a mixing bowl and add the chia seeds; mix well.

2. Divide the pudding mixture between 4 individual serving bowls, glasses, or small ramekins.

3. Chill in the refrigerator for 1 to 2 hours or overnight to allow the chia seeds to bloom and the pudding to set; overnight is ideal.

4. When ready to serve, remove from the refrigerator and sprinkle with cinnamon and a few pumpkin seeds, if desired.

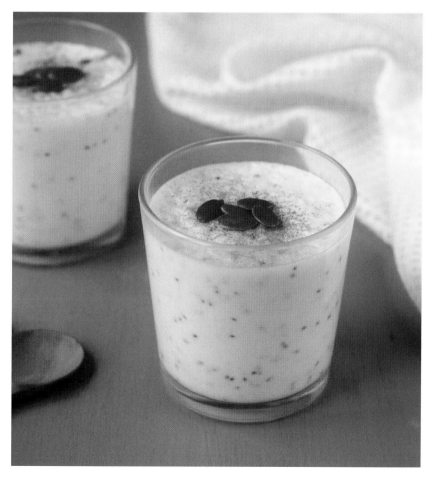

MACRONUTRIENTS (per serving)				
Fat	Protein	Carbs	Fiber	Energy
27.7g	4.5g	6g	4.5g	291 cal
86%	6%	8%		

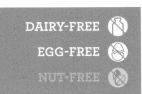

DAIRY-FREE

EGG-FREE

NUT-FREE

Chocolate Mint
Mousse

Prep Time: 5 minutes, plus time to chill
Yield: 4 servings

1½ cups (12 ounces/340 g) coconut cream (see note, page 108)

1½ cups (12 fluid ounces/350 ml) almond milk

2 tablespoons unsweetened cocoa powder

½ teaspoon liquid stevia

¼ teaspoon vanilla extract

2 to 4 drops peppermint extract, to taste

Pinch of sea salt

1½ teaspoons chopped fresh mint, plus 4 small sprigs for garnish

3 tablespoons chia seeds

1. In a blender, blend the cream, milk, cocoa powder, stevia, extracts, salt, and chopped mint. Pour into a mixing bowl and add the chia seeds; mix well. Divide the mixture between 4 individual serving bowls, glasses, or ramekins.

2. Chill in the refrigerator for 1 to 2 hours or overnight to allow the chia seeds to bloom and the mousse to set; overnight is ideal.

3. When ready to serve, remove the mousse from the refrigerator and garnish with the mint sprigs.

note

If you forget to chill the cans of coconut milk ahead of time (allowing the cream to separate from the milk), you can use the same amount of room-temperature full-fat coconut milk. The mousse will have a slightly higher carb content when made with coconut milk.

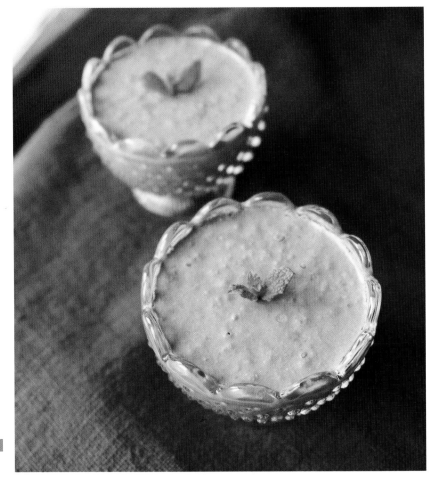

MACRONUTRIENTS
(per serving)

Fat	Protein	Carbs	Fiber	Energy
20g	4g	7g	4.5g	216 cal
80%	7%	13%		

Cinnamon Custard

DAIRY-FREE

EGG-FREE

NUT-FREE

Prep Time: **10 minutes** | Cook Time: **1 hour**
Yield: **2 servings**

1 cup (8 ounces/225 g) coconut cream (see note, page 108)

1 cup (8 fluid ounces/240 ml) almond milk

1 egg

1 tablespoon erythritol or powdered stevia (optional)

1 teaspoon vanilla extract

½ teaspoon liquid stevia

¼ teaspoon ground Ceylon cinnamon or regular cinnamon

¼ teaspoon ground nutmeg (optional)

Pinch of sea salt

1 or 2 drops almond extract, to taste

1. Preheat the oven to 325°F (163°C).

2. In a blender, blend all the ingredients until smooth.

3. Place two 1-cup (240-ml) ramekins in a deep ovenproof baking dish. Divide the custard between the ramekins. Pour boiling water into the baking dish until it comes about halfway up the sides of the ramekins.

4. Bake for 1 hour, until set but still a bit jellylike in the center. Let cool slightly and then serve warm, or place in the refrigerator to chill before serving.

note

If you forget to chill the cans of coconut milk ahead of time (allowing the cream to separate from the milk), you can use the same amount of room-temperature full-fat coconut milk. The custard will have a slightly higher carb content when made with coconut milk.

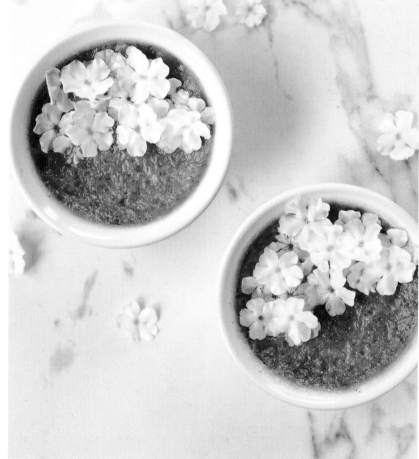

MACRONUTRIENTS
(using erythritol and liquid stevia)

Fat	Protein	Carbs	Fiber	Energy
24g	6.5g	9.5g	6.5g	251 cal
77%	9%	14%		

MACRONUTRIENTS
(using liquid stevia only)

Fat	Protein	Carbs	Fiber	Energy
24g	6.5g	4g	1g	259 cal
85%	10%	5%		

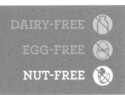

DAIRY-FREE

EGG-FREE

NUT-FREE

Lemon Curd

Prep Time: 15 minutes, plus time to chill | **Cook Time:** 7 minutes
Yield: 8 servings

This is one of the most popular recipes on my blog. With only seven ingredients, it is such an easy dessert to make, but the shot glasses are a wow factor for entertaining. Try different sweeteners if you prefer. Most of the carbs in this recipe come from the erythritol, which I count; however, many people do not count the carbs in erythritol, as it is a fiber-based sweetener. I understand this logic; however, because erythritol is made from sugar in a chemical process, in my opinion it's important to count those carbs.

6 egg yolks

¾ cup (6 fluid ounces/175 ml) freshly squeezed lemon juice

½ cup (4 ounces/115 g) erythritol, ground in a small food processor until powdery

½ to 1 teaspoon liquid stevia, to taste

⅛ teaspoon fine sea salt

½ cup (4 ounces/115 g) unsalted butter, cut into ½-inch (1.25-cm) cubes

2 teaspoons grated lemon zest

tip

For an even prettier presentation, top the lemon curd with some shredded coconut and fresh berries.

1. In a small heavy saucepan, whisk together the egg yolks, lemon juice, erythritol, stevia, and salt. Cook over medium heat, whisking constantly, until it coats the back of a wooden spoon, 6 to 7 minutes.

2. Remove the pan from the heat and add the butter, stirring as it melts.

3. Pour the curd into eight 2-ounce (30-ml) shot glasses, 8 small ramekins, or a serving bowl and place in the refrigerator to chill completely, 1 to 2 hours or overnight. Store in the refrigerator for up to 5 days.

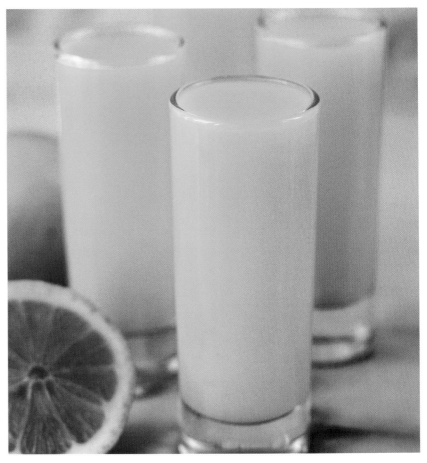

MACRONUTRIENTS
(per serving)

Fat	Protein	Carbs	Fiber	Energy
15g	2.3g	2.9g	3.3g	148 cal
87%	6%	7%		

No-Bake Cookie Dough

Prep Time: 10 minutes, plus 30 to 60 minutes to chill
Yield: 4 servings

This is a fantastic no-bake recipe that you can throw together in just a few minutes. If you're like me and you love store-bought cookie dough, this recipe is going to be a new favorite! You can now enjoy cookie dough in a healthy way—guilt-free. I love vanilla, so I usually add closer to 2 teaspoons of vanilla extract and closer to ½ teaspoon of salt to suit my taste buds. You can sweeten it according to your preference, too; start with a little bit of sweetener, taste, and then add more if desired. For the chocolate, I use 100 percent dark chocolate (aka unsweetened baking chocolate) broken into chocolate chip–sized chunks or sugar-free chocolate chips, which are made from cocoa liquor.

4 ounces (125 g) cream cheese, softened

4 ounces (125 g) mascarpone cheese, room temperature, or 4 more ounces cream cheese, softened

¼ cup plus 2 tablespoons (3 ounces/85 g) coconut butter, homemade (page 344) or store-bought, room temperature

¼ cup plus 2 tablespoons (3 ounces/85 g) unsalted butter, softened

2 tablespoons coconut oil

2 teaspoons granulated stevia

¼ to 1 teaspoon liquid stevia, to taste

1 teaspoon vanilla extract

¼ teaspoon baking soda

¼ teaspoon fine sea salt

2½ ounces (70 g) unsweetened chocolate (100% cacao), broken into small pieces, or sugar-free chocolate chips

1. Place all the ingredients except the chocolate in the bowl of a stand mixer or in a metal mixing bowl. Whip until well blended.

2. Fold in the chocolate pieces or chips.

3. Transfer to a mason jar or bowl and refrigerate for 30 to 60 minutes to firm up to the consistency of store-bought cookie dough.

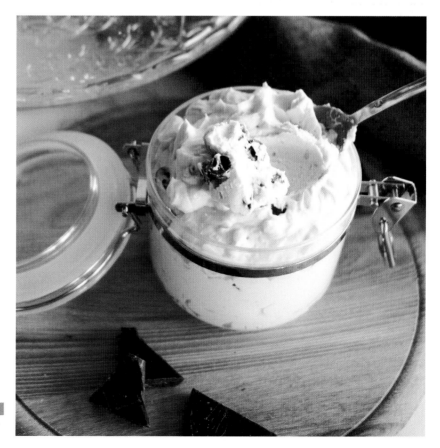

MACRONUTRIENTS
(per serving)

Fat	Protein	Carbs	Fiber	Energy
52g	7.8g	8g	0g	531 cal
88%	6%	6%		

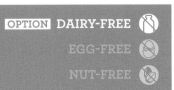

Decadent
Keto Brownies

Prep Time: **20 minutes** | Cook Time: **30 minutes**
Yield: **5 servings**

I like to add pecans or walnuts when making this recipe in maintenance mode or for guests. Adjust the amount of stevia as desired; it can be an acquired taste. Start with ¼ or ½ teaspoon and increase to up to 1 teaspoon based on what you like.

½ cup (4 ounces/115 g) butter or butter-flavored coconut oil

2 (1¾-ounce/50-g) bars dark chocolate (99% cacao), or 3½ ounces (100 g) unsweetened baking chocolate (100% cacao), chopped

½ cup (2 ounces/55 g) almond flour or almond meal

2 tablespoons coconut flour

½ teaspoon baking powder

¼ cup (2 ounces/57 g) erythritol, ground in a small food processor until powdery

¼ cup (2 fluid ounces/60 ml) filtered water

2 whole eggs

1 egg yolk

½ cup (4 ounces/115 g) coconut cream (see note, page 108)

1 teaspoon liquid stevia

¼ teaspoon vanilla extract

Pinch of sea salt

¼ cup (1 ounce/28 g) raw walnuts or pecans, chopped (optional)

1. Preheat the oven to 350°F (177°C). Grease a 9 by 5-inch (23 by 13-cm) loaf pan with coconut oil spray.

2. In a heavy saucepan or double boiler over very low heat, melt the butter and chocolate. When almost melted, remove from the heat and stir to blend.

3. In a medium bowl, whisk together the almond flour, coconut flour, baking powder, and erythritol until well combined.

4. Add the melted chocolate mixture to the dry ingredients, stirring with a whisk. Add the water, whole eggs, egg yolk, coconut cream, stevia, vanilla, and salt and blend into a thick batter. Fold in the nuts, if using.

5. Pour the batter into the prepared loaf pan and bake for 20 to 30 minutes, until a toothpick inserted in the center comes out clean. Let cool in the pan before serving; the brownies will firm up as they cool. Cut into 5 pieces and serve.

MACRONUTRIENTS
(per serving)

Fat	Protein	Carbs	Fiber	Energy
45.4g	9.2g	6.8g	3.4g	474 cal
87%	8%	5%		

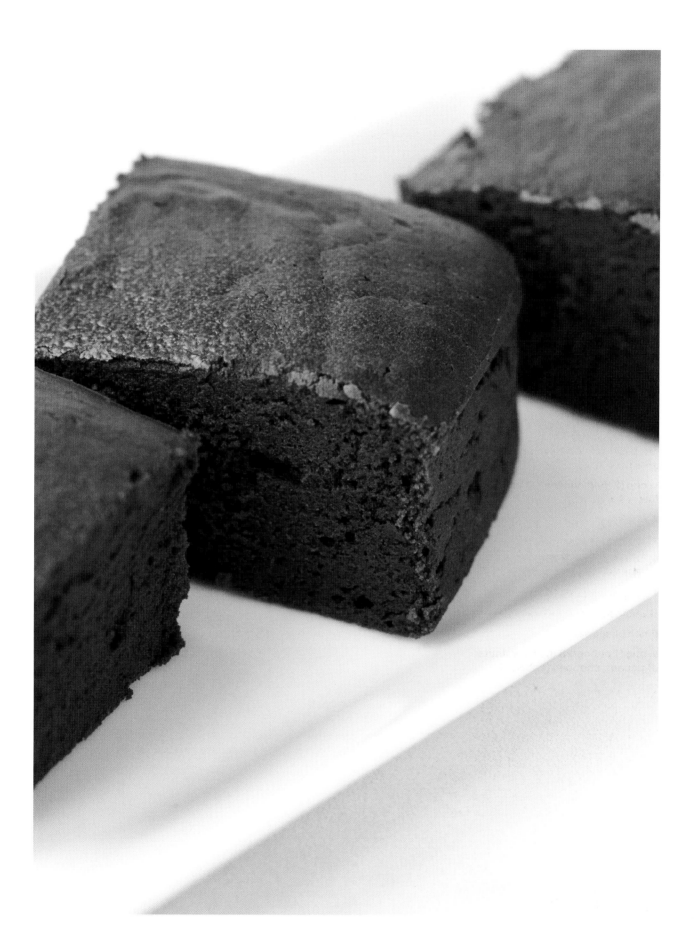

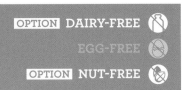

OPTION DAIRY-FREE

EGG-FREE

OPTION NUT-FREE

Ketogenic Girl
Cheesecake

Prep Time: 20 minutes, plus time to chill | **Cook Time:** 55 minutes
Yield: one 9-inch (23-cm) cake (12 servings)

Most of the low-carb cheesecake recipes I've tried use almond flour or ground almonds for the crust, but pecans have a more favorable macronutrient profile, as they are higher in fat and lower in carbohydrate than almonds. For this reason, I have included pecans as well as almond flour in my crust. If you are dairy-sensitive or in weight-loss mode, you can make this cheese-cake dairy-free and nut-free by using coconut butter in place of the cream cheese in the filling, omitting the sour cream from the filling, and leaving off the crust. Use vanilla extract for a traditional cheesecake flavor or substitute your preferred flavoring—my favorite is blueberry!

CRUST:

12 ounces (340 g) raw pecans

½ cup (2 ounces/55 g) almond flour or raw almonds

1 tablespoon coconut flour (optional)

½ cup (4 ounces/115 g) butter or coconut oil

1 teaspoon baking powder

Pinch of sea salt

FILLING:

3 (8-ounce/225-g) packages cream cheese, softened, or 3 cups (24 ounces/680 g) coconut butter, room temperature

1 cup (8 ounces/225 g) sour cream (omit for dairy-free)

4 egg yolks

¼ cup (1¾ ounces/50 g) erythritol or powdered stevia

1 teaspoon liquid stevia

1 teaspoon vanilla extract or other flavored extract of choice

Pinch of sea salt

¼ cup (1 ounce/28 g) raw pecan halves, some left whole and some crushed, for garnish (optional)

1. Preheat the oven to 350°F (177°C). Grease a 9-inch (23-cm) springform pan with butter or coconut oil.

2. Make the crust: Place the crust ingredients in a food processor and pulse to combine. Press into the bottom of the prepared pan and bake for 10 to 12 minutes, until browned, being careful not to let it burn. Remove from the oven and let cool in the pan.

3. Meanwhile, make the filling: Beat the cream cheese and sour cream in the bowl of a stand mixer. Add the egg yolks one at a time, beating well after each addition. Beat in the sweeteners and vanilla and finally the salt.

4. Pour the filling into the cooled crust and bake for 30 to 45 minutes, until the center is firm. Let cool in the pan, then place in the refrigerator to chill for 4 hours or overnight.

5. Just before serving, run a knife or offset spatula around the sides of the cake. Gently remove the side of the springform pan and place the cake on a plate. If desired, decorate the top of the cake with pecan halves and crushed pecans, as shown. Store in the refrigerator for up to 5 days.

MACRONUTRIENTS
(per serving, without pecans)

Fat	Protein	Carbs	Fiber	Energy
54g	9.3g	8.4g	4.5g	552 cal
87%	7%	6%		

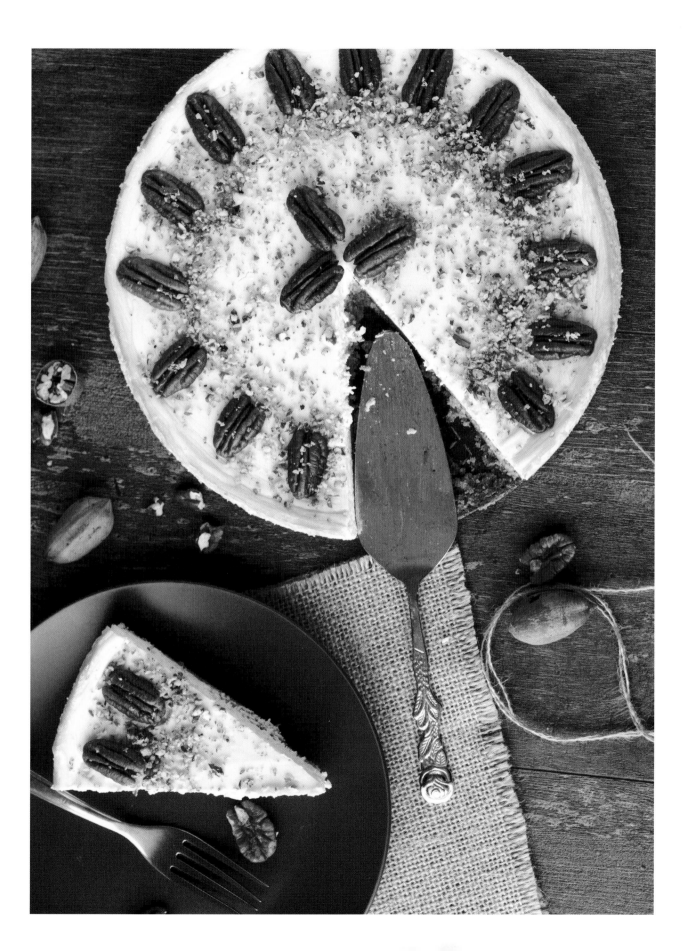

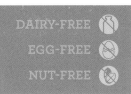

DAIRY-FREE
EGG-FREE
NUT-FREE

Coconut "Carrot" Cake

Prep Time: 15 minutes, plus 1 hour to cool | **Cook Time:** 35 minutes
Yield: One single-layer, 9-inch (23-cm) cake (10 servings)

Carrot cake is everyone's favorite indulgence, mostly because it sounds like a healthy treat. Here I've remade the classic using an unusual substitute for the carrots: daikon. Give it a taste; I bet it will become your new favorite dessert!

CAKE:

½ cup plus 2 tablespoons (2½ ounces/70 g) almond flour or meal

2 tablespoons coconut flour

2 tablespoons flax meal

2 teaspoons ground Ceylon cinnamon or regular cinnamon

½ teaspoon baking powder

½ teaspoon baking soda

½ teaspoon fine sea salt

4 whole eggs

2 egg yolks

¾ cup (6 ounces/170 g) coconut oil or butter, melted but not hot

¼ cup (2 fluid ounces/60 ml) walnut oil

1 cup plus 2 tablespoons (6 ounces/170 g) shredded daikon or zucchini (measured after being patted dry with paper towels)

¾ cup (2 ounces/55 g) unsweetened shredded coconut

¾ cup (3¼ ounces/95 g) raw pecans, chopped

2 teaspoons vanilla extract

¼ cup (2 ounces/57 g) erythritol

½ to 1 teaspoon liquid stevia

½ cup (4 fluid ounces/120 ml) almond milk

FROSTING:

1 (8-ounce/225-g) package cream cheese, softened

½ cup (4 ounces/115 g) butter, softened

1 teaspoon vanilla extract

1 tablespoon erythritol, ground in a small food processor until powdery (optional)

½ teaspoon liquid stevia

1. Preheat the oven to 350°F (177°C). Grease a 9-inch (23-cm) round cake pan.

2. In a small bowl, use a fork to combine the almond flour, coconut flour, flax meal, cinnamon, baking powder, baking soda, and salt.

3. In a medium bowl, whisk together the whole eggs, egg yolks, coconut oil, walnut oil, daikon, shredded coconut, pecans, vanilla, erythritol, and stevia.

4. Use a wooden spoon to stir the dry ingredients into the daikon mixture. Add the milk and combine into a thick but moist batter.

5. Pour the batter into the prepared cake pan and smooth out the top. Bake for 30 to 35 minutes, until cooked through and springy in the middle (when done, a toothpick inserted in the center will come out clean). Let cool in the pan for 1 to 2 hours.

6. Meanwhile, make the frosting: Combine all the ingredients in a small bowl and beat with a hand mixer until creamy and fluffy. Refrigerate for 1 to 2 hours while the cake cools.

7. Gently run a knife or offset spatula around the sides of the cooled cake to loosen, then invert the cake onto a clean surface Frost the top and sides with the frosting.

note

For a fun touch, add unsweetened shredded coconut to the frosting. Try decorating the cake with pumpkin seeds, pecans, toasted shredded coconut, thin strips of lemon zest, and/or edible flowers for a beautiful presentation!

MACRONUTRIENTS
(per serving)

Fat	Protein	Carbs	Fiber	Energy
44.6g	8.2g	12.3g	9.2g	452 cal
83%	7%	10%		

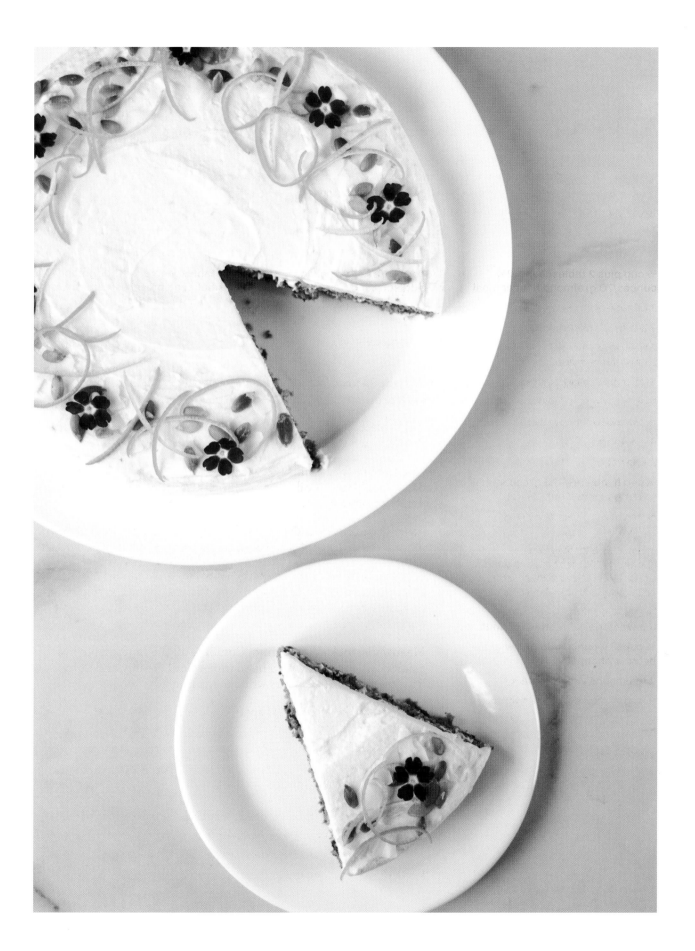

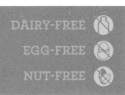

DAIRY-FREE
EGG-FREE
NUT-FREE

Easy Vanilla Cupcakes

Prep Time: 15 minutes, plus 20 minutes to cool | **Cook Time:** 20 minutes
Yield: 10 cupcakes (1 per serving)

What's not to love about sweet, fluffy cupcakes topped with a creamy frosting? This amazing version is ketogenic with all the satiety but none of the guilt!

CUPCAKES:

1 cup (4 ounces/115 g) almond flour

2 tablespoons coconut flour

1 teaspoon baking powder

½ teaspoon fine sea salt

1 cup (8 fluid ounces/240 ml) heavy whipping cream

2 whole eggs

4 egg yolks

¼ cup (1¼ ounces/36 g) erythritol or granulated or powdered stevia

½ teaspoon liquid stevia

½ teaspoon vanilla bean paste, or 1 teaspoon vanilla extract

FROSTING:

½ cup (4 ounces/115 g) butter, softened

2 tablespoons coconut oil, softened

2 tablespoons granulated stevia or erythritol, ground in a small food processor until powdery

½ teaspoon liquid stevia

½ teaspoon vanilla bean paste, or 1 teaspoon vanilla extract

1. Preheat the oven to 350°F (177°C). Line 10 wells of a standard-size 12-well muffin pan with paper liners.

2. In a medium bowl, use a fork to stir together the almond flour, coconut flour, baking powder, and salt until well blended. Set aside.

3. Using a stand mixer or handheld mixer, whip the cream until stiff peaks form. Add the whole eggs and egg yolks, one at a time, beating after each addition. Add the powdered sweetener, liquid stevia, and vanilla and mix to combine.

4. Using a wooden spoon, fold the flour mixture into the cream mixture and combine well.

5. Fill each cupcake liner about three-quarters full with the batter. Bake for 20 minutes, until a toothpick inserted in the center of a cupcake comes out clean. Let cool in the pan for 20 minutes before frosting.

6. While the cupcakes are cooling, make the frosting: Using a stand mixer or handheld mixer, whip together all the frosting ingredients until creamy and fluffy.

7. When the cupcakes are cool, scoop the frosting into a piping bag and pipe the frosting evenly onto the cupcakes. Alternatively, use a knife to spread frosting on each cupcake.

tips

Almond flour is similar to almond meal, but is much more finely ground; you can make it at home by grinding raw almonds in a food processor to a near-powdery texture. Be careful not to process it for too long, though, or you'll end up with almond butter!

Half of the carbs in this recipe are from the erythritol.

MACRONUTRIENTS (per cupcake)				
Fat	Protein	Carbs	Fiber	Energy
31g	5.3g	11g	8.9g	309 cal
82%	6%	12%		

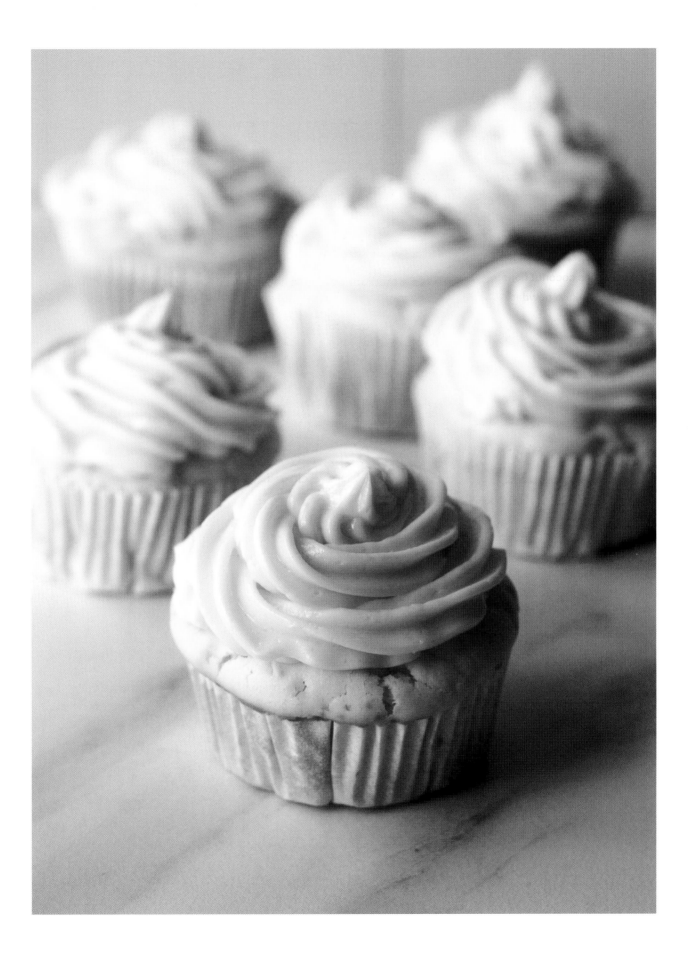

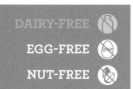

DAIRY-FREE

EGG-FREE

NUT-FREE

Ketogenic Girl
Macaroons

Prep Time: 20 minutes | **Cook Time: 20 minutes**
Yield: 20 cookies (1 per serving)

I love coconut in every form: unsweetened coconut chips, coconut oil, coconut milk, coconut cream, and coconut butter. All of it is perfect for a keto diet—dairy-free, high in saturated fat, and low in protein and carbohydrate. Coconut is such a versatile food for creating all kinds of heavenly desserts. I love using it to make macaroons!

This recipe has a higher percentage of carbs and is lower in fat due to the erythritol, which has 4 grams of carbohydrate per teaspoon. If you use powdered stevia instead of erythritol, it has nearly zero carbs, making it closer to 80 percent fat, 15 percent protein, and 5 percent carbohydrate.

These cookies are delicious on their own or with melted sugar-free chocolate drizzled on top. My Chocolate Hazelnut Spread (page 342) is great for dipping or drizzling on these!

6 egg whites

1 teaspoon vanilla extract

½ teaspoon baking soda

2 tablespoons erythritol

2 cups (7 ounces/195 g) unsweetened shredded coconut

½ cup (2 ounces/55 g) almond meal

1. Preheat the oven to 325°F (160°C). Line a baking sheet with parchment paper.

2. In the bowl of a stand mixer or in a metal mixing bowl with a hand mixer, whip the egg whites, vanilla, and baking soda until well blended, 4 to 5 minutes.

3. Slowly pour in the erythritol, 1 tablespoon at a time. Whip until stiff peaks form.

4. Remove the beaters and gently fold in the coconut and almond meal.

5. Drop the batter by rounded tablespoons onto the lined cookie sheet, spacing them ½ to 1 inch (1.25 to 2.5 cm) apart. (Macaroons don't rise or spread during baking, so you can put them close together.)

6. Bake for about 20 minutes, until golden brown. Turn off the oven, open the door slightly, and let the macaroons sit in the oven until cool; this keeps the moisture content down, helping the macaroons hold their shape and extending their shelf life.

7. Store in an airtight container at room temperature for up to a week.

MACRONUTRIENTS
(per cookie)

Fat	Protein	Carbs	Fiber	Energy
9.5g	2.6g	3.8g	3.8g	108 cal
78%	9%	13%		

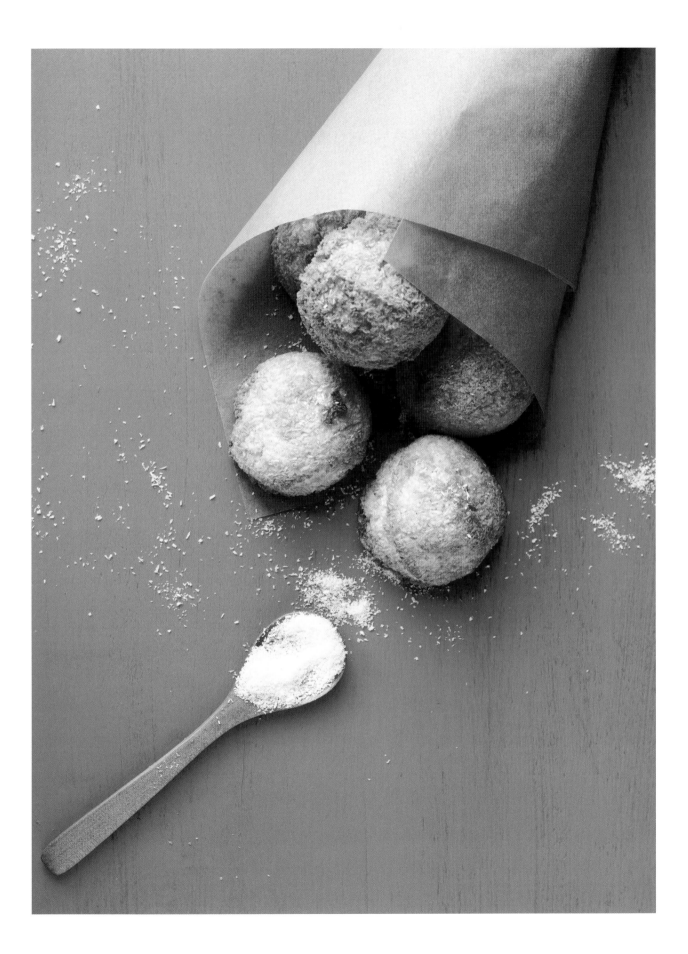

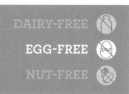

DAIRY-FREE
EGG-FREE
NUT-FREE

Easy Keto
Hot Fudge Sundaes

Prep Time: **10 minutes** | Cook Time: **5 minutes**
Yield: **4 servings**

This is one of my favorite go-to desserts: a fast-and-easy faux ice cream sundae made with sweetened whipped cream—no need to make ice cream! At close to 90 percent fat, it makes a great fat bomb as well.

1¼ cups (10 fluid ounces/300 ml) heavy whipping cream

¾ teaspoon liquid stevia, divided

3½ ounces (100 g) unsweetened baking chocolate (100% cacao)

1 tablespoon butter

Pinch of sea salt

¼ cup (2 ounces/55 g) raw walnuts, chopped

1. In a medium mixing bowl or the bowl of a stand mixer, combine the cream and up to ¼ teaspoon of the stevia, depending on how sweet you like your whipped cream. Whip until stiff peaks form, about 5 minutes.

2. In a heavy saucepan or double boiler over low heat, melt the chocolate, remaining ½ teaspoon of stevia, butter, and salt. When almost melted, remove from the heat and stir to blend.

3. Divide the sweetened whipped cream between 4 serving bowls or glasses. Top evenly with the melted chocolate and walnuts.

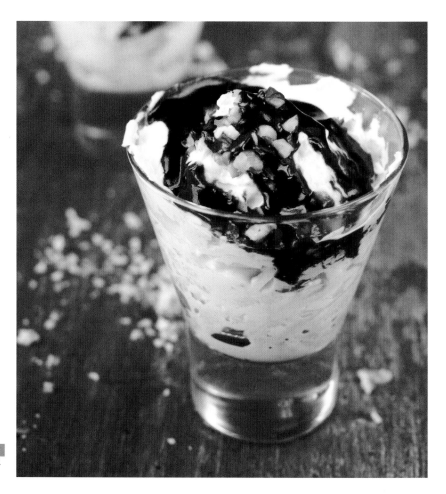

MACRONUTRIENTS
(per serving)

Fat	Protein	Carbs	Fiber	Energy
47.5g	4.8g	8g	4.8g	506 cal
89%	4%	7%		

Viennese Coffee

Prep Time: 15 minutes
Yield: 4 servings

This drink is wonderful in the morning with brunch, or for dessert after dinner with decaf espresso and a bit of sweetener. You can make this recipe using a stand mixer with a whipping attachment, a handheld mixer, or a whipped cream dispenser. (I found my whipped cream dispenser in a gourmet cooking shop.) One cup of heavy whipping cream will yield about 2 cups of whipped cream. The key is to stop whipping when it becomes whipped cream—just before it becomes butter!

1 cup (8 fluid ounces/240 ml) heavy whipping cream

2 or 3 drops liquid stevia, to taste

Hot espresso or brewed coffee (enough for 4 servings)

1. In a medium mixing bowl or the bowl of a stand mixer, combine the cream and stevia. Whip until stiff peaks form, about 5 minutes.

   Alternatively, use a whipped cream dispenser. Insert a cartridge into the dispenser and pour the cold cream and stevia mixture into the cylinder. Close, turn upside down, and shake.

2. Spoon or dispense about one-quarter of the whipped cream (about ½ cup/1 ounce/32 g) onto each serving of espresso or coffee.

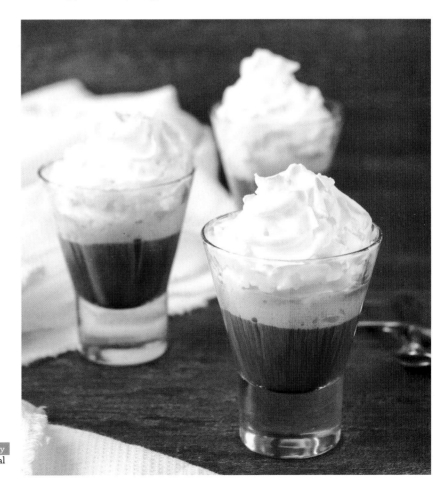

MACRONUTRIENTS (per serving)				
Fat	Protein	Carbs	Fiber	Energy
22g	1.3g	1g	0g	205 cal
96%	3%	1%		

Chapter 15
Sauces & Kitchen Staples

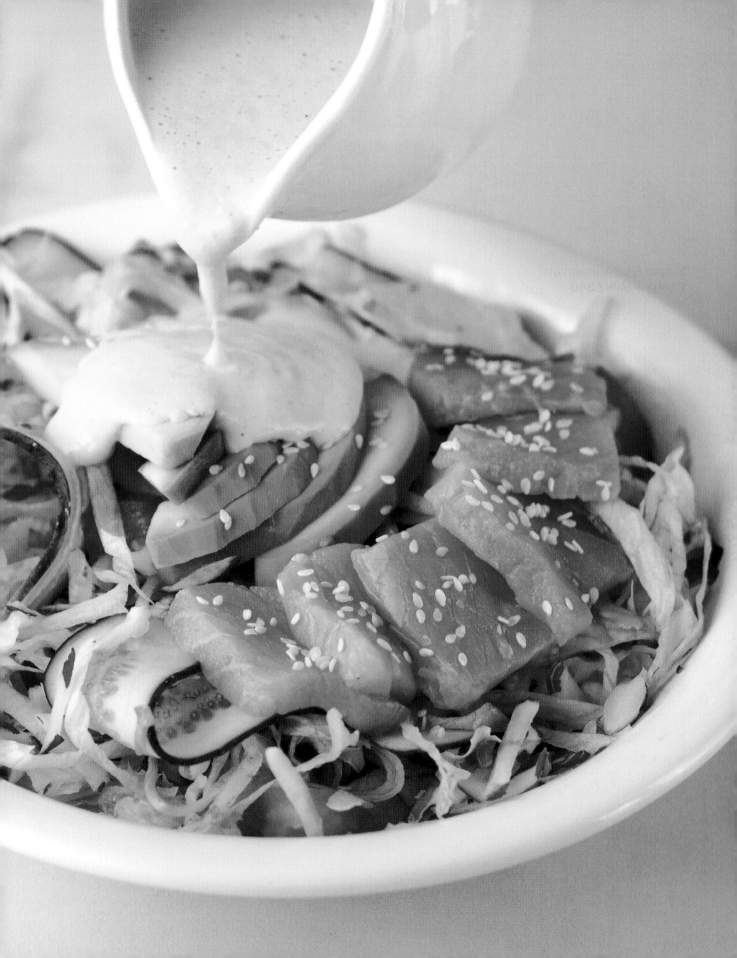

DAIRY-FREE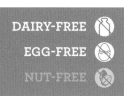

EGG-FREE

NUT-FREE

Sugar–Free
Almond or Cashew Milk

Prep Time: 10 minutes
Yield: 6 cups (48 fluid ounces/1.4 L) (1 cup/8 fluid ounces/240 ml per serving)

I love making my own almond or cashew milk. It is so easy and fun! I always used to soak the nuts overnight, but once I decided not to bother with that extra step. I discovered that other than needing to strain the milk a bit more because it doesn't blend as smoothly, the result is very similar. It's your choice whether you want to soak overnight or not.

½ cup (2½ ounces/70 g) skinless raw almonds or cashews

6 cups (48 fluid ounces/1.4 L) filtered water, plus 1 cup more if soaking nuts

½ teaspoon vanilla extract (optional; see note)

1 or 2 drops liquid stevia, to taste (optional)

Pinch of sea salt

1. If desired, soak the nuts in 1 cup (8 fluid ounces/240 ml) of water; refrigerate overnight.

2. Place the nuts in a blender (if using soaked nuts, drain them first). Add the 6 cups of water, vanilla (if using), stevia (if using), and salt and puree until smooth.

3. Strain through cheesecloth or a fine-mesh strainer. You can use the strained nuts to blend again and make more milk.

note

Do not add vanilla to the nut milk if you plan to use it in savory recipes.

MACRONUTRIENTS (using almonds)				
Fat	Protein	Carbs	Fiber	Energy
6g	2.5g	2.6g	1.5g	69 cal
72%	14%	14%		

MACRONUTRIENTS (using cashews)				
Fat	Protein	Carbs	Fiber	Energy
4g	1.7g	2.7g	0.3g	54 cal
67%	13%	20%		

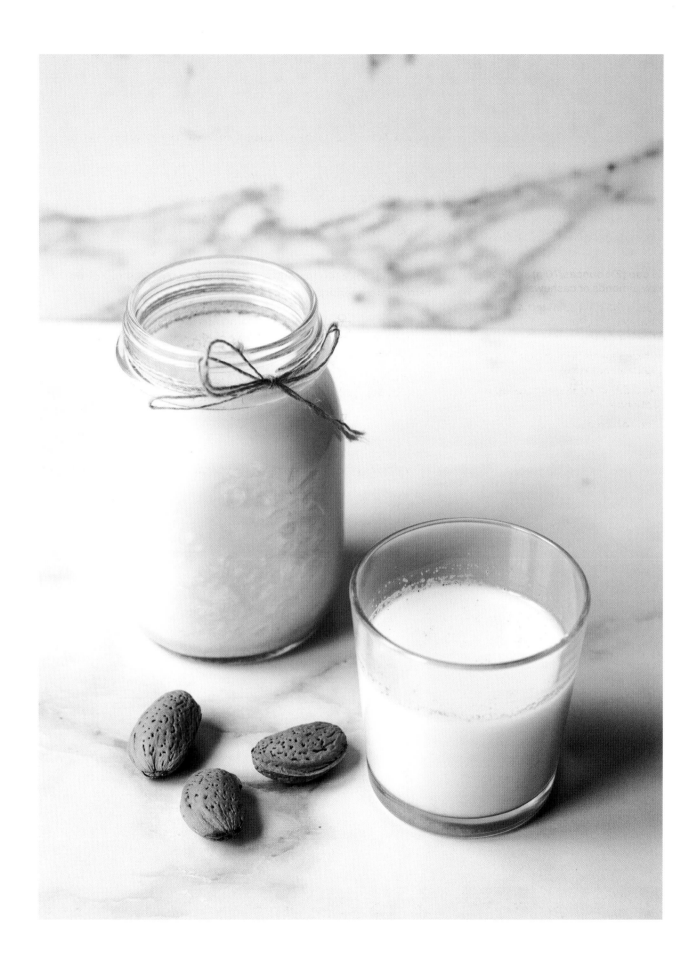

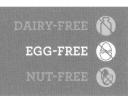

DAIRY-FREE

EGG-FREE

NUT-FREE

Ketogenic Girl
Chocolate Hazelnut Spread

Prep Time: 5 minutes | **Cook Time: 5 minutes**
Yield: 1½ cups (16½ ounces/470 g) (15 servings)

I grew up on Nutella; it was my favorite breakfast food. Putting it on buttered toast was ab-solute heaven. The funny thing is, I always thought of it as a healthy nut spread until a few years ago when I noticed that "sugar," and not "hazelnuts," comes first in the ingredient list. I was pretty shocked—sugar as the first ingredient! Followed by palm oil, and then hazelnuts in third. After going keto, I wanted to figure out how to make a healthy low-carb version of my favorite childhood treat. I love this spread on protein bread, alone as a snack, or heated up and drizzled on Ketogenic Girl Macaroons (page 334) or Vanilla Ice Cream (page 318). Hazelnut butter and flavoring add an incredible flavor, but the spread tastes just as great without those ingredients.

2 tablespoons unsalted butter or coconut oil

¼ cup (¾ ounce/20 g) unsweetened cocoa powder

2 tablespoons unsweetened hazelnut butter

¾ cup (6 fluid ounces/180 ml) heavy whipping cream

¼ cup (1 ounce/28 g) powdered stevia or erythritol

1 teaspoon hazelnut–flavored or plain liquid stevia

½ teaspoon hazelnut flavoring or almond extract

½ teaspoon vanilla extract

⅛ teaspoon fine sea salt

1. In a heavy saucepan over very low heat, melt the butter. Add the cocoa powder and stir with a whisk.

2. Add the hazelnut butter and whisk together, then pour in the cream while continuing to whisk. Add the sweeteners and stir to combine.

3. Increase the heat to medium-low and cook for 2 to 3 minutes, until the mixture develops a nice thick consistency.

4. Remove from the heat. Add the hazelnut flavoring and vanilla and stir well. Let cool, then transfer to a mason jar or bowl. Enjoy warm or let cool to room temperature. Store in the refrigerator for up to a week.

MACRONUTRIENTS
(per serving)

Fat	Protein	Carbs	Fiber	Energy
5.1g	0.6g	1.5g	1.5g	49 cal
84%	4.5%	11.5%		

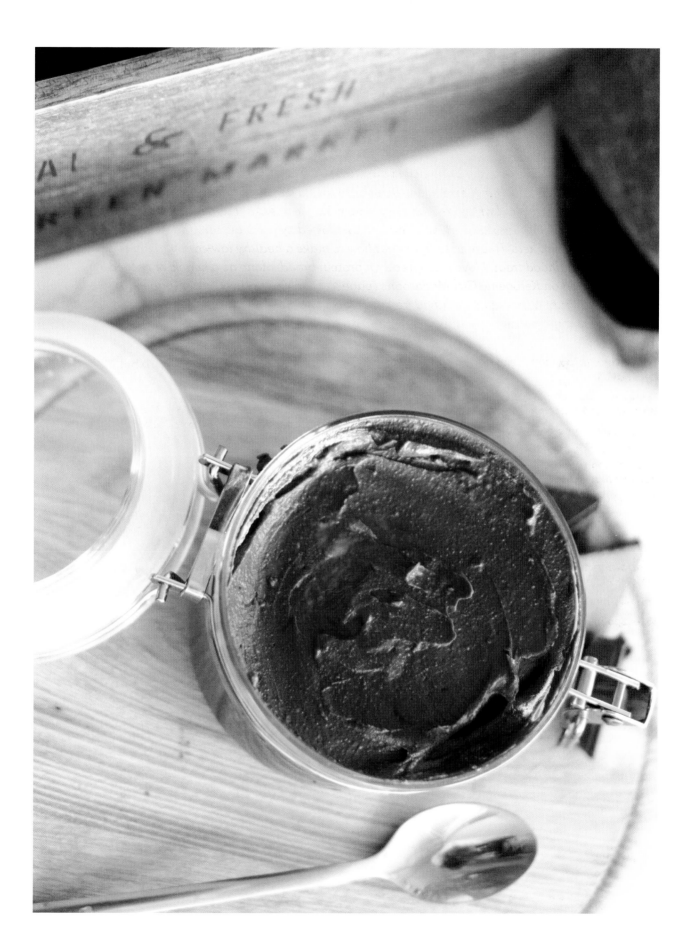

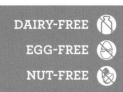

DAIRY-FREE

EGG-FREE

NUT-FREE

Creamed Coconut Butter

Prep Time: 15 minutes with a food processor or 7 minutes with a heavy-duty blender
Yield: about 1¼ cups (10 ounces/285 g) (1 tablespoon per serving)

Between coconut oil, coconut milk, coconut cream, and creamed coconut butter, what can the coconut NOT do? Unsweetened coconut butter costs only 2 to 3 dollars per jar to make, instead of 10 to 20 dollars per jar to buy at health food stores, and it is so easy to whip up. The trick to this recipe is patience, but one lick of a spoon of your own delicious creamed coconut and you'll understand that it's worth the time required. A spoonful or two makes a nice little fat bomb or treat!

4 cups plus 2 tablespoons (9 ounces/250 g) unsweetened coconut flakes

1. In a food processor or heavy-duty blender, process the coconut flakes, scraping down the sides periodically. A food processor will require 15 to 20 minutes of processing; a blender will require 7 to 10 minutes. If using a blender, rather than pouring in all the flakes at once, it is best to blend the flakes about 1 cup at a time, adding another cup of flakes once the previous portion is blended.

2. The coconut will initially turn into a thick paste, then eventually process into a smooth, liquid-like state.

3. Transfer to a mason jar or other container and store in the refrigerator for up to a week.

note

For a smoother, soft treat, warm for 20 to 30 seconds in a toaster oven or microwave before enjoying. I like to also warm up coconut butter and add a little bit of vanilla extract, stevia, and sea salt for an even more heavenly combo!

MACRONUTRIENTS
(per serving)

Fat	Protein	Carbs	Fiber	Energy
16.5g	1.6g	6.6g	3.3g	181 cal
82%	4%	15%		

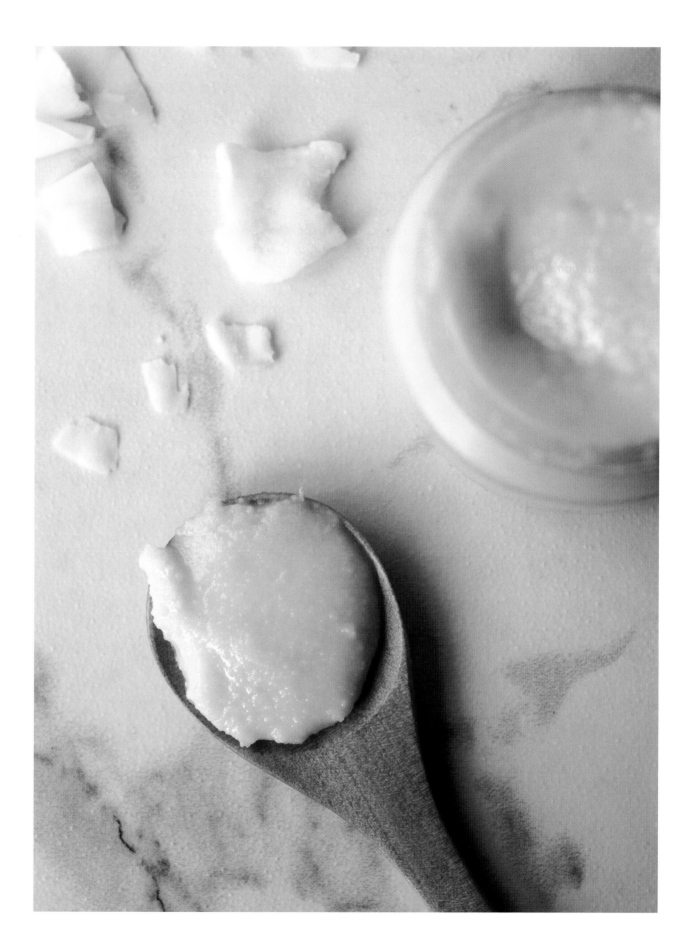

DAIRY-FREE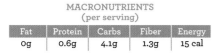
EGG-FREE
NUT-FREE

Sugar-Free
Cranberry Sauce

Prep Time: 15 minutes, plus 3 hours to set | **Cook Time:** 15 minutes
Yield: about 1¾ cups (18 ounces/510 g) (2⅓ tablespoons per serving)

I love to stay on track with my keto lifestyle over the holidays, and with all the available sweeteners to reduce the natural sourness of cranberries, it has never been easier! Can you believe that most cranberry sauce recipes are made with a whole cup of sugar? And the canned versions are basically corn syrup with some cranberries—pretty much the same as putting candy on your turkey.

Keto or not, a holiday dinner isn't the same to me without delicious thick gravy and the tangy sweetness of cranberry sauce. This sauce is so quick to make, and the Ceylon cinnamon is great for lowering blood sugar. (If Ceylon cinnamon isn't available, just use regular cinnamon.) Fruit is not typically keto, but berries are the most acceptable on keto, and of all the fruits and berries, cranberries are the lowest in sugar. If you're not a fan of stevia, use your favorite sweetener, such as erythritol and/or monk fruit. Everyone has varying degrees of sensitivity to sweeteners; if you know you are sensitive, taste the sauce as you sweeten it. Combining the erythritol and stevia makes the sauce extra sweet, which works well as cranberries are quite sour. This recipe is all carbohydrates so I have not provided the ratios, however you could also add coconut oil or butter to this recipe if you would like to.

1 (12-ounce/340-g) bag fresh
cranberries, rinsed and drained

1½ cups (12 fluid ounces/350 ml)
filtered water, divided

1 tablespoon unflavored gelatin

2 tablespoons erythritol

¼ teaspoon liquid stevia

Grated zest of 1 medium orange
(about 1 teaspoon)

½ teaspoon ground Ceylon
cinnamon or regular cinnamon

1. Place the cranberries and 1 cup (8 fluid ounces/240 ml) of the water in a medium saucepan; bring to a boil over high heat.

2. Meanwhile, pour the remaining ½ cup (4 fluid ounces/120 ml) of water into a small bowl; sprinkle the gelatin evenly over the water. (There's no need to mix the gelatin into the water.)

3. Once the cranberry mixture is boiling, reduce the heat to very low and simmer for about 10 minutes, stirring frequently. Add the erythritol and stevia to the cranberries. The berries will pop and the sauce will thicken gradually as the pectin from the berries is released. Remove from the heat.

4. Add the gelatin mixture to the cranberry mixture and blend well. Add the zest and cinnamon. Taste for sweetness and add more sweetener, if needed.

5. Pour the sauce into a mold or serving bowl. Refrigerate for 3 to 4 hours, until set. It will thicken as it cools.

note

I like my cranberry sauce nice and thick with crushed berries throughout, which is what this recipe makes. If you prefer a smooth consistency, after removing the cooked sauce from the heat in Step 3, pour into a food processor and process to cut up the berry chunks. Pour through a strainer for a perfectly smooth sauce.

MACRONUTRIENTS
(per serving)

Fat	Protein	Carbs	Fiber	Energy
0g	0.6g	4.1g	1.3g	15 cal

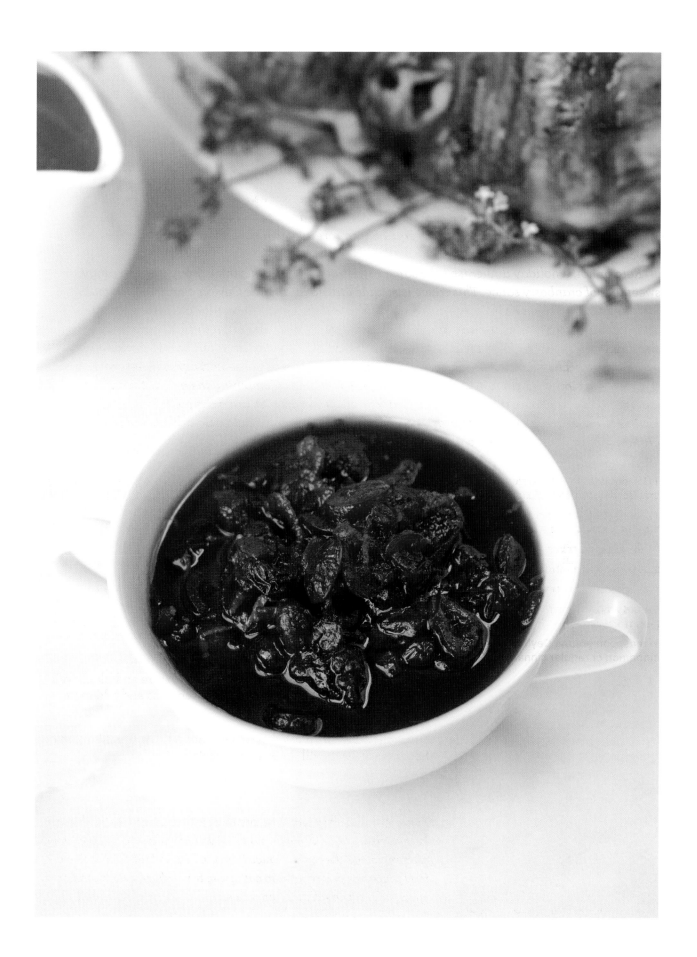

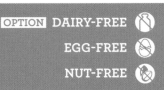

OPTION DAIRY-FREE

EGG-FREE

NUT-FREE

Holiday Gravy

Prep Time: **5 minutes, plus 15 minutes to reconstitute mushrooms**
Cook Time: **10 to 25 minutes** | Yield: **6 servings**

For me, gravy makes the meal at special occasion feasts; the celebration doesn't feel complete without it. This holiday gravy brings the turkey, stuffing, cranberry sauce, Brussels sprouts, and sides together, and it's the ultimate comfort sauce for all the holiday gatherings throughout the year!

½ cup (1¼ ounces/40 g) dried porcini mushrooms

1 cup (8 fluid ounces/240 ml) filtered water

½ cup (4 ounces/115 g) unsalted butter or butter–flavored coconut oil

1 clove garlic, minced

Pan drippings from turkey or beef roast (optional)

2 cups (16 fluid ounces/475 ml) turkey or chicken bone broth

1 tablespoon coconut flour

¼ cup (2 fluid ounces/60 ml) heavy whipping cream or coconut milk

1 teaspoon Dijon mustard

1 teaspoon fine sea salt

Pinch of black or white peppercorns

1 to 2 sprigs fresh thyme

1. In a small bowl, combine the mushrooms and water; let sit for 10 to 15 minutes to reconstitute. Drain and chop the mushrooms.

2. In a medium saucepan over low heat, melt the butter; simmer until lightly browned, swirling the pan to prevent burning. (If using butter-flavored coconut oil, simply melt the oil.)

3. Add the garlic and cook for 1 to 2 minutes. Add the pan drippings, if using, and mushrooms. Stir until well combined.

4. Whisk in the broth, then add the coconut flour. Whisk until well blended. Depending on how thick you like your gravy, simmer over low heat for 5 to 20 minutes. (I like to simmer mine for only 5 minutes.)

5. Remove from the heat and add the cream, mustard, salt, peppercorns, and thyme sprigs. Using an immersion blender, blend until the gravy is smooth; strain through a mesh strainer before serving.

MACRONUTRIENTS
(per serving)

Fat	Protein	Carbs	Fiber	Energy
27.5g	2.8g	1g	0.3g	263 cal
94%	4%	2%		

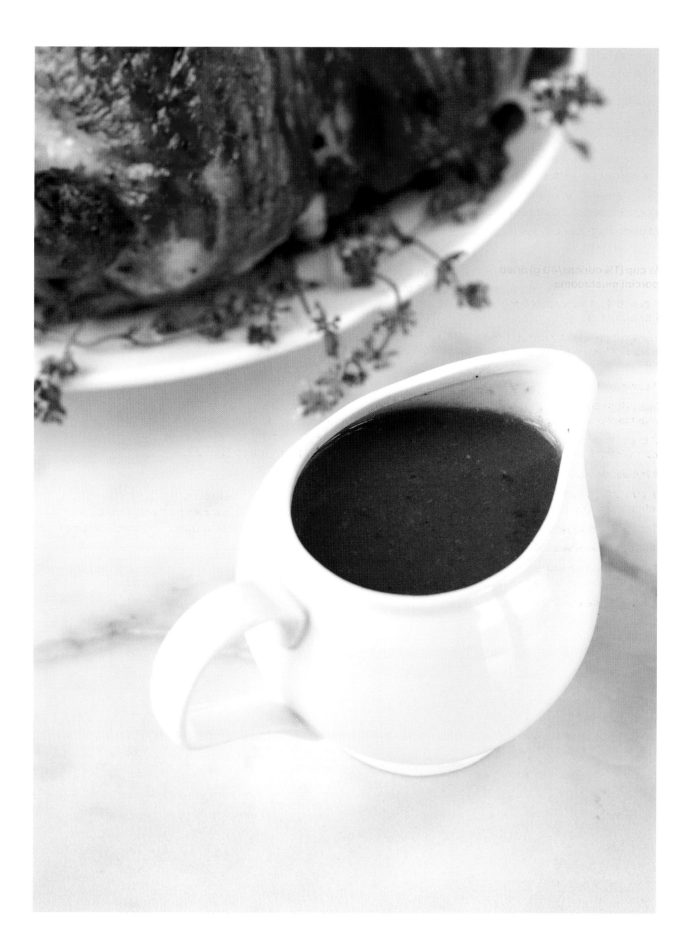

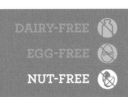

DAIRY-FREE

EGG-FREE

NUT-FREE

Béarnaise Sauce

Prep Time: 10 minutes | **Cook Time: 10 minutes**
Yield: about 1¼ cups (10 fluid ounces/300 ml) (3⅓ tablespoons per serving)

I adapted this keto-friendly version from Julia Child's original recipe. Béarnaise sauce is simply hollandaise taken a step further, so if you have any leftover hollandaise on hand, use it as a base to make béarnaise. Pour this sauce liberally over steak or other prepared meats for a decadent and satisfying dish! If it starts to separate, just whisk in a tablespoon of ice water to bring it back together.

¼ cup (2 fluid ounces/60 ml) white wine vinegar or apple cider vinegar

1 tablespoon minced shallots

1 tablespoon dried tarragon

6 egg yolks from pasteurized eggs

¾ cup (6 ounces/170 g) butter, melted, or room-temperature MCT oil

2 tablespoons freshly squeezed lemon juice

1 tablespoon Dijon mustard

½ teaspoon fine sea salt

¼ teaspoon ground black pepper

½ teaspoon chopped fresh dill

1. In a small saucepan, boil the vinegar, shallots, and tarragon until the liquid is reduced to about 2 tablespoons. Strain and set aside.

2. Place the egg yolks in a tall immersion blender container or a wide and tall mason jar. Add the melted butter, lemon juice, mustard, salt, and pepper.

3. Insert the immersion blender so that it is at the bottom of the container. Turn on the blender and don't move it for 15 to 30 seconds. Gradually start moving it up as the sauce becomes creamy and blended; the hot butter will cook the egg yolks as the sauce emulsifies. While continuing to blend, slowly pull the immersion blender up and out of the container.

4. Add the dill and blend to combine. Add the reduced vinegar mixture and blend once more.

5. Store in the refrigerator for up to 5 days. To reheat, pour the sauce into a bowl, set the bowl over a pan of simmering water, and whisk constantly until warmed through.

note

Always use pasteurized eggs when making béarnaise or any other recipe in which the eggs are not fully cooked.

MACRONUTRIENTS (per serving)				
Fat	Protein	Carbs	Fiber	Energy
26.5g	2.7g	0.8g	0g	257 cal
94%	5%	1%		

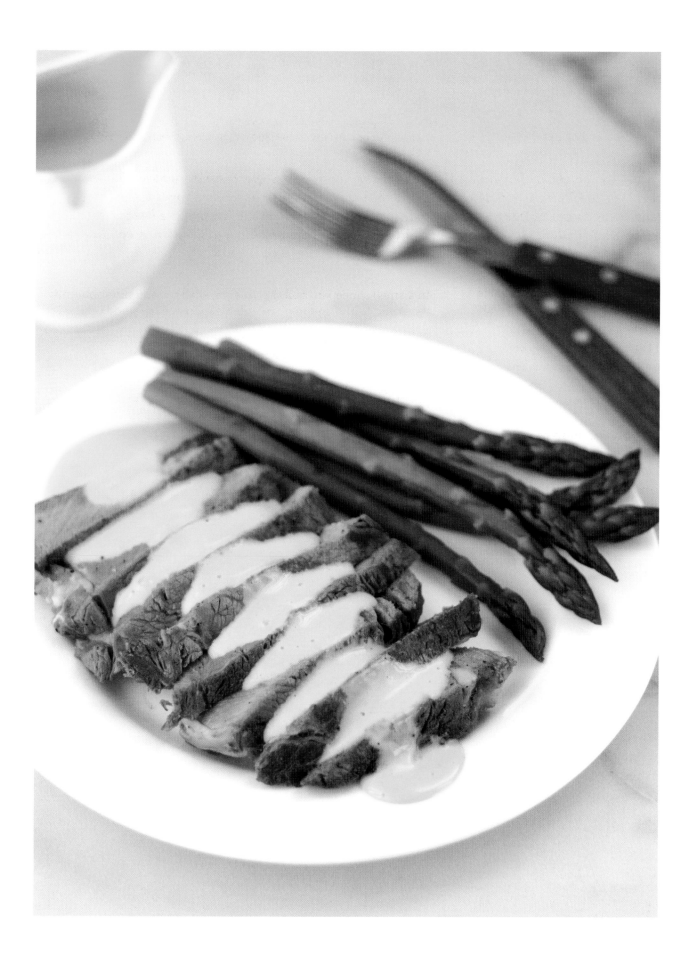

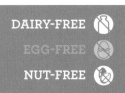

DAIRY-FREE

EGG-FREE

NUT-FREE

Aioli

Prep Time: 10 minutes, plus 30 minutes to chill
Yield: 1 scant cup (7½ ounces/210 g) (1 tablespoon per serving)

This is the easiest homemade aioli for dipping. It pairs really well with fried calamari (see page 258) and other dishes. You can choose which oil you use. For an omega-3 oil, use a combination of flaxseed or walnut oil and extra-light olive oil. For a flavor profile most closely resembling that of store-bought mayo, go for GMO-free canola oil. Avocado oil is a fantastically keto choice also.

3 cloves garlic

¾ cup (6 fluid ounces/180 ml) oil of choice (see note above)

1 egg yolk from a pasteurized egg

1 tablespoon freshly squeezed lemon juice

¾ teaspoon fine sea salt

½ teaspoon ground white or black pepper

1. Crush the garlic in a garlic press. Use a fork to mash the garlic into a paste.

2. Pour the oil into a tall immersion blender container or a wide and tall mason jar.

3. Add the egg yolk and let it settle to the bottom.

4. Add the garlic paste, lemon juice, salt, and pepper.

5. Insert the immersion blender so that it is at the bottom of the container. Turn on the blender and don't move it for 15 to 30 seconds. Gradually start moving it up as the sauce becomes creamy and blended; the hot butter will cook the egg yolks as the sauce emulsifies into aioli. While continuing to blend, slowly pull the immersion blender up and out of the container.

6. Transfer the aioli to an airtight container and refrigerate for at least 30 minutes before serving. Store in the refrigerator for up to 5 days.

note

Always use a pasteurized egg yolk for this recipe.

MACRONUTRIENTS
(per serving)

Fat	Protein	Carbs	Fiber	Energy
11g	0.3g	0.3g	0g	100 cal
98%	1%	1%		

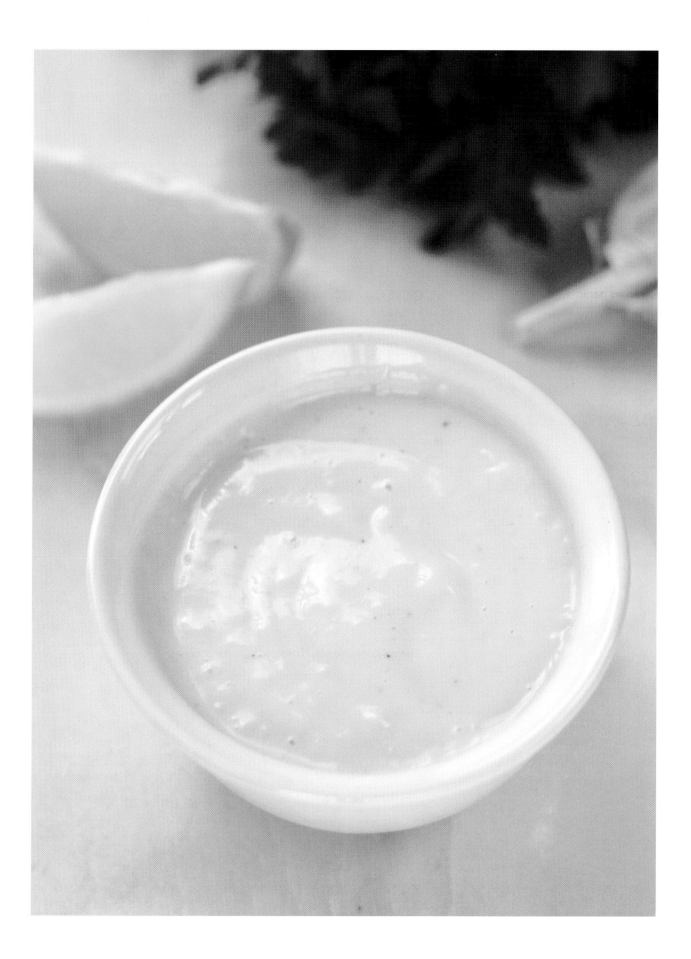

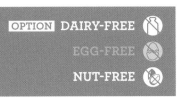

OPTION **DAIRY-FREE** 🚫

~~EGG-FREE~~ 🚫

NUT-FREE 🚫

Hollandaise

Prep Time: 5 minutes
Yield: about 1⅓ cups (10⅔ fluid ounces/315 ml) (about 3½ tablespoons per serving)

This delicious sauce has so many tasty applications, from rich eggs Benny breakfasts to decadent healthy fish dinners. It can be stored in the fridge for 4 to 6 days; if it starts to separate, just whisk in a tablespoon of ice water to bring it back together.

6 egg yolks from pasteurized eggs

¾ cup (6 ounces/170 g) butter, melted, or room-temperature MCT oil

1 tablespoon Dijon mustard

1 tablespoon freshly squeezed lemon juice

½ teaspoon fine sea salt

¼ teaspoon ground black pepper

½ teaspoon chopped fresh dill

notes

This is my super-easy immersion-blender version of basic hollandaise. To see the method in action, check out the video on my Ketogenic Girl YouTube channel. Always use pasteurized eggs for this recipe.

1. Place the egg yolks in a tall immersion blender container or a wide and tall mason jar. Add the melted butter, mustard, lemon juice, salt, and pepper.

2. Insert the immersion blender so that it is at the bottom of the container. Turn on the blender and don't move it for 15 to 30 seconds. Gradually start moving it up as the sauce becomes creamy and blended; the hot butter will cook the egg yolks as the sauce emulsifies into hollandaise. While continuing to blend, slowly pull the immersion blender up and out of the container. Add the dill and blend to combine.

3. Store in the refrigerator for up to 5 days. To reheat, pour the sauce into a bowl, set the bowl over a pan of simmering water, and whisk constantly until warmed through.

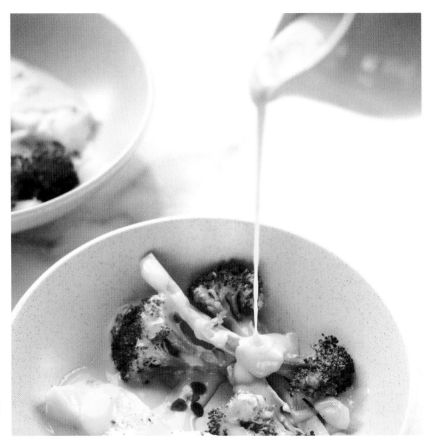

	MACRONUTRIENTS			
	(per serving)			
Fat	Protein	Carbs	Fiber	Energy
26.5g	2.7g	0.8g	0g	257 cal
94%	5%	1%		

Homemade
Mayonnaise

Prep Time: 5 minutes
Yield: 1¼ cups (10 ounces/285 g) (1 tablespoon per serving)

DAIRY-FREE

EGG-FREE

NUT-FREE

This is the easiest homemade mayonnaise, and you can make it any time. You get to choose which oil to use, as you do with Aioli (page 352). You may add more flavors to the mayo and customize it to your taste; some options are your favorite herbs, hot sauce, or spices.

1 cup (8 fluid ounces/240 ml) oil of choice (see note above)

1 pasteurized egg

1 teaspoon freshly squeezed lemon juice

1 teaspoon Dijon mustard

½ teaspoon fine sea salt

¼ teaspoon ground white or black pepper

note

Always use a pasteurized egg for this recipe.

1. Pour the oil into a tall immersion blender container or a wide and tall mason jar.

2. Add the egg yolk and let it settle to the bottom.

3. Add the lemon juice, mustard, salt, and pepper.

4. Insert the immersion blender so that it is at the bottom of the container. Turn on the blender and don't move it for 30 to 45 seconds. Gradually start moving the blender around, until the mixture becomes creamy. While continuing to blend, slowly pull the immersion blender up and out of the container.

5. Use immediately or transfer to an airtight container and store in the refrigerator for up to 5 days.

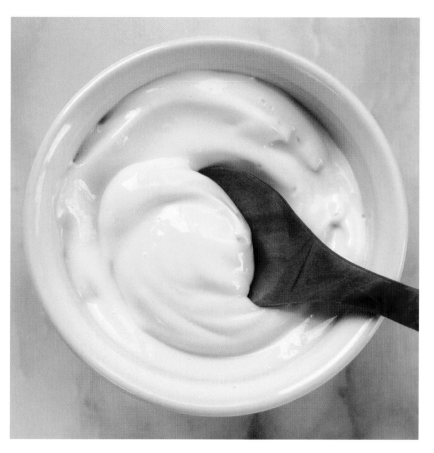

MACRONUTRIENTS (per serving)				
Fat	Protein	Carbs	Fiber	Energy
11.5g	0.3g	0g	0g	108 cal
99%	1%	0%		

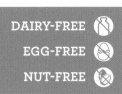

DAIRY-FREE

EGG-FREE

NUT-FREE

Homemade
Worcestershire Sauce

Prep Time: **5 minutes** | Cook Time: **3 minutes**
Yield: **about ⅔ cup (5⅓ fluid ounces/160 ml) (1 tablespoon per serving)**

I love making sauces at home with no hidden sugars or preservatives. This flavor-packed sauce is used in several recipes throughout this book, and it will give a boost to many of your favorite foods.

¼ cup (2 fluid ounces/60 ml) apple cider vinegar

¼ cup (2 fluid ounces/60 ml) tamari

2 tablespoons filtered water

½ teaspoon Dijon mustard

¼ teaspoon ground Ceylon cinnamon or regular cinnamon

¼ teaspoon ginger powder

¼ teaspoon ground nutmeg

¼ teaspoon garlic powder

¼ teaspoon onion powder

⅛ teaspoon ground black pepper

1 teaspoon erythritol

2 to 4 drops liquid stevia, to taste

Place all the ingredients in a saucepan and bring to a boil over medium heat. Boil for about 1 minute, then remove from the heat and let cool. Store in a glass jar in the refrigerator for up to 6 days.

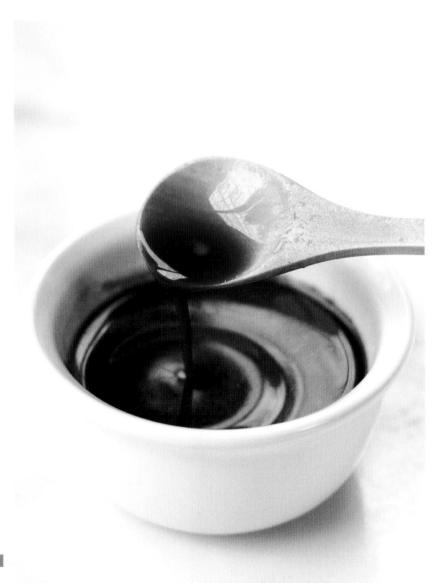

MACRONUTRIENTS
(per serving)

Fat	Protein	Carbs	Fiber	Energy
0g	.8g	.4g	.1g	6.3 cal
0%	67%	33%		

Blue Cheese Dressing

DAIRY-FREE
EGG-FREE
NUT-FREE

Prep Time: 5 minutes
Yield: 1¼ cups (10 fluid ounces/300 ml) (1 tablespoon per serving)

This creamy, steakhouse-inspired dressing is ideal for the Bacon Wedge Salad (page 164), Cobb Salad (page 165), or Hot Wings (page 246).

1 cup (8 ounces/225 g) mayonnaise

½ cup (2 ounces/55 g) crumbled blue cheese

½ cup (4 fluid ounces/120 ml) heavy whipping cream

1 teaspoon freshly squeezed lemon juice

½ teaspoon Homemade Worcestershire Sauce (opposite)

½ teaspoon garlic powder

¼ teaspoon paprika

Place all the ingredients in a bowl and whisk to combine. Use immediately or store in the refrigerator for up to 3 days.

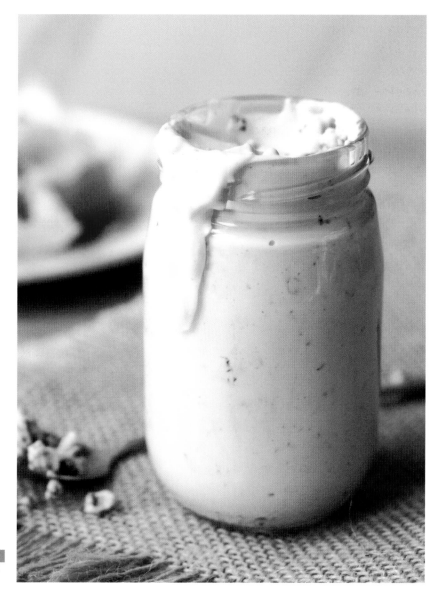

MACRONUTRIENTS (per serving)				
Fat	Protein	Carbs	Fiber	Energy
11.9g	1.3g	0.3g	0g	114 cal
94%	5%	1%		

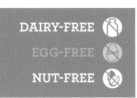

DAIRY-FREE

EGG-FREE

NUT-FREE

Ketogenic Girl
"Honey"-Mustard Dressing

Prep Time: 5 minutes
Yield: ¾ cup (6 fluid ounces/180 ml) (1½ tablespoons per serving)

This take on classic honey-mustard dressing contains mustard but no honey. I promise you won't miss it in this versatile dressing!

¼ cup (2 ounces/55 g) mayonnaise

2 tablespoons prepared yellow mustard

¼ teaspoon onion powder

1 to 3 drops liquid stevia, to taste

Place all the ingredients in a bowl and whisk to combine. Use immediately or store in the refrigerator for up to 4 days.

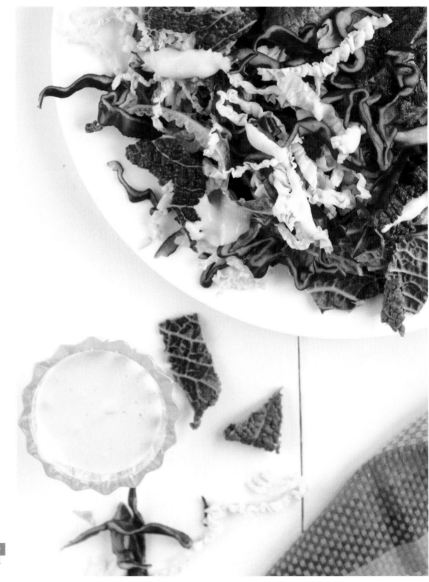

MACRONUTRIENTS
(per serving)

Fat	Protein	Carbs	Fiber	Energy
20g	4g	7g	4.5g	216 cal
82%	5%	13%		

Ranch Dressing

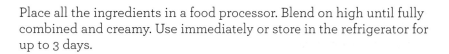

DAIRY-FREE

EGG-FREE

NUT-FREE

Prep Time: 10 minutes
Yield: just over 1½ cups (12 fluid ounces/350 ml) (1⅔ tablespoons per serving)

This dressing is great for a Cobb Salad (page 165) or as a substitute for the vinaigrette in the Niçoise Salad (page 176). The store-bought versions of ranch dressing are full of carbs and sugars; this one has zero carbs.

1 cup (8 ounces/225 g) mayonnaise

½ cup (4 ounces/115 g) sour cream

1 teaspoon minced fresh chives

1 teaspoon finely chopped fresh parsley

1 teaspoon finely chopped fresh dill

½ teaspoon paprika

½ teaspoon fine sea salt

¼ teaspoon ground black pepper

¼ teaspoon garlic powder

¼ teaspoon onion powder

Place all the ingredients in a food processor. Blend on high until fully combined and creamy. Use immediately or store in the refrigerator for up to 3 days.

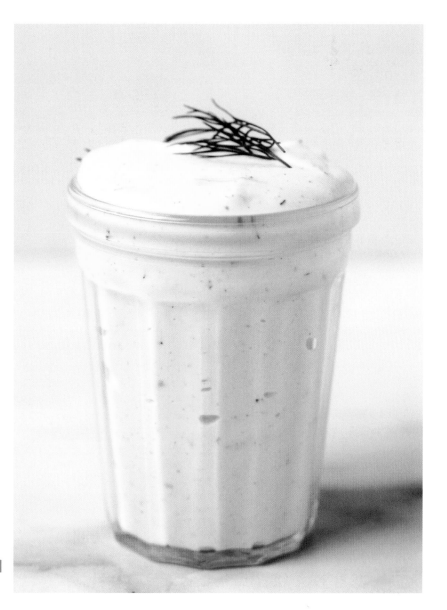

MACRONUTRIENTS
(per serving)

Fat	Protein	Carbs	Fiber	Energy
13.7g	0.3 g	0.2g	0g	126 cal
98%	1%	1%		

DAIRY-FREE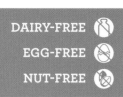
EGG-FREE
NUT-FREE

Creamy
Poppy Seed Dressing

Prep Time: 5 minutes
Yield: 1 cup (8 fluid ounces/240 ml) (¼ cup/2 fluid ounces/60 ml per serving)

I use stevia in this luscious recipe, but you may use any keto-friendly sweetener, such as erythritol or monk fruit, or combine them with the stevia. Start with just a couple of drops of liquid stevia and adjust to your desired sweetness.

⅔ cup (5⅓ fluid ounces/160 ml) MCT oil

¼ cup (2 fluid ounces/60 ml) apple cider vinegar

1 tablespoon Dijon mustard

1 teaspoon freshly squeezed lemon juice

1 teaspoon onion powder

½ teaspoon fine sea salt

¼ teaspoon garlic powder

¼ teaspoon liquid stevia

2 tablespoons poppy seeds

1. Place all the ingredients, except the poppy seeds, in a food processor. Pulse until well combined. Stir in the poppy seeds.

2. Store in an airtight container in the refrigerator for up to a week.

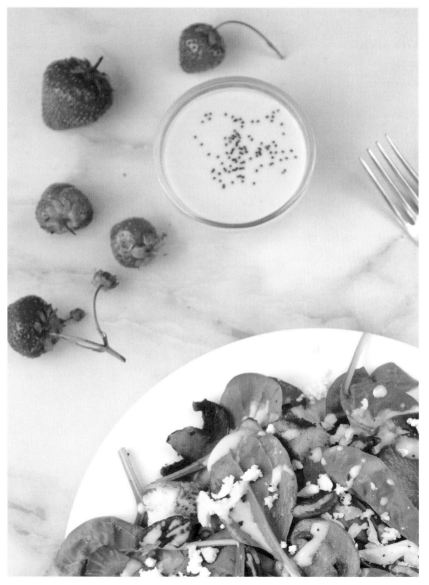

MACRONUTRIENTS
(per serving)

Fat	Protein	Carbs	Fiber	Energy
41.5g	0.8g	2g	0.8g	388 cal
97%	1%	2%		

Restaurant-Style Keto
Japanese Ginger Dressing

Prep Time: 10 minutes
Yield: ¾ cup (6 fluid ounces/180 ml) (6 tablespoons/3 fluid ounces/90 ml per person)

You'll find a ton of uses for this Japanese restaurant-inspired dressing. It's amazing on proteins, greens, or seaweed, but sometimes I'm tempted to just eat it with a spoon!

¼ cup (2 fluid ounces/60 ml) MCT oil

2 tablespoons mayonnaise

2 tablespoons peanut oil

2 tablespoons apple cider vinegar

2 tablespoons tamari

2 tablespoons minced celery

1 to 2 tablespoons sugar-free ketchup

1 tablespoon ginger juice, or 1 (1-inch/2.5-cm) piece fresh ginger, peeled and minced

1 tablespoon filtered water

1 teaspoon freshly squeezed lemon juice

1 tablespoon powdered stevia or erythritol

¼ to ½ teaspoon liquid stevia, to taste

¼ teaspoon garlic powder

¼ teaspoon onion powder

¼ teaspoon fine sea salt

Ground black pepper, to taste

1. Place all the ingredients in a food processor or blender. Blend on high until almost liquefied.

2. Chill in the refrigerator for 5 minutes before serving. Store in an airtight container in the fridge for up to 3 days.

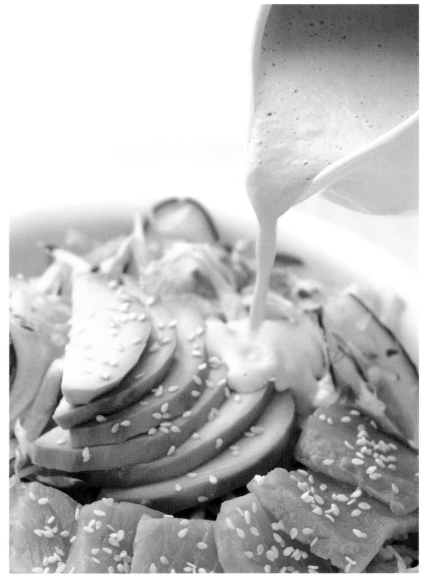

MACRONUTRIENTS
(per serving)

Fat	Protein	Carbs	Fiber	Energy
56g	2.5g	2.5g	0g	535 cal
96%	2%	2%		

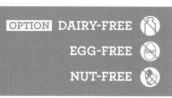

OPTION DAIRY-FREE

EGG-FREE

NUT-FREE

Sweet Balsamic Glaze

Prep Time: **5 minutes**
Yield: **10 tablespoons (5 fluid ounces/150 ml) (1 tablespoon per serving)**

This rich and flavor-packed glaze is perfect for drizzling over many dishes. If you prefer to eliminate all sugar from this recipe, you can use apple cider vinegar or another vinegar of your choice, such as sherry or white or red wine vinegar, in place of the balsamic.

½ cup (4 fluid ounces/120 ml) balsamic vinegar

½ teaspoon guar gum or xanthan gum

½ teaspoon liquid stevia and/or 1 tablespoon granulated stevia

¼ cup (2 ounces/55 g) coconut oil or butter, melted (optional)

1. Place the vinegar, guar gum, stevia, and coconut oil, if using, in a tall immersion blender container or a wide and tall mason jar.

2. Using an immersion blender, blend the ingredients together until they form a thick syrup or cream. To thicken the glaze, add more guar gum. To thin it, add more vinegar. Use immediately or store in the refrigerator for up to 3 days.

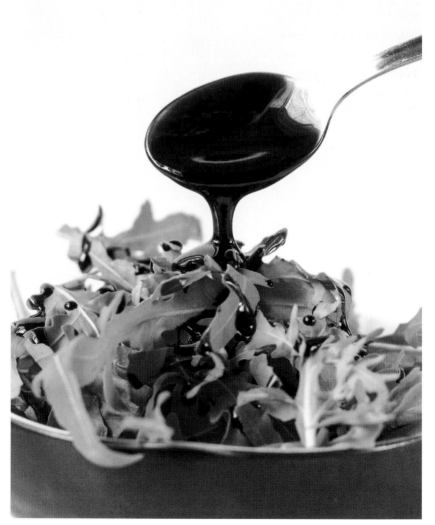

MACRONUTRIENTS
(per serving)

Fat	Protein	Carbs	Fiber	Energy
11.2g	0.3g	4.8g	0g	121 cal
83%	1%	16%		

Special Burger Sauce

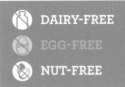

DAIRY-FREE

EGG-FREE

NUT-FREE

Prep Time: 8 minutes
Yield: about ⅓ cup (2⅔ fluid ounces/75 g) (2½ tablespoons per serving)

This is hands-down my most popular recipe. You'll never eat a burger again without a generous coating of this savory sauce!

¼ cup (2 ounces/55 g) mayonnaise

1 teaspoon medium–hot hot sauce or sugar–free ketchup

1 teaspoon prepared yellow mustard

1 teaspoon apple cider vinegar

2 fermented sugar–free pickles, finely chopped

1 tablespoon finely chopped onions

½ teaspoon fine sea salt

½ teaspoon onion powder

¼ teaspoon garlic powder

¼ teaspoon paprika

3 or 4 drops liquid stevia, to taste (omit if using ketchup)

In a bowl, combine all the ingredients, mixing well. Use immediately or store in the refrigerator for up to 4 days.

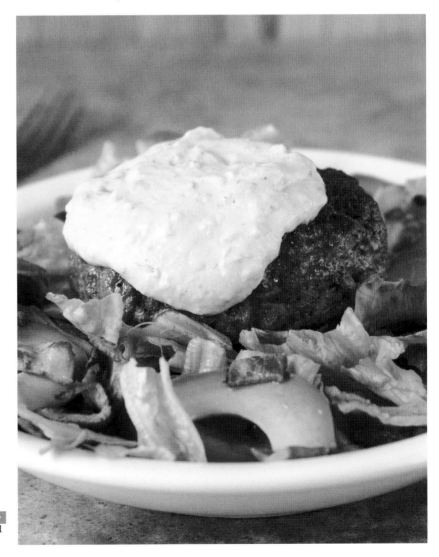

MACRONUTRIENTS
(per serving)

Fat	Protein	Carbs	Fiber	Energy
22g	0g	2g	0g	208 cal
96%	0%	4%		

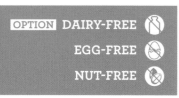

Sugar-Free Glaze

Prep Time: 5 minutes
Yield: ½ cup (1 tablespoon per serving)

Unlike the Sweet Balsamic Glaze (page 362), which contains concentrated grape must, this glaze is completely keto and 100 percent sugar-free.

3 ounces (85 g) unsalted butter or coconut oil

2 tablespoons powdered stevia

½ teaspoon baking powder

½ teaspoon liquid stevia

½ teaspoon vanilla extract (optional)

Pinch of sea salt

1. In a saucepan over medium heat, bring the butter to a boil, watching it closely to ensure that it doesn't burn. When it reaches a boil, remove from the heat and quickly whisk in the powdered stevia, baking powder, liquid stevia, vanilla (if using), and salt.

2. Use immediately or store in the refrigerator for up to 3 days.

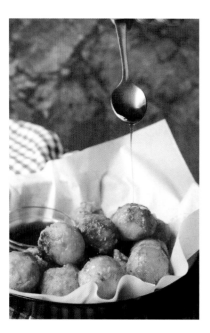

MACRONUTRIENTS
(per serving)

Fat	Protein	Carbs	Fiber	Energy
11.2g	0g	0.2g	0.2g	100 cal
99%	0%	1%		

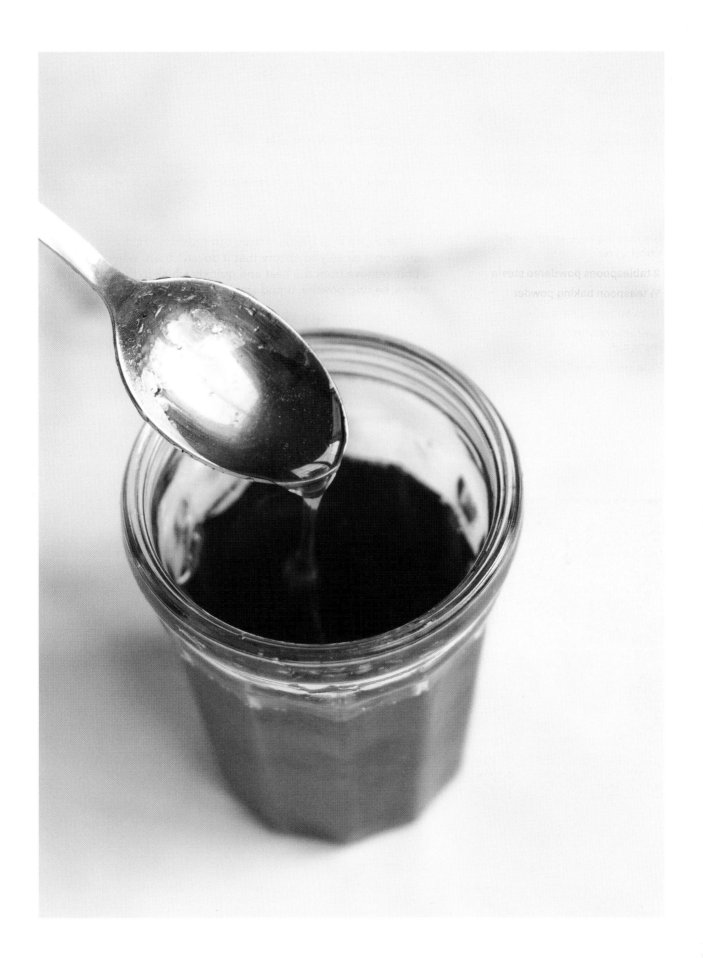

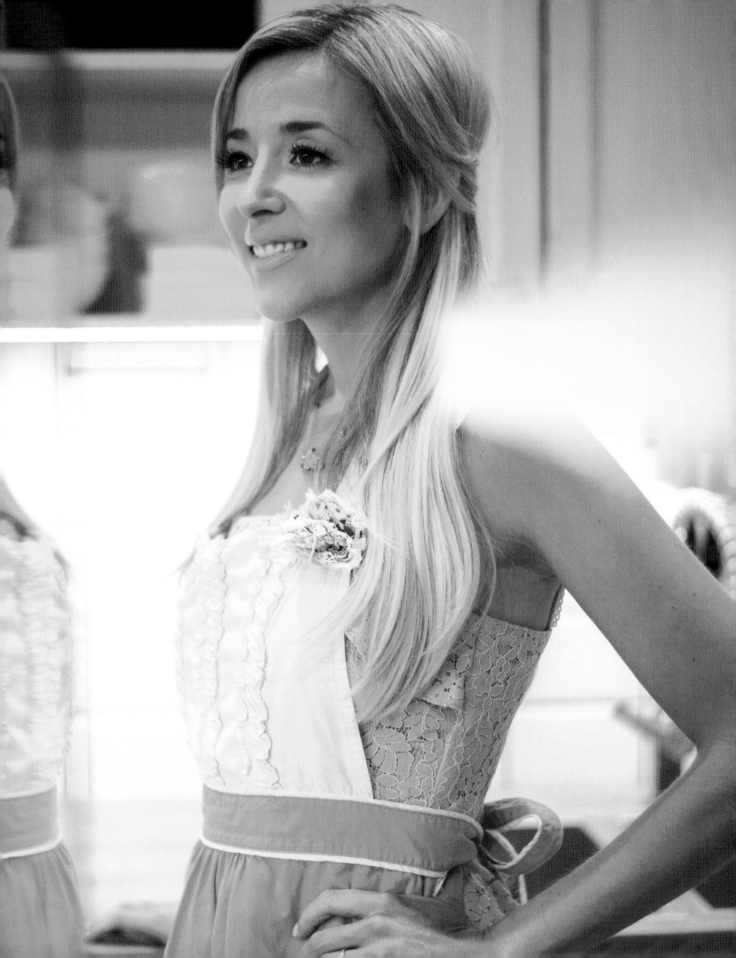

Chapter 16

7-Day Meal Plans for Healing and Weight Loss

When your body is in nutritional ketosis, it is burning fat for fuel. This state is called *ketosis* because it causes the body to produce what are known as *ketone bodies*. My 7-Day Meal Plans are designed to help you get all the benefits from being in ketosis with ease, while teaching you how to do keto long-term.

My meal plans use recipes from this book to get you started without needing to track macronutrients on your own. These plans are designed to heal your body and restore homeostasis by emphasizing whole foods and providing you with the nourishment your body needs. I recommend following the plan as written and then testing your blood sugar and ketones to determine whether you are in nutritional ketosis (see page 66). Because these plans are based on my proven macronutrient distributions, they will get the majority of people into ketosis. However, if you are not getting the results you want, you might need to tweak the program by increasing or reducing portion sizes and testing your blood sugar and ketones while you do so.

We all have different taste preferences, as well as different thresholds for carbohydrates and protein. For example, some very active men with a high ratio of lean body mass to body fat (less than 10 percent body fat) can consume anywhere from 50 to 100 grams of carbohydrates and up to 200 grams of protein a day and still get into nutritional ketosis. However, I more commonly see people whose health is not where they want it to be and who have followed "healthy" high-carb and low-fat diets for years. As a result, they have impaired insulin sensitivity or even insulin resistance that is caused by a bombardment of excessive carbs, leading to perpetually circulating insulin—even during sleep because they often snack all day and stay up late. This gradual building of insulin resistance leads to carb sensitivity, which means that their bodies are triggered by the slightest amount of carbohydrates for hours afterward. This sensitivity knocks the body out of fat-burning mode and back into glucose-burning mode. My meal plans are designed with these more insulin-resistant people in mind.

Many people fail to get into nutritional ketosis because they use the "net carbs" approach and subtract grams of fiber from grams of carbohydrate. This leads many people to eat 40 to 50 grams of total carbohydrates per day and subtract the fiber to get a net carb total of around 20 grams. For this reason, I focus on total carbs instead of net carbs. See page 65 for more on the net carbs approach.

The meals laid out in these plans are designed to be eaten to satiety, with no snacking between meals. The intermittent fasting that occurs between meals and outside of the eating window (that is, during the longer period of fasting between dinner and breakfast) facilitates fat burning in the absence of circulating insulin. This is why it is so important not to graze or snack between meals and instead eat to fullness at each meal.

Grazing

While humans and cows are both mammals, we differ greatly in terms of how we digest food. Cows are herbivores and eat a lot of carbs—grass. With four stomachs, they are designed to graze for most of the day and are in a constant consumption-and-digestion mode. Humans have only one stomach and are not designed to graze, especially not on grass or other high-carb foods. You need only look at the current state of health in Western societies to see why a culture of grazing has made us none the healthier.

The Meal Plans

On the following pages I have a meal plan for maintenance and meal plans for healing and fat loss. The more advanced fat-burning plans utilize three meals instead of four, and you have a choice between a savory third meal and a sweet one. Note that most of the recipe in these plans make more than one serving, so if you're using these meal plans just for yourself, you should plan for leftovers or make less than a full batch of some recipes. Better yet, encourage your family and friends to join you on your keto journey by sharing these delicious meals.

These plans should serve as a guide to beginning a ketogenic way of life!

Basic Meal Plan for Maintenance

	DAY 1	DAY 2	DAY 3	DAY 4	DAY 5	DAY 6	DAY 7
Meal 1	Breakfast Crêpes P122	Avocado Bacon Deviled Eggs P118	Eggs Benedict Royale P130	Breakfast Muffins P123	Instant Chia Pudding P321	Eggs, Bacon, and Roasted Rosemary Radishes P127	Eggs with Sausage Stuffing P126
Macros & Energy Value	fat: 23.3g protein: 11.3g carbs: 3.7g cal: 227	fat: 53g protein: 28g carbs: 4g cal: 610	fat: 56.5g protein: 37.5g carbs: 2g cal: 677	fat: 34.5g protein: 25g carbs: 3.5g cal: 432	fat: 27.7g protein: 4.5g carbs: 6g cal: 291	fat: 59g protein: 18.5g carbs: 5.5g cal: 496	fat: 61g protein: 25g carbs: 9g cal: 684
Meal 2	Deconstructed Bacon Burger Salad P174	Fully Loaded Gourmet Hot Dogs P305	White Truffle Fettuccine Alfredo P206	Green Thai Pork Curry P300	Bacon Wedge Salad P164	Keto Bacon "Potato" Salad P225	Cobb Salad P165
Macros & Energy Value	fat: 66g protein: 37g carbs: 8g cal: 724	fat: 35.8g protein: 12.5g carbs: 3.8g cal: 390	fat: 52.5g protein: 15g carbs: 6g cal: 550	fat: 45.5g protein: 38g carbs: 10g cal: 608	fat: 59g protein: 21.5g carbs: 5g cal: 639	fat: 39g protein: 18g carbs: 4.6g cal: 445	fat: 67g protein: 46.5g carbs: 8.5g cal: 831
Meal 3	Keto Shepherd's Pie P274	Teriyaki Chicken P250	Steak on "Honey"-Mustard Slaw P281	Spicy Shrimp Cocktail P256	Lemon Chicken P240	Ginger Beef P294	Shrimp Hollandaise Avocado Stacks P257
Macros & Energy Value	fat: 47g protein: 27.5g carbs: 12.5g cal: 577	fat: 60g protein: 40.5g carbs: 11.5g cal: 721	fat: 60.5g protein: 24g carbs: 10.5g cal: 631	fat: 44g protein: 9g carbs: 3.3g cal: 450	fat: 49.8g protein: 38.8g carbs: 11.7g cal: 631	fat: 33.5g protein: 23.5g carbs: 7.5g cal: 435	fat: 31.5g protein: 13.5g carbs: 4.5g cal: 345
Optional Sweet Snack	Cheesecake Fat Bomb P320	Cinnamon Custard P323	Chocolate Mint Mousse P322	Cinnamon Muffins P160	Crème Brûlée P316	Easy Keto Hot Fudge Sundaes P336	Instant Chia Pudding P321
Macros & Energy Value	fat: 30.8g protein: 4g carbs: 2g cal: 319	fat: 24g protein: 6.5g carbs: 4g cal: 259	fat: 20g protein: 4g carbs: 7g cal: 216	fat: 34.3g protein: 11g carbs: 9.3g cal: 386	fat: 23.8g protein: 5g carbs: 10.1g cal: 252	fat: 47.5g protein: 4.8g carbs: 8g cal: 506	fat: 27.7g protein: 4.5g carbs: 6g cal: 306
Daily Totals	fat: 167.1g protein: 79.8g carbs: 26.2g cal: 1,847	fat: 172.8g protein: 87.8g carbs: 23.3g cal: 1,980	fat: 189.5g protein: 80.5g carbs: 25.5g cal: 2,074	fat: 158.3g protein: 83g carbs: 26.1g cal: 1,876	fat: 160.3g protein: 69.8g carbs: 32.8g cal: 1,813	fat: 179g protein: 64.8g carbs: 25.6g cal: 1,882	fat: 187.2g protein: 89.5g carbs: 28g cal: 2,166

Meal Plan for Healing and Fat Loss with a Savory Option

	DAY 1	DAY 2	DAY 3	DAY 4	DAY 5	DAY 6	DAY 7
Meal 1	Breakfast Crêpes P122	Avocado Bacon Deviled Eggs P118	Eggs Benedict Royale P130	Breakfast Muffins P123	Instant Chia Pudding P321	Savory Brie, Spinach, and Mushroom Crêpes P124	Eggs with Sausage Stuffing P126
Macros & Energy Value	fat: 23.3g protein: 11.3g carbs: 3.7g cal: 277	fat: 53g protein: 28g carbs: 4g cal: 610	fat: 56.5g protein: 37.5g carbs: 2g cal: 677	fat: 34.5g protein: 25g carbs: 3.5g cal: 432	fat: 27.7g protein: 4.5g carbs: 6g cal: 291	fat: 65.5g protein: 28g carbs: 11g cal: 729	fat: 61g protein: 25g carbs: 9g cal: 684
Meal 2	Deconstructed Bacon Burger Salad P174	Fully Loaded Gourmet Hot Dogs P305	White Truffle Fettuccine Alfredo P206	Green Thai Pork Curry P300	Bacon Wedge Salad P164	Keto Bacon "Potato" Salad P225	Cobb Salad P165
Macros & Energy Value	fat: 66g protein: 37g carbs: 8g cal: 724	fat: 35.8g protein: 12.5g carbs: 3.8g cal: 390	fat: 52.5g protein: 15g carbs: 6g cal: 550	fat: 45.5g protein: 38g carbs: 10g cal: 608	fat: 59g protein: 21.5g carbs: 5g cal: 639	fat: 39g protein: 18g carbs: 4.6g cal: 445	fat: 67g protein: 46.5g carbs: 8.5g cal: 831
Meal 3 (Savory Option)	Keto Shepherd's Pie P274	Teriyaki Chicken P250	Steak on "Honey" Mustard Slaw P281	Spicy Shrimp Cocktail P256	Lemon Chicken P240	Ginger Beef P294	Shrimp Hollandaise Avocado Stacks P257
Macros & Energy Value	fat: 47g protein: 27.5g carbs: 12.5g cal: 577	fat: 60g protein: 40.5g carbs: 11.5g cal: 721	fat: 60.5g protein: 24g carbs: 10.5g cal: 631	fat: 44g protein: 9g carbs: 3.3g cal: 450	fat: 49.8g protein: 38.8g carbs: 5.7g cal: 631	fat: 33.5g protein: 23.5g carbs: 7.5g cal: 435	fat: 31.5g protein: 13.5g carbs: 4.5g cal: 346
Daily Totals	fat: 136.3g protein: 75.8g carbs: 24.2g cal: 1,578	fat: 148.8g protein: 81g carbs: 19.3g cal: 1,721	fat: 169.5g protein: 76.5g carbs: 25.5g cal: 1,858	fat: 124g protein: 72g carbs: 16.8g cal: 1,490	fat: 136.5g protein: 64.8g carbs: 16.7g cal: 1,561	fat: 138g protein: 69.5g carbs: 23.1g cal: 1,609	fat: 159.5g protein: 85g carbs: 22g cal: 1,861

Meal Plan for Healing and Fat Loss with a Sweet Option

	DAY 1	DAY 2	DAY 3	DAY 4	DAY 5	DAY 6	DAY 7
Meal 1	Breakfast Crepes P122	Avocado Bacon Deviled Eggs P118	Eggs Benedict Royale P130	Breakfast Muffins P123	Instant Chia Pudding P321	Eggs, Bacon, and Roasted Rosemary Radishes P127	Eggs with Sausage Stuffing P126
Macros & Energy Value	fat: 23.3g protein: 11.3g carbs: 3.7g cal: 277	fat: 53g protein: 28g carbs: 4g cal: 610	fat: 56.5g protein: 37.5g carbs: 2g cal: 677	fat: 34.5g protein: 25g carbs: 3.5g cal: 432	fat: 27.7g protein: 4.5g carbs: 6g cal: 291	fat: 59g protein: 18.5g carbs: 5.5g cal: 618	fat: 61g protein: 25g carbs: 9g cal: 684
Meal 2	Deconstructed Bacon Burger Salad P174	Fully Loaded Gourmet Hot Dogs P305	White Truffle Fettuccine Alfredo P206	Green Thai Pork Curry P300	Bacon Wedge Salad P164	Keto Bacon "Potato" Salad P225	Cobb Salad P165
Macros & Energy Value	fat: 66g protein: 37g carbs: 8g cal: 724	fat: 35.8g protein: 12.5g carbs: 3.8g cal: 390	fat: 52.5g protein: 15g carbs: 6g cal: 550	fat: 45.5g protein: 38g carbs: 10g cal: 608	fat: 59g protein: 21.5g carbs: 5g cal: 639	fat: 39g protein: 18g carbs: 4.6g cal: 445	fat: 67g protein: 46.5g carbs: 8.5g cal: 831
Meal 3 (Sweet Option)	Cheesecake Fat Bombs P320	Decadent Keto Brownies P326	Dark Chocolate and Coconut Energy Bars P116	Cinnamon Muffins P160	Crème Brûlée P316	Easy Keto Hot Fudge Sundaes P336	Instant Chia Pudding P321
Macros & Energy Value	fat: 30.8g protein: 4g carbs: 2g cal: 319	fat: 45.4g protein: 9.2g carbs: 6.8g cal: 474	fat: 27.9g protein: 7.2g carbs: 6.1g cal: 298	fat: 34.3g protein: 11g carbs: 9.3g cal: 386	fat: 23.8g protein: 5g carbs: 10.1g cal: 252	fat: 47.5g protein: 4.8g carbs: 8g cal: 506	fat: 27.7g protein: 4.5g carbs: 6g cal: 291
Daily Totals	fat: 120.1g protein: 52.3g carbs: 13.7g cal: 1,320	fat: 134.2g protein: 59.7g carbs: 14.6g cal: 1,474	fat: 136.9g protein: 59.7g carbs: 14.1g cal: 1,525	fat: 114.3g protein: 74g carbs: 22.8g cal: 1,426	fat: 110.5g protein: 31g carbs: 21.1g cal: 1,182	fat: 145.5g protein: 41.3g carbs: 18.1g cal: 1,569	fat: 155.7g protein: 76g carbs: 23.5g cal: 1,806

Allergen Index

RECIPES	PAGE	DAIRY-FREE	EGG-FREE	NUT-FREE
Avocado Smoothie	108	✓	✓	
Omega-3 Keto "Oatmeal"	110	✓	✓	
Omega-3 Seed and Nut Mix	112	✓	✓	
Omega-3 Portable Seed and Nut Energy Bar	114	OPTION		
Dark Chocolate and Coconut Energy Bars	116	OPTION	✓	
Avocado Bacon Deviled Eggs	118	✓		✓
Baked Eggs Benedict Casserole	120			
Breakfast Crêpes	122	OPTION		
Egg, Bacon, Sun-Dried Tomato, and Feta Breakfast Muffins	123			✓
Savory Brie, Mushroom, and Spinach Crêpes	124			
Eggs with Sausage Stuffing	126	OPTION		✓
Eggs, Bacon, and Roasted Rosemary Radishes	127	✓		✓
Eggs Benedict	128			✓
Eggs Benedict Royale	130			✓
Deep-Fried Goat Cheese Balls with Sugar-Free Glaze	134			
Fried Eggplant Mozzarella Balls	136			
Prosciutto Baked Brie	138		✓	✓
Keto Antipasto Plate	140		✓	✓
Prosciutto Mozzarella Sticks with Pesto Dipping Sauce	142		✓	
Guacamole with Cabbage "Chips"	143	✓	✓	✓
Spinach, Kale, and Artichoke Dip	144			✓
Sun-Dried Tomato Dip	146			✓
Ketogenic Girl Hummus	147	✓	✓	✓
Keto Baba Ghanoush	148	✓	✓	✓
Tzatziki Dip	150		✓	✓
Avocado Tzatziki Dip	151		✓	✓
Stuffed Mushrooms	152			
Stuffed Tomatoes	153	✓		✓
Eggplant Cherry Tomato Pizzas	154		✓	✓
Keto Bread Loaf	156	✓		✓
Keto Chive and Onion "English Muffins"	158			✓
Cinnamon Muffins	160			✓
Bacon Wedge Salad	164			✓
Cobb Salad	165			✓
Spinach Gomae Salad	166	✓	✓	
Fennel, Asparagus, and Goat Cheese Salad	168		✓	
Spinach, Goat Cheese, Pecan, and Strawberry Salad	170			
Oriental Salad	172	✓		
Deconstructed Bacon Burger Salad	174	✓		✓
Keto Gado-Gado Bowl	175	✓		
Niçoise Salad	176	✓		OPTION
Seaweed Salad	177	✓	✓	✓
Superfood Buddha Bowl	178	✓		✓
French Onion Soup with Keto Croutons	180		✓	✓
Lobster Bisque	182		✓	✓
Keto "Kulajda" Dill and Poached Egg Soup	184			✓
Tom Yum Koong (Thai Shrimp Soup)	186	✓	✓	✓
Tom Kha Gai (Thai Chicken Coconut Soup)	188	✓	✓	✓
Three-Cheese Macaroni with Bacon au Gratin	192		✓	
Bacon Pesto Pasta	194		✓	
Pasta Bolognese	196		✓	✓
Fettuccine Alfredo with Grilled Shrimp	198		✓	✓
Shrimp Pad Thai	200	✓		
Pasta Carbonara	202			✓
Sun-Dried Tomato Fettuccine	204			
White Truffle Fettuccine Alfredo	206	✓		
Shrimp Fried Rice	208	✓		✓
Truffle, Leek, and Mushroom Risotto	210			✓

RECIPES	PAGE	🚫 DAIRY-FREE	🚫 EGG-FREE	🚫 NUT-FREE
"Honey"-Mustard Slaw	214	✓		✓
Creamy Keto Slaw	215			✓
Braised Red Cabbage	216	OPTION	✓	✓
Creamed Spinach	217		✓	
Loaded Cauliflower Bake	218			✓
Avocado Fries	220	✓	✓	✓
Broccoli Stem Fries	221	✓	✓	✓
Toasted Coconut Chips	222	✓	✓	✓
Broccoli Mash	223	OPTION	✓	
Cauliflower Mash	224	OPTION	✓	
Keto Bacon "Potato" Salad	225	✓		✓
Roasted Eggplant with Tahini-Almond Sauce	226		✓	
Deep-Fried Brussels Sprouts with Tangy Sauce	228	✓		✓
Duck Fat–Roasted Rosemary Radishes	230	✓	✓	✓
Zucchini Chips	231		✓	✓
Cauliflower Sausage Herb Stuffing	232	OPTION		✓
Thai Chicken Satay	236	✓	✓	
Pesto Chicken Skewers	238	✓	✓	
Lemon Chicken	240	✓	✓	OPTION
Chicken and Bacon Pâté	242			✓
No-Bake Chicken and Bacon Pâté	244			✓
Hot Wings with Blue Cheese and Celery	246			✓
Spicy Chicken Fajitas	248		✓	✓
Teriyaki Chicken	250	OPTION	✓	✓
Duck Rillettes	252	✓	✓	✓
Ceviche with Spicy Mayo Dressing	253	✓		✓
Crab Cakes with Garlic-Dill Cream	254			
Spicy Shrimp Cocktail	256	✓		✓
Shrimp Hollandaise Avocado Stacks	257			✓
Crispy Calamari with Aioli	258	✓		✓
Keto–Moules "Frites" (Mussels and "Fries")	260		✓	✓
Easy Baked Lobster Tails with Herb Butter	262		✓	✓
One-Pan Salmon	264	✓		✓
Smoked Salmon Blini with Dill Cream	265	OPTION		
Salmon Avocado Poke	266	✓	✓	✓
Salmon Rillettes on Cucumber Rounds	267			✓
One-Pan Cod with Broccolini and Mint Hollandaise	268	OPTION		✓
Easy Keto Meatloaf	272			
Keto Shepherd's Pie	274	OPTION	✓	✓
Steak with Béarnaise Sauce	276	OPTION		✓
Steak with Mushroom Sauce	278		✓	✓
Steak and Keto Tabbouleh	280	OPTION	✓	✓
Steak on "Honey"-Mustard Slaw	281	✓		✓
Steak with Green Peppercorn Sauce	282		✓	✓
Trio of Beef Sliders	284			✓
Zucchini Lasagna	286			✓
Feta-Stuffed Meatballs	288			
Keto Moussaka	290			✓
Stuffed Peppers	292		✓	✓
Ginger Beef	294	✓	✓	✓
Easy Keto Casserole	296		✓	✓
Bacon Poutine	298		✓	✓
Green Thai Pork Curry	300	✓	✓	OPTION
Pork Gyro Lettuce Wraps	302		✓	✓
Asparagus with Prosciutto and Hollandaise	304			✓
Fully Loaded Gourmet Hot Dogs	305	OPTION		✓
Pork Belly with Caramelized Zucchini	306		✓	✓
Pork Terrine	308	OPTION	✓	✓
Spicy Pork Skewers with Hollandaise	310			✓
Pulled Pork	311		✓	OPTION
Pulled Pork and Avocado Boats	312		✓	OPTION

RECIPES	PAGE	🥛 DAIRY-FREE	🥚 EGG-FREE	🥜 NUT-FREE
Pulled Pork with Keto Slaw	313			OPTION
Crème Brûlée	316	OPTION		
Vanilla Ice Cream	318			
Cheesecake Fat Bombs	320		✓	✓
Instant Chia Pudding	321	✓		
Chocolate Mint Mousse	322	✓	✓	
Cinnamon Custard	323	✓		
Lemon Curd	324			✓
No-Bake Cookie Dough	325		✓	✓
Decadent Keto Brownies	326	OPTION		
Ketogenic Girl Cheesecake	328	OPTION		OPTION
Coconut "Carrot" Cake	330			
Easy Vanilla Cupcakes	332			
Ketogenic Girl Macaroons	334		✓	✓
Easy Keto Hot Fudge Sundaes	336	✓		
Viennese Coffee	337	✓		✓
Sugar-Free Almond or Cashew Milk	340	✓	✓	
Ketogenic Girl Chocolate Hazelnut Spread	342	✓		
Creamed Coconut Butter	344	✓	✓	✓
Sugar-Free Cranberry Sauce	346	✓	✓	✓
Holiday Gravy	348	OPTION	✓	✓
Béarnaise Sauce	350			✓
Aioli	352	✓		✓
Hollandaise	354	OPTION		✓
Homemade Mayonnaise	355	✓		✓
Homemade Worcestershire Sauce	356	✓	✓	✓
Blue Cheese Dressing	357			✓
"Honey"-Mustard Dressing	358	✓		✓
Ranch Dressing	359			✓
Creamy Poppy Seed Dressing	360	✓	✓	✓
Restaurant-Style Keto Japanese Ginger Dressing	361	✓		✓
Sweet Balsamic Glaze	362	OPTION	✓	✓
Special Burger Sauce	363	✓		✓
Sugar-Free Glaze	364	OPTION	✓	✓

Recipe Index

Breakfast

Avocado Smoothie

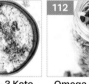

Omega-3 Keto Porridge

Omega-3 Seed and Nut Mix

Omega-3 Portable Seed and Nut Energy Bars

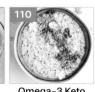

Dark Chocolate and Coconut Energy Bars

Avocado Bacon Deviled Eggs

Baked Eggs Benedict Casserole

Breakfast Crêpes

Egg, Bacon, Sun-Dried Tomato, and Feta Breakfast Muffins

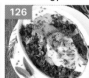

Savory Brie, Spinach, and Mushroom Crêpes

Eggs with Sausage Stuffing

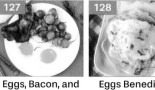

Eggs, Bacon, and Roasted Rosemary Radishes

Eggs Benedict

Eggs Benedict Royale

Appetizers, Snacks & Breads

134
Deep-Fried Goat Cheese Balls

136
Fried Eggplant Mozzarella Balls

138
Prosciutto Baked Brie

140
Keto Antipasto Plate

142
Prosciutto Mozzarella Sticks

143
Guacamole with Cabbage "Chips"

144
Spinach, Kale, and Artichoke Dip

146
Sun-Dried Tomato Dip

147
Ketogenic Girl Hummus

148
Keto Baba Ghanoush

150
Tzatziki Dip

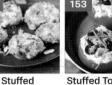
151
Avocado Tzatziki Dip

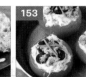
152
Stuffed Mushrooms

153
Stuffed Tomatoes

154
Eggplant Cherry Tomato Pizzas

156
Keto Bread Loaf

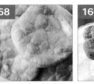
158
Keto Chive and Onion "English Muffins"

160
Cinnamon Muffins

Salads & Soups

164
Bacon Wedge Salad

165
Cobb Salad

166
Spinach Gomae Salad

168
Fennel, Asparagus, and Goat Cheese Salad

170
Spinach, Goat Cheese, Pecan, and Strawberry Salad

172
Oriental Salad

174
Deconstructed Bacon Burger Salad

175
Keto Gado-Gado Bowl

176
Niçoise Salad

177
Seaweed Salad

178
Superfood Buddha Bowl

180
French Onion Soup with Keto Croutons

182
Lobster Bisque

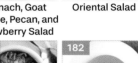

184
Keto "Kulajda" Dill and Poached Egg Soup

186
Tom Yum Koong (Thai Shrimp Soup)

188
Tom Kha Gai (Thai Chicken Coconut Soup)

Noodles & Rice

192 Three-Cheese Macaroni with Bacon au Gratin

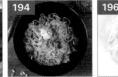
194 Bacon Pesto Pasta

196 Pasta Bolognese

198 Fettuccine Alfredo with Grilled Shrimp

200 Shrimp Pad Thai

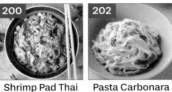
202 Pasta Carbonara

204 Sun-Dried Tomato Fettuccine

206 White Truffle Fettuccine Alfredo

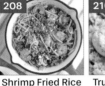
208 Shrimp Fried Rice

210 Truffle, Leek, and Mushroom Risotto

Sides

214 "Honey"-Mustard Slaw

215 Creamy Keto Slaw

216 Braised Red Cabbage

217 Creamed Spinach

218 Loaded Cauliflower Bake

220 Avocado Fries

221 Broccoli Stem Fries

222 Toasted Coconut Chips

223 Broccoli Mash

224 Cauliflower Mash

225 Keto Bacon "Potato" Salad

226 Roasted Eggplant with Tahini-Almond Sauce

228 Deep-Fried Brussels Sprouts with Tangy Sauce

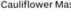
230 Duck Fat–Roasted Rosemary Radishes

231 Zucchini Chips

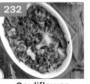
232 Cauliflower Sausage Herb Stuffing

Poultry & Seafood

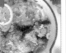
236 Thai Chicken Satay

238 Pesto Chicken Skewers

240 Lemon Chicken

242 Chicken and Bacon Pâté

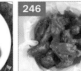
244 No-Bake Chicken and Bacon Pâté

246 Hot Wings with Blue Cheese and Celery

248 Spicy Chicken Fajitas

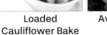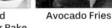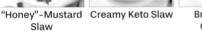

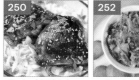
Teriyaki Chicken

Duck Rillettes

Ceviche with Spicy Mayo Dressing

Crab Cakes with Garlic-Dill Cream

Spicy Shrimp Cocktail

Shrimp Hollandaise Avocado Stacks

Crispy Calamari with Aioli

Keto–Moules "Frites" (Mussels and "Fries")

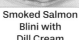
Easy Baked Lobster Tails with Herb Butter

One-Pan Salmon

Smoked Salmon Blini with Dill Cream

Salmon Avocado Poke

Salmon Rillettes on Cucumber Rounds

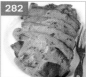
One-Pan Cod with Broccolini and Mint Hollandaise

Beef & Pork

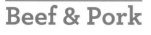

Easy Keto Meatloaf

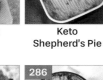
Keto Shepherd's Pie

Steak with Béarnaise Sauce

Steak with Mushroom Sauce

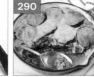
Steak and Keto Tabbouleh

Steak on "Honey"–Mustard Slaw

Steak with Green Peppercorn Sauce

Trio of Beef Sliders

Zucchini Lasagna

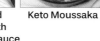
Feta-Stuffed Meatballs with Greek Tomato Sauce

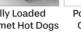

Keto Moussaka

Stuffed Peppers

Ginger Beef

Easy Keto Casserole

Bacon Poutine

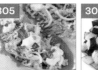
Green Thai Pork Curry

Pork Gyro Lettuce Wraps with Quick Pickled Red Onions

Asparagus with Prosciutto and Hollandaise

Fully Loaded Gourmet Hot Dogs

Pork Belly with Caramelized Zucchini

Pork Terrine

Spicy Pork Skewers with Hollandaise

Pulled Pork

Pulled Pork and Avocado Boats

Pulled Pork with Keto Slaw

Desserts

 316
Crème Brûlée

 318
Vanilla Ice Cream

 320
Cheesecake Fat Bombs

 321
Instant Chia Pudding

 322
Chocolate Mint Mousse

 323
Cinnamon Custard

324
Lemon Curd

 325
No-Bake Cookie Dough

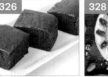 326
Decadent Keto Brownies

328
Ketogenic Girl Cheesecake

 330
Coconut "Carrot" Cake

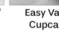 332
Easy Vanilla Cupcakes

 334
Ketogenic Girl Macaroons

 336
Easy Keto Hot Fudge Sundaes

 337
Viennese Coffee

Sauces & Kitchen Staples

 340
Sugar-Free Almond or Cashew Milk

 342
Ketogenic Girl Chocolate Hazelnut Spread

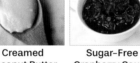 344
Creamed Coconut Butter

 346
Sugar-Free Cranberry Sauce

 348
Holiday Gravy

 350
Béarnaise Sauce

352
Aioli

 354
Hollandaise

 355
Homemade Mayonnaise

 356
Homemade Worcestershire Sauce

 357
Blue Cheese Dressing

  358
Ketogenic Girl "Honey"-Mustard Dressing

  359
Ranch Dressing

   360
Creamy Poppy Seed Dressing

 361
Restaurant-Style Keto Japanese Ginger Dressing

 362
Sweet Balsamic Glaze

  363
Special Burger Sauce

 364
Sugar-Free Glaze

Compliant Food List

FAT	serving size
Avocado oil	1 Tbsp
Bacon fat	1 Tbsp
Butter	1 Tbsp
Butter-flavored coconut oil	1 Tbsp
Coconut oil	1 Tbsp
Duck fat	1 Tbsp
Lard	1 Tbsp
Mayonnaise (make sure it has no added sugar)	1 Tbsp
MCT oil	1 Tbsp
Olive oil	1 Tbsp

MEAT AND POULTRY	srv. size	total carbs	fiber	protein
Bacon★	4 oz	0 g	44 g	32 g
Beef, ground	4 oz	0 g	4 g	24 g
Chicken breast, skinless	4 oz	0 g	3 g	28 g
Chicken drumstick	4 oz	0 g	7 g	21 g
Chicken thigh, skin-on	4 oz	0 g	18 g	28 g
Cornish hen	4 oz	0 g	8 g	12 g
Duck	4 oz	0 g	4 g	32 g
Egg	1 large	0 g	5 g	6 g
Goose	4 oz	0 g	12 g	40 g
Ham★	4 oz	2 g	4 g	18 g
Lamb	4 oz	0 g	24 g	28 g
Ostrich	4 oz	0 g	4 g	32 g
Pheasant	4 oz	0 g	12 g	36 g
Pork tenderloin	4 oz	0 g	8 g	32 g
Pork belly	4 oz	0 g	60 g	12 g
Quail	4 oz	0 g	16 g	28.5 g
Ribs, beef	4 oz	0 g	32 g	24 g
Ribs, pork	4 oz	0 g	8 g	8 g
Steak, porterhouse	4 oz	0 g	8 g	32 g
Steak, rib-eye	4 oz	0 g	32 g	24 g
Steak, rump	4 oz	0 g	4 g	24 g
Turkey breast	4 oz	0 g	0 g	24 g
Turkey, ground, 99% lean	4 oz	0 g	0 g	28 g
Veal	4 oz	0 g	0 g	28 g
Venison	4 oz	0 g	3 g	31 g

★Opt for uncured with no sugar added

SEAFOOD	srv. size	total carbs	fiber	protein
Clams	4 oz	2.5 g	1.5 g	14 g
Cod	4 oz	0 g	0 g	17 g
Crabmeat	4 oz	0 g	1.2 g	10 g
Flounder	4 oz	1 g	2 g	25 g
Halibut	4 oz	0 g	16 g	16 g
Herring	4 oz	16 g	8 g	12 g
Lobster	4 oz	1 g	1 g	11 g
Mussels★★	4 oz	2.5 g	1.5 g	19 g
Oysters★★	4 oz	6 g	3 g	11 g
Salmon	4 oz	0 g	12 g	24 g
Sardines	4 oz	0 g	16 g	24 g
Scallops	4 oz	6 g	2 g	21 g
Shrimp	4 oz	0 g	0 g	18 g
Sole	4 oz	0 g	0 g	20 g
Squid	4 oz	0 g	1 g	16 g
Tilapia	4 oz	0 g	3 g	20 g
Trout	4 oz	0 g	16 g	24 g
Tuna	4 oz	0 g	4 g	28 g

★★Limit mussels and oysters to 4 ounces per day

KETO VEGGIES	srv. size	total carbs	fiber
Alfalfa sprouts	1 cup	1 g	1 g
Artichoke hearts (marinated)	½ cup	9 g	2 g
Artichoke quarters (in water)	10 drained	5 g	3 g
Artichoke, whole	1	13 g	7 g
Arugula	½ cup	0.4 g	0.2 g
Asparagus (cooked)	6 stalks	4 g	2 g
Avocado, Haas	½	8.5 g	6.7 g
Beet greens (cooked)	½ cup	3.9 g	2.1 g
Bell pepper, green, chopped	½ cup	3.4 g	1.2 g
Bell pepper, red, chopped	½ cup	4.5 g	1.5 g
Bok choy (cooked)	½ cup	1.5 g	0.8 g
Broccoli (cooked)	½ cup	3.4 g	1.6 g
Broccoli rabe (cooked)	½ cup	3 g	2 g
Broccolini (cooked)	3 stalks	6.3 g	2.4 g
Brussels sprouts (cooked)	½ cup	4 g	1.65 g
Button mushrooms	½ cup	1.1 g	0.4 g
Cabbage (cooked)	½ cup	3 g	1 g
Cauliflower (cooked)	½ cup	3 g	1 g
Celery	1 stalk	1.4 g	0.6 g
Cherry tomatoes	10	6.6 g	2 g
Chicory greens	½ cup	0.7 g	0.6 g
Collard greens (cooked)	½ cup	1 g	0.6 g
Cucumber, sliced	½ cup	1.9 g	0.3 g
Daikon, grated	½ cup	2.6 g	1.1 g
Eggplant (cooked)	½ cup	2 g	1 g
Endive	½ cup	0.8 g	0.8 g
Escarole	½ cup	3.2 g	2.9 g
Fennel	½ cup	3.1 g	1.3 g
Garlic, minced	2 Tbsp	6 g	0 g
Green beans (cooked)	½ cup	4.9 g	2 g
Green onions, chopped	½ cup	3.6 g	1.3 g
Heart of palm	1	1.5 g	0.8 g
Jicama	½ cup	5.7 g	3.2 g
Kale (cooked)	½ cup	3.3 g	0.7 g
Kohlrabi (cooked)	½ cup	4 g	2 g
Leeks (cooked)	2 Tbsp	2 g	0.2 g
Lettuce	½ cup	0.8 g	0.3 g
Okra (cooked)	½ cup	3.5 g	1.6 g
Olives, black	5	1 g	0.5 g
Olives, green	5	1 g	0 g
Pickle, dill	1	3.1 g	1.6 g
Portobello mushroom (cooked)	1	4.2 g	1.3 g
Pumpkin, mashed (cooked)	½ cup	6 g	1.35 g
Radicchio	½ cup	0.9 g	0.2 g
Radish	1	0.3 g	0.1 g
Red/white onions, chopped	2 Tbsp	2.6 g	0.5 g
Rhubarb	½ cup	2.7 g	1.1 g
Sauerkraut (drained)	½ cup	3 g	1.8 g
Shallots, chopped	2 Tbsp	3.3 g	0 g
Spinach	½ cup	0.5 g	0.3 g
Spinach (cooked)	½ cup	1.1 g	0.7 g
Sprouts, mung beans	½ cup	3 g	1 g
Swiss chard (cooked)	½ cup	1 g	0 g
Tomato	1 small	3.5 g	1.1 g
Tomato (cooked)	½ cup	5 g	1 g
Turnip (cooked)	½ cup	3.9 g	2.4 g
Turnip greens (cooked)	½ cup	3.1 g	2.5 g
Watercress	½ cup	0.2 g	0.1 g
Zucchini (cooked)	½ cup	3 g	1 g

HERBS AND SPICES	srv. size	total carbs	fiber
Basil	1 Tbsp	0 g	0 g
Black pepper	1 tsp	1.4 g	0.7 g
Cayenne pepper	1 Tbsp	1 g	0 g
Chives (fresh or dried)	1 Tbsp	0.1 g	0.1 g
Cilantro	1 Tbsp	0 g	0 g
Dill	1 Tbsp	0 g	0 g
Ginger, grated	1 Tbsp	3.8 g	0.7 g
Oregano	1 Tbsp	0.6 g	0.4 g
Parsley	1 Tbsp	0.2 g	0.1 g
Rosemary, dried	1 Tbsp	2.1 g	1.4 g
Sage, ground	1 tsp	1.2 g	0.8 g
Tarragon	1 Tbsp	0.9 g	0.1 g

SAUCES	srv. size	total carbs	fiber
Balsamic vinegar	1 Tbsp	2.6 g	0 g
Blue cheese	2 Tbsp	1 g	0 g
Caesar dressing	2 Tbsp	1 g	0 g
Hollandaise or béarnaise sauce	2 Tbsp	0 g	0 g
Italian dressing, creamy	2 Tbsp	3 g	0 g
Lemon juice	2 Tbsp	1.9 g	0 g
Lime juice	2 Tbsp	3 g	0 g
Ranch dressing	2 Tbsp	2 g	0 g

Special Thanks

This book is dedicated to my awe-inspiring husband, Peter, and my wonderful parents, Marilyn and Robert, and is in loving memory of my grandfather, Ronald T. Wash.

Peter, the abiding love, support, and faith you provide me with is what allows me to spread my wings and soar. Your patience and encouragement never wavers. You have taught and inspired me by the person you are with your strong character and big heart, and I thank you with all my heart for the hero that you are to me every day in both small and big ways.

Mother and Papa, you always support me and all my crazy ideas no matter how out there they are. Thank you for imparting your strong work ethic and your passion for travel, adventure, and fearlessly following your dreams! I love you both more than words can express. *Je vous adore avec tout mon coeur. Merci.*

To my dear grandpa, I miss you every day and cherish our memories. Thank you for imparting your love of writing and creativity to me. So many of the ethics and values that you lived by shaped my perspective of life and I thank you for that. I dedicate this book to your honor and legacy.

To my second parents, Ilona and Vlady, thank you for all your loving support and patience with my never-ending tirades about sugar! I am so thankful for all your encouragement and recognition of my work in building something I love. Thank you, Christine, my brilliant sister, for your love and support! You are each so wonderful, and I am so blessed to have you as my parents and sister. I love you both very much!

To my best friend, Jessica Green, you are the most kind, generous, and supportive friend–my dream bestie. You have supported me on every step of this journey. I appreciate you and Cody for all your advice, mentoring, and guidance! Cody, thank you for being a mentor to me and for getting me to take that first bite of steak. ;) Love you guys!

To my fabulous teammates, Monica and Kathy, I don't know what I would do without you. You are both such wonderful, hardworking, kind, and caring people. Your hard work enabled me to focus on this book in the past year and a half, and I love and appreciate you both so much!

To Amber, thank you for all your love and support—and for being the first official purchaser of this book! I love you.

To my brother, Mathieu, thank you for your support and sharing your fantastic ideas with me! I love you!

To my dedicated photographer, Diana, thank you for your patience and hard work! I appreciate you so much for your beautiful contributions to this book. You are so talented and a lovely soul. Thank you to Lucie for your stunning photos and contributions!

A *huge* thank you to the incredible and tireless team at Victory Belt, including Lance, Erich, Susan, Pam, Holly, Cindy, Donna, Justin, Kathy, and Rick and other amazing support staff!

Thank you to Dr. Jeffry Gerber, Dr. John Limansky, Megan Ramos, Martina Slajerova, and Leanne Vogel for their endorsements of my work.

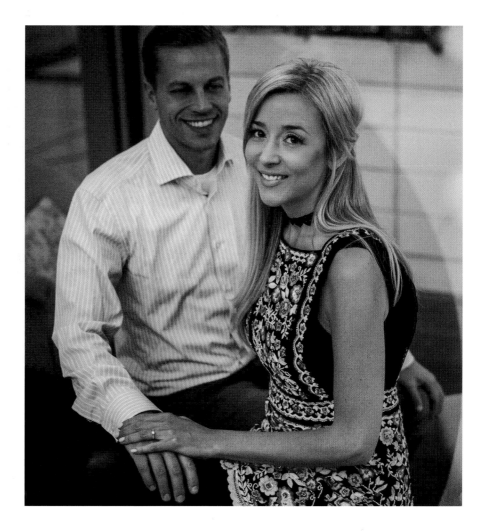

Index